History of Suicide

HISTORY OF SUICIDE

Voluntary Death in Western Culture

GEORGES MINOIS

TRANSLATED BY
Lydia G. Cochrane

The Johns Hopkins University Press
BALTIMORE AND LONDON

The translation was prepared with the generous assistance of the
French Ministry of Culture.

Originally published as *Histoire du suicide: La société occidentale face
à la mort volontaire,* © Libraire Arthème
Fayard, 1995

Johns Hopkins Paperbacks edition, 2001
2 4 6 8 9 7 5 3 1

The Johns Hopkins University Press
2715 North Charles Street
Baltimore, Maryland 21218-4363
www.press.jhu.edu

Library of Congress Cataloging-in-Publication Data will be
found at the end of this book.
A catalog record for this book is available from the
British Library.

ISBN 0-8018-6647-2 (pbk.)

To be, or not to be: that is the question.
Whether 'tis nobler in the mind to suffer
The slings and arrows of outrageous fortune,
Or to take arms against a sea of troubles,
And by opposing end them. To die; to sleep;
No more; and by a sleep to say we end
The heart-ache and the thousand natural shocks
That flesh is heir to. 'Tis a consummation
Devoutly to be wish'd. To die; to sleep;—
To sleep? Perchance to dream! Ay, there's the rub;
—Shakespeare, *Hamlet,* act 3, scene 1

CONTENTS

History of Suicide

Introduction

In the great studies of death in past times by Michel Vovelle, François Lebrun, Pierre Chaunu, Philippe Ariès, John McManners, and many others who left their mark on the historiography of the 1970s and 1980s, voluntary death is conspicuously absent. It almost never appears in works as weighty and remarkable as Vovelle's *La mort et l'Occident: De 1300 à nos jours,* Lebrun's *Les hommes et la mort en Anjou aux XVIIᵉ et XVIIIᵉ siècles,* Chaunu's *La mort à Paris: XVIᵉ, XVIIᵉ et XVIIIᵉ siècles,* Ariès's *L'homme devant la mort,* and McManners's *Death and the Enlightenment.*[1]

The first reason for this omission is documentary: The sources of information on voluntary death are different from the ones that record natural deaths. Parish registers are of no help because suicides had no right to religious burial. Since voluntary death was considered a crime, historians have to consult judicial archives; because those sources are highly fragmentary, they must be supplemented by a broad variety of other, but hardly abundant, sources, such as memoirs and chronicles, private journals, and works of literature. Voluntary death was in itself an exception to the rule (there were only a few hundred cases per year in France, for example), which means that it is nearly insignificant in statistical, demographic, or sociological studies.

A more strictly substantive problem joins these methodological ones: Suicide cannot be studied in precisely the same way as the ravages of plague or tuberculosis; voluntary death is significant for philosophic, religious, moral, and cultural reasons, rather than demographic ones. The silence and dissimulation that accompanied suicide surrounded it with a climate of discomfort.

After the publication of Émile Durkheim's *Suicide* in 1897, sociologists, psychologists, psychoanalysts, and physicians took up the study of suicide, using contemporary statistics and viewing it from the standpoint of their various disciplines. Historical studies of suicide before the end of the ancien régime have for the most part concentrated on one or more particular aspects of the question or on a limited number of famous examples. For classical antiquity, for example, we have Yolande Grisé's fine book, *Le suicide dans la Rome antique,* a work that relies primarily on literary sources. Jean-Claude Schmitt takes up problems of methodology concerning the Middle Ages in a remarkable article, "Le Suicide au Moyen Age." Bernard Paulin's *Du couteau à la plume: Le suicide dans la littérature anglaise de la Renaissance (1580–1625),* originally his doctoral dissertation, covers a far greater range than its title indicates. Perhaps the best documented study, and the one whose conclusions strike most deeply, is Michael MacDonald and Terence R. Murphy's *Sleepless Souls: Suicide in Early Modern England.* Thus far there has been only one overall study of the history of suicide, Albert Bayet's *Le suicide et la morale* (1922), a work published several decades ago, but one that is still a mine of information.[2]

Scholars today investigate all domains of human experience: Should not everything that has shaped humankind be studied without prejudice or taboo? As Jean Baechler reminds us, what could be more specifically human than voluntary death?[3] Animal "suicides" are in the realm of myth; human-kind alone is capable of reflecting on its own existence and deciding to prolong life or put an end to it. Humanity has existed thus far because humans have found sufficient reason to remain alive, but nonetheless a certain number of individuals decide that life is no longer worth living and prefer to depart voluntarily before being sent on their way by illness, old age, or war. Some think them mad. Cato, Seneca, Henry de Montherlant, Bruno Bettelheim, and many others have regarded the specifically human act of voluntary death as the supreme proof of liberty, of the freedom to decide one's own being or nonbeing. As Raymond Aron asks, "By killing oneself, does one capitulate before a difficulty or attain the highest mastery over one's life?"[4]

In 1600 William Shakespeare posed the fundamental question in its full and terrible simplicity with Hamlet's "To be or not to be?" We can take that question as our guide. Why, in a given period, did some people choose not to be? They had their particular reasons, and it is important to try to understand what they were because they reflect an attitude that reveals society's most vital values and engages both the individual and the group. Albert Camus put it best:

There is but one truly serious philosophical problem, and that is suicide. Judging whether life is or is not worth living amounts to answering the fundamental question of philosophy. All the rest—whether or not the world has three dimensions, whether the mind has nine or twelve categories—come afterwards. These are games; one must first answer. . . . The worm is in man's heart. That is where it must be sought. One must follow and understand this fatal game that leads from lucidity in the face of existence to flight from light.[5]

From remotest antiquity to today, some men and women have chosen death. Society has never been indifferent to that choice. On rare occasions acclaimed as an act of heroism, suicide has more often been subject to social reprobation because it was considered an insult to God, who gave us life, and to society, which provides for the well-being of its members. Refusing God's gift and the company of our fellows at the banquet of life is a dual offense that the agents of religion, who dispense divine largesse, and those of politics, who organize the social banquet, find intolerable.

"To be or not to be?" they insist, is by no means the question. If we exist it is because we must exist in order to glorify God and to make ourselves useful in society. Anyone who rejects that rule deserves punishment, both of the dead body and in the afterlife. This attitude reigned supreme and uncontested in Europe throughout the Middle Ages. It began to change in the early Renaissance, toward the end of the fifteenth century, when a first challenge emerged, expressed in joking tones and indirectly through madness. Contestation increased rapidly until by 1600 the question, "To be or not to be?" was posed openly, giving rise to a debate that grew increasingly bitter as Europe faced a series of crises of conscience. In the age of the Enlightenment, challenge became open defiance.

The very term *suicide,* which replaced the expression *self-murder* shortly before 1700, is a sign of that change. Resistance on the part of the authorities did not disappear, but from the sixteenth to the eighteenth century, Hamlet's question gradually came to be raised publicly. Some dared to claim that individuals should be free to answer it as they saw fit, which meant that those who held power were forced to adopt a more flexible attitude. That crucial change in ways of thinking in Western Europe has thus far been insufficiently studied. It is what I intend to examine in these pages.

PART I

Tradition

A Repressed Question

ONE

Suicide in the Middle Ages

Nuances

A Chronicle of Ordinary Suicide

1249 Pietro Della Vigna, a jurist, poet, and minister to Frederick II, committed suicide. Dante pictures him in hell in the *Inferno*.

1257 A Parisian jumped into the Seine. When he was rescued, he took communion before he died. His family claimed the body, arguing that he had died in a state of grace, but because he had attempted suicide and had been in his right mind, as shown by his repentance, the court sentenced his corpse to torture.

1238, 1266 Two women who had lived within the jurisdiction of the Abbey of Sainte-Geneviève in Paris committed suicide. Their bodies were buried without ceremony *(enfouis)*.

1274 Pierre Crochet of Boissy-Saint-Léger killed himself while under suspicion of murder. The judicial arm of the Abbey of Saint-Maur-des-Fossés sentenced the body to be dragged through the streets, then hanged.

1278 A man committed suicide in Reims. The monks of Saint-Rémi had the body dragged and hanged, but the Parlement de Paris ordered them to hand over the cadaver to the archbishop, who alone held the right to hang criminals.

1278 Philippe Testard, a man a hundred years old who had been *prévôt* to the archbishop of Paris, got up in the night to urinate out the window and threw himself down to the street below. Brought back to his bed, he received the Eucharist but then stabbed himself. His heirs pleaded his insanity to avoid confiscation of his estate. During the trial twelve witnesses attested to his odd behavior: "He did so many silly things that everyone said he was out of his senses."

1288   A man living within the jurisdiction of the Abbey of Sainte-Geneviève in Paris committed suicide, and the abbey had his body hanged. Soon after, the royal *prévôt* ordered the abbey to repeat the execution, first "dragging the said murderer" through the streets behind a horse, a rite that the abbey had neglected to perform.

1293   Adam Le Yep, a freeholder in Worcestershire, was reclassified a serf because of his extreme poverty. Rejecting the social demotion, he drowned himself in the Severn.

1302   Raoul de Nesles rushed headlong into the melee during the Battle of the Golden Spurs at Courtrai, preferring certain death to the humiliation of defeat.

1358   Jacquet de Fransures, a peasant in revolt, strangled himself in prison "with the rope that tied him around the shoulders, and murdered himself in desperation."

1382   Several persons were executed following Charles VI's return to Paris. "The wife of one of these," Jean Juvénal des Ursins tells us, "who was great with child, threw herself from the window of her house and killed herself."

1387   When soldiers pushed him to desperation by their rapacious demands, Jean Lunneton, a tenant farmer of the Abbey of Chaalis, hanged himself. The abbey ordered confiscation of his estate, but eventually permitted his wife to inherit, "in consideration of the fact that one cannot know for sure if the said event occurred because of the desperation of her said late husband or otherwise."

1394   After several days of illness, Jean Masstoier decided to drown himself in the river. Saved in time but still suffering from "melancholy of the head," he threw himself down a well.

1399   A pious and wealthy burgher in Strasbourg, Hugelinus Richter, confessed, took communion, then jumped into the Bruche River.

1418   When his wife fell ill, Pierre le Vachier, a retired butcher from Sarcelles who had been ruined by the civil war and had lost two of his children, not only was left destitute but also felt totally abandoned. He "went to hang himself from a tree, where he died and strangled himself." The chronicle adds that he was obviously "tempted by the enemy [the devil]."

1421   "By the temptation of the enemy and on the occasion of his said madness and illness," Denisot Sensogot, a Paris baker who had contracted an infectious disease, hanged himself. His case was brought to trial to determine whether his act was to be attributed to the influence of the devil (in which case his body would be dragged, hanged, and deprived of Christian burial, and his goods would be confiscated) or to madness *(frénésie)*, which would exculpate him. His widow, pregnant and the mother of a year-old daughter, petitioned that he be declared mad, as "it would be a very hard thing for the said widow . . . to lose their goods and chattels by such a decision; moreover their relatives and friends, people of note and of good family, would be vilified if the body of the deceased were executed."

1423   Michelet le Cavelier, a Paris embroiderer stricken by an illness that brought him terrible suffering, threw himself out of the window.

1426   Jeannette Mayard, a shoemaker's wife and a good Catholic but given to drink and jealousy, hanged herself.

1447   A woman known to be insane got up in the middle of the night. "Her husband asked her where she was going and she answered that she wanted to go relieve herself. Thus the said woman went about the house stark naked, then threw herself into a well a good thirteen armwidths deep."

1460   Philippe Braque, a barrister of the Parlement de Paris and a man some fifty years of age, committed suicide in the basement of his house.

1484   A journeyman in Metz hanged himself after a quarrel over a girl.

Fragmentary though it is, this rapid survey of the suicides of ordinary people in the Middle Ages, drawn from memoirs, journals kept by clerics and burghers, and surviving judiciary records,[1] shows that suicide was practiced in all social categories and by both men and women. Voluntary death was seen as the result of diabolic temptation induced by despair or as mad behavior. The act, condemned as murder, led to savage punishment inflicted on the dead body and to confiscation of the estate of the deceased. At times the judges showed a degree of indulgence by taking into account the circumstances of the death and the family's situation. Civil and ecclesiastical justice collaborated to repress suicide. Suicides had a variety of reasons for taking their own lives: poverty, illness, physical suffering, fear of punishment, honor, reaction to humiliation, love, and jealousy.

Only an insignificant number of cases appear in chronicles and court records, however. In a ground-breaking article Jean-Claude Schmitt discusses fifty-four cases of suicide over a period of nearly three centuries. As Schmitt remarks, such a "limited and heterogeneous" sampling "cannot be subjected to the statistical manipulations devised by sociologists."[2] Establishing a suicide rate for medieval Europe that might permit comparison with other ages seems an impossible dream.

Without going as far as Félix Bourquelot, who stated in 1842 that in the twelfth century "a mania for suicide penetrated all classes of society,"[3] we can say that there seems to be no evidence that voluntary death occurred any less often in the Middle Ages than in any other period. To the contrary, the many laws that were passed, both canon and civil, the number of philosophical and theological pronouncements made on the subject, the absence of expressions of surprise in the chronicles, and the dockets of court cases regarding voluntary homicide all show that suicides occurred with some regularity. Moreover, recent sociological studies have shown that the suicide rate remains stable in all types of society.

Noble Substitutes for Suicide

Even though the Middle Ages (unlike pagan classical antiquity) stand out as having almost no illustrious suicides, it seems improbable that medieval society was an exception to the rule. There was no medieval Lucretius, no Brutus, Cato, or Seneca, and the discredit that an omnipresent Catholicism cast on a practice it considered cowardly quite certainly had an effect on the elites—social circles restricted to limited numbers and profoundly marked by clerical influence. The way of life of the warrior aristocracy, however, did include behaviors that substituted for suicide and were an indirect means of suicide: Tournaments might in many ways be likened to "gaming suicides," as could judiciary duels and the various forms of the judgment of God. Omnipresent war was both an essential safety valve for suicidal impulses and a deterrent to direct suicide. It is known that the suicide rate declines sharply in times of war, when group cohesion is reinforced and a sense of solidarity, shared emotions, and a desire for victory give life purpose and enhance a taste for existence.

One of the time-honored psychological explanations for suicide is that in the majority of cases individuals turn against themselves aggressive impulses that could not be directed at others in civilized societies. The Merovingian warrior, the knight of the age of chivalry, and later the mercenary soldier were by no means inhibited by pacifist prohibitions, and free expression of violence against their contemporaries served to diminish their own self-destructive tendencies.

We can see from many examples how the interplay between an externalized aggression and the risking of one's life on a permanent and voluntary basis produced an effective substitute for direct suicide. Jean Froissart tells us that in the fourteenth century ninety knights chose slaughter on the battlefield over retreat before enemy forces. Similarly, the *Chroniques de Flandre* recount that at Courtrai in 1302, Raoul de Nesles declared that "he no longer wanted to live when he saw all the flower of Christendom dead." The rules of the chivalric Order of the Estoile founded by King John II (Jean le Bon) forbade flight from battle.

The Crusades provide a long list of similar events. Guibert de Nogent notes that many Christians drowned themselves rather than be taken by the Turks, "preferring to choose their manner of death." Jean de Joinville witnessed similar scenes, which at times involved ecclesiastics. The bishop of Soissons refused to accept defeat and threw himself at the Turks, meeting certain death. Louis IX's queen, Marguerite de Provence, asked an aged knight to cut off her head should the Saracens threaten to take her. When Joinville and his companions were about to be taken prisoner, one cleric exclaimed, "I am for letting us all be killed if we are going right to heaven!" His suggestion was not taken, but it illustrates the attitudes of chivalry, when knights refused to see voluntary martyrdom as suicide. The same frame of mind can be seen in certain religious orders: In Seville in the thirteenth century, for instance, Franciscans taunted Muslims by shouting insults about Mohammed.[4]

Medieval chronicles are full of indirect warrior suicides of the sort. At times knights even directly murdered one another. The *Miracles de Saint Benoît* tells us that Aimo, the archbishop of Bourges, and his companions ran one another through with their swords when they were defeated by Eudes, the seigneur de Déols.[5] Prisoners, too, might prefer death to humiliation: Regnault, comte de Boulogne, was one; another was Jean de la Rivière, who declared, "No, I will not see the Paris rabble enjoying my ignominious death."[6]

The chronicles also report cases of suicide after a rape that recall the death of Lucretia. Examples include the wife of Jean de Carrouges,[7] as well as some women raped by the Normans.[8] Other women took their own lives out of loyalty to their husbands, still others out of a sense of duty or in an attempt to save the lives of relatives.[9] The self-sacrifice of the burghers of Calais in 1347 also bears all the signs of altruistic suicide. Even the pious Blanche of Castile flirted with the idea of suicide after the death of her husband, Louis VIII. At the death of Charles VII in 1461, the rumor circulated that he had deliberately stopped eating. Some claimed that he had been poisoned, but the king, weakened by an abscess on the brain, was in such a sorry state that there probably would have been little point to hastening his death.

Joan of Arc presents a more troubling case. At one point during her imprisonment (and for reasons not clarified) she threw herself from a high tower. During her interrogation she declared that "she would rather die than live after such a destruction of good folk" (an allusion to a massacre of civilians in Compiègne); on another occasion she responded that "she would have preferred to die rather than fall into the hands of the English, her enemies." She later contradicted these statements to declare that she had no intention of killing herself. Still, one of the accusations against her was an attempted self-homicide out of despair.

Thus the practice of voluntary death was known in the Middle Ages, but it occurred in very different ways in different social categories. The peasant or the craftsman hanged himself to escape poverty and suffering; the knight or the cleric arranged to get himself killed to escape humiliation and to deprive "the infidel" of a victory. In the first instance we have direct suicide of what the sociologists call the "egotistic" type; in the second, indirect and "altruistic" suicide. The goal was the same, the means and motivations differed.

The dominant morality (that is, the morality of the elite) sanctioned this difference in motivation and means. Direct, egotistic suicide was considered a cowardly act of avoidance and was severely punished by torturing the corpse, by refusing the body burial in consecrated ground, by promising eternal damnation to the soul, and by confiscating the estate of the deceased. Indirect, altruistic suicide was considered an act of courage in conformity with chivalric honor, or it was set up as a model and an example of unyielding faith unto martyrdom. Medieval society, which was governed by a military and priestly caste, was consistent with itself when it established the chivalric ideal and the quest for Christian sacrifice as the moral norm.

Voluntary Death in Literature

Literature illustrates the same dual vision of suicide, condemned in some cases and praised in others. Writers (who tended to be clerics or troubadours) usually condemned voluntary death in the name of Christian principles. There is no lack of warnings against suicide in literature. Albert Bayet lists a great many of them.[10] In *Le conte de la belle Maguelonne,* Pierre de Provence, unhappy in love, contemplates killing himself, "but as he was a true Catholic, he immediately took hold of himself and turned to the embrace of conscience." In the prose version of *Lancelot,* Galehaut (Galahad), who has decided to starve himself to death, is warned by priests "that if he died in that fashion his soul would be lost and damned"; the Lady of the Lake warns Lancelot that it would be a "grievous sin" if he killed himself. In *Fergus,* when Galiene threatens to throw herself off a high tower rather than marry a prince she does not love, God intervenes, not wishing to lose a soul. Similarly, the lady for whom Guillaume au Faucon wants to die warns him, "Your soul will be lost." Many courtly romances—*La Charette, Yvain, Beaudous, Floriant et Florete, Ipomédon, Éracles, L'Escoufle, Manekine,* and *Amadis et Idoine*—express horror at the idea of suicide.

In popular drama, mystery and miracle plays directly expressed the Church's moral position in an incontrovertible condemnation of suicide. Works such as *Les miracles de Notre Dame* present suicide as the result of a despair inspired by the devil. In *Les miracles de Sainte Geneviève,* for example, a nun declares: "Je me tuerais volontiers, / Mais c'est d'enfer le droit sentier. / Dieu, gardez-moi du désespoir!" (I would willingly kill myself, but that is the direct path to hell. Lord, deliver me from despair!).

In Rutebeuf's *Miracle de Théophile* the protagonist, a wicked character, wonders aloud, "Shall I go drown myself or hang myself?" Three suicides (or supposed suicides), Judas Iscariot, Herod Antipas, and Pontius Pilate, were archetypal villains, true antiheroes who met with damnation in all such plays. In *Le mystère de la Passion* the archangel Gabriel declares that Herod (who has stabbed himself) "has died an impetuous, ugly, abominable, and shameful death."

A quite different climate reigns in the chansons de geste. Suicide, of course, remains a sign of failure, whatever its immediate cause or circumstances. People kill themselves because of an impossible love, out of deeply felt sorrow, remorse, or shame, or else to avoid the humiliation that follows defeat. In short, they kill themselves because they have been vanquished and find it unbearable. The fatal act is prompted by anger or by a fit of jealousy or despair, hence by a sin. Moreover, it is above all the wicked who commit suicide, as does Gaumadrus in *Garin de Montglane,* who summons demons as he kills himself. It is often the way defeated infidels die. When this is the case, they are not accorded any admiration: The Muslim who kills himself to avoid captivity, as in *La chanson d'Antioche* or *Guy de Bourgogne,* is presented as beneath contempt.

Certain chansons de geste go so far as to recommend that the Christian knight flee rather than put up a desperate resistance. In his *Chronique rimée* Geoffroy de Paris presents such heroic behavior as tantamount to suicide: "I hold it, to the contrary, as homicide." In *Florent et Octavian* two clerics state that war is a form of voluntary death. In other stories (*La Châtelaine de Vergy*, for example) leaving for a crusade is presented as a worthy alternative to suicide: In this instance the duke, who has killed his wife, leaves in despair for the Holy Land. In real life the long and perilous journey that was like a "death" for the lord separated from his family and his lands undoubtedly often served as a compensatory act, thus helping to reduce the number of actual suicides in chivalry.

Although at first sight the general tone of the chansons de geste seems hostile to suicide in any form, they repay closer scrutiny. Albert Bayet states that "among the celebrated heroes of the best known chansons, not one is himself the artisan of his own death." To illustrate his point, Bayet lists the examples of Roland, who fights to the death with no thought of killing himself; Ogier, who asks Turpin to cut off his head when he is taken prisoner because he is loath to strike himself; Braminonde, who cries out for someone to kill him; Florence, who pleads with Miles, "Cut off my head soon"; Jérôme, who, overwhelmed with shame at having involuntarily wounded Huon, tells him, "Take my sword; cut my head"; Garsion, who asks the same service when he mistakenly kills his own brother; and Galienne, who cries out to Charlemagne, "Kill me!"[11] None of these warriors kills himself directly, but in asking for death at the hands of someone else, are they not all committing indirect suicide? The difference is one of pure form: The intention is the same, and the result is the same; the would-be suicide simply makes use of someone else's hand to commit the deed. All these episodes elicited the admiration of both the author of the work and the medieval listener.

The chansons de geste even include some honorable direct suicides. In *Auberi* Gauteron hangs himself in his father's stead; after her son's death and her husband's banishment, Béatrice throws herself from a high tower in *Daurel et Beton;* Dieudonné drowns himself in *Charles le Chauve;* Florent jumps out of a window in *Hernaut de Beaulande;* Doraine and Aye d'Avignon kill themselves to escape dishonor in *Charles le Chauve* and *Aye d'Avignon.* Moreover, these examples do not include all the heroes who simply express a desire to commit suicide rather than live on after defeat.

There are many altruistic suicides in courtly literature as well. One such is Lambègue, a knight who delivers himself to the enemy to save a city under siege; another is Perceval's sister, who dies after giving her blood to save a leper woman. In *Lancelot* Galehaut starves to death after learning that his friend has killed himself, and the author salutes his death as heroic. Lancelot tries to impale himself on his sword and is saved in extremis by a messenger from the Lady of the Lake. Ritually, almost instinctively, the characters in the romances of the Round Table speak of killing themselves whenever misfortune catches up with them. Tristan throws himself off a cliff rather than submit to torture, and Yseut asks Sandret to kill her rather than allowing herself to be handed over to the lepers. Suicide for love is even an obligatory gesture when a hero is faced by an insurmountable obstacle: Yvain, banished from his lady's sight, announces his intention to kill himself with his sword, declaring,

> Qui perd la joie et le plaisir
> par sa faute et par son tort,
> moult se doit bien haïr de mort,
> haïr et occir se doit

(Whoever loses happiness and comfort because of his own wrongs should hate himself to death. He should kill himself.)[12]

Aucassin announces that he will crack his head open against a wall if Nicolette is taken from him; Gloriandre throws herself from a window rather than marry Clodoveus's son; Pyrame and Thisbé die together, prefiguring Romeo and Juliet; the lady of Coucy starves herself to death; a lady in *Lancelot* jumps off a cliff rather than live on after her lover's death; when Lancelot believes Geneviève is dead, he prepares to die, passing a rope attached to his saddle pommel around his neck. Innumerable women prefer death to dishonor.

All these suicides, of course, exhibit failure behaviors, and we must agree with Jean-Claude Schmitt that "in literature as well [as life], suicide was a supremely doleful act that could only be dictated by insurmountable grief."[13] Yet in all these aristocratic works suicide appears as a heroic and admirable act, one that the author does not seek to condemn. Heroes make the supreme sacrifice when it is the only way to compensate for a shameful fault or to overcome an obstacle insurmountable by human means. Through suicide they surpass their mortal condition and rise above ordinary humanity. A Roland who sought to save his skin by fleeing or who handed over his sword to the Saracens would never have become the immortal worthy of the medieval epic. Here real-life conduct and literature were in total agreement on the distinction between noble suicide and a suicide deserving of scorn: More than the act itself, what counted were the personality and the motivation of the person committing the act. Both in romance and in life, the peasant who hanged himself as a way out of his misery was a coward whose corpse deserved to be subjected to torture and whose soul was relegated to hell; the impetuous knight who chose death over surrender on the battlefield was a hero deserving of both civil and religious honors. We cannot find a single instance of judiciary punishment meted out to the corpse of a noble who died by his own hand during the Middle Ages.

To Each Class Its Own Suicide

Suicide in the Middle Ages had two faces. It seems to have been rampant among commoners but to have spared nobles, who had compensatory behaviors that enabled them to avoid "self-homicide." Tourneys, hunting, wars, and crusades offered them opportunities to expose themselves to death or to sublimate their suicidal tendencies, but peasants and craftsmen had only the rope or the river if they wished to end their woes. Hence direct suicide was much more frequent among the lower classes.

This distinction can also be traced in the law and in theoretical works on morality. The noble's indirect suicide, whether he sacrificed himself for the cause he was defending or killed himself for love, in a fit of anger, or because he was afflicted by madness, was seen as altruistic. In all cases it was excusable. What is more, suicide for love and suicide in warfare were both connected with the noble's social function and involved his social entourage, thus diluting his personal responsibility. Since noble suicide was a social act, it was to some extent honorable. The peasant's suicide, on the other hand, was an isolated act born of egotism and cowardice: When the countryman went off to hang himself in secret, he was fleeing his responsibilities; his motivation was despair, a fatal vice inspired in him by the devil. The noble faced his responsibilities by going to a glorious death.

Allegorical representations in manuscript illuminations, stained-glass windows, cathedral statuary, and frescoes present this same dual view. For the most part these images illustrate the *Psychomachia,* an allegorical poem by Prudentius composed in the early fifth century in which Ira (anger) plunges a sword into her own body because she is unable to get the better of Patientia (patience, forbearance).[14] In medieval depictions, however, Desperatio (despair) is the chief cause of suicide, and Anger is shown either defeated by Patience or displaying her frustration by such violent gestures as tearing her clothing. Details in Giotto's decorations for the Arena Chapel in Padua, for example, show Desperatio hanging herself and Ira ripping her dress. In treatises on moral philosophy, as in manuscript illuminations, anger—a "noble" vice—rarely leads to suicide. Except in cases of madness or "frenzy," suicide arose out of despair.

Ecclesiastical suicides were a separate category. The texts tell us that priests and monks rarely committed suicide, but many such cases were undoubtedly concealed or made to seem accidental deaths or deaths by natural causes in order to avoid scandal. Bernard Paulin states, "People talk about epidemics of suicide in monasteries. Religious of both sexes are said to have fled this world in large numbers, either inspired by mysticism or by despair—the famous *acedia*. The phenomenon probably existed, but nothing permits us to state that it reached those proportions."[15] Among the clergy solidarity, a strong group cohesion, and a relatively privileged status probably all helped limit the number of priestly suicides, but a certain number of examples are attested, even among the high clergy, as with the death of Jacques de Chastel, bishop of Soissons during the reign of Louis IX.

The body of a cleric who had committed suicide was not subject to execution by civil justice. In the late fourteenth century the jurist Jean le Coq declared that if a cleric put an end to his days, his corpse must be handed over to the local bishop, even if the suicide had been in possession of his senses. He added, speaking of a prior of Sainte-Croix who had just committed suicide, "He should not have been hanged, because he was a priest."[16] In 1412 a typical case occurred in Rouen: Jean Mignot, a cleric, hanged himself. To stifle scandal the judge of the diocesan court *(official)* gave orders for his body to be buried in the cemetery by night. This was done, but when the affair was discovered, the body had to be disinterred and the cemetery, which had been polluted, had to be reconsecrated. The body was reburied in unconsecrated ground, but the corpse was not dragged or hanged.[17]

Confrontations between civil and ecclesiastical justice did at times arise, especially concerning confiscation of the estate of the deceased, as local custom demanded. Thus a question came up in Anjou concerning a priest, Jean Ambroys, who had stabbed himself to death in Montreuil-Bellay. The bishop of Poitiers and the comte de Tancarville both laid claim to his estate. The 1463 redaction of the *Ancienne Coutume d'Anjou* seemed to favor the count's claims:

Any person who is homicide of himself must be dragged, then hanged; all his goods and holdings are confiscate to the lord, baron, castellan, or others with rights of justice and entitled to the said confiscation where the said offense was committed and perpetrated—to wit, whoever has full [powers of] justice over his land. Furthermore, the said custom makes no difference according to the estate [social standing] of the person or to whether he dies intestate or not. Declared by my lord the comte de

Tancarville, lord of Montreuil-Bellay, concerning a priest named M. Jean Ambroys, resident in Montreuil-Bellay, who killed himself with a knife, whose goods monsignor of Poitiers attempted to put into question, saying that they belonged to him inasmuch as [the deceased] is a man of the church and died intestate.[18]

Suicide among Jews and Heretics

Some Jews and heretics were among the suicides of the Middle Ages. It was usually Christian persecution that drove Jews to suicide, particularly in the periods of general excitement preceding and during the crusades. This was the case in Mainz in 1065, as the chronicler Albert d'Aix tells us:

The Jews, seeing the Christians take up arms as enemies against them and their children with no respect for the weakness of old age, armed themselves as well against one another, against their co-religionists, against their wives, their children, their mothers, and their sisters, and massacred one another. It was horrible! Mothers grasped knives to cut the throats of their nursing babes, and they knifed their other children as well, preferring to destroy themselves by their own hands rather than succumb under the blows of the uncircumcised.[19]

Other mass suicides recalling the massacre at Masada are recorded in 1069, in twelfth-century England, and again in 1320 and 1321.[20]

Heretics committed suicide either because of persecution or as a result of their own particular beliefs. Examples of voluntary immolation following a refusal to abjure or arising from fear of torture are numerous. Rodulfus Glaber notes several instances during the eleventh century: One occurred in Orléans, where a band of heretics voluntarily went to the stake.[21]

This scene was repeated on several occasions during the Albigensian crusade—for example, when seventy-four Cathar knights threw themselves into the flames.[22] The leaders of the crusade were so persuaded of the Albigensians' steadfastness in their faith that they pushed them to suicide to spare themselves the responsibility for their deaths. The chronicler Pierre de Cernay tells us that Arnaud d'Amoury, abbot of Cîteaux, "keenly desired the death of Christ's enemies" after the capture of a group of heretics at Minerve, "but as he was a monk and a priest, he did not dare put them to death." Arnaud offered his prisoners a choice between death and abjuration, knowing well (as he himself told Simon de Montfort) that they would choose death.[23] Although the voluntary self-sacrifice of the Christian martyrs of the heroic centuries was held to be admirable, the Albigensians who marched joyfully to the stake were granted no merit, since their audacity was held to be inspired by the devil: Their acts were identical, but the souls of the early Christian martyrs were saved, while those of the Albigensian heretics were damned.

The Cathars also had a suicidal ritual, the *endura*—a hunger strike that followed receiving *consolamentum*, or "heretication." With the *consolamentum* a Cathar became "perfect" and was expected to die, thus obtaining eternal salvation and avoiding a return under the power of evil by prolonging this terrestrial life. The rite was usually administered when the individual was gravely ill and death seemed imminent. Emmanuel Le Roy Ladurie gives several examples of death by *endura* in Montaillou in the late thirteenth century. He has also shown that the practice was by no means systematic and that many people abandoned their hunger strike before reaching the point of death. "With all the good will in the world, and no matter how good a Cathar they may have been, there are good suicides but no delightful ones," Le Roy Ladurie concludes.[24]

Thus the medieval vision of suicide, far from being a monolithic condemnation of suicide, offers various nuances. The personality and social origin of the suicide and his or her motives mattered more than the act itself. Theory and law, of course, were extremely rigorous, but their application displays an astonishing flexibility. Condemnation of suicide in principle is neither obvious nor original in Christian civilization, and the religious sources of Christianity are either silent or highly ambiguous regarding suicide.

Suicide in the Hebraic World

The Old Testament offers a strictly neutral report of several voluntary deaths. After Saul had lost a battle with the Philistines, he first asked his armor-bearer to kill him; when the man refused, Saul fell on his sword, an event that the Book of Samuel reports without comment: "So Saul took his own sword, and fell upon it" (1 Sam. 31.4). When Abimelech's skull was fractured by part of a millstone thrown down at him by a woman, he told his armor-bearer, "Draw your sword and dispatch me, lest they say of me that a woman killed me" (Judges 9.54). Samson committed suicide by bringing the Philistines' palace down on his own head and theirs. Eleazar, son of Mattathias, "exposed himself to deliver his people and to get himself an everlasting name" at the battle of Beth-zachariah by throwing himself under an elephant in the army of Antiochus V, slitting the beast's belly, and being crushed as it fell (1 Macc. 6.43). Fleeing before Nicanor's troops, Razis found a spectacular way to kill himself:

Razis, now caught on all sides, turned his sword against himself, preferring to die nobly rather than fall into the hands of vile men and suffer outrages unworthy of his noble birth. In the excitement of the struggle he failed to strike exactly. . . . Still breathing, and inflamed with anger, he got up and ran through the crowd, with blood gushing from his frightful wounds. Then, standing on a steep rock, as he lost the last of his blood, he tore out his entrails and flung them with both hands into the crowd, calling upon the Lord of life and of spirit to give these back to him again. Such was the manner of his death. (2 Macc. 14.41–46)

When Tirzah was besieged, Zimri set fire to the royal palace and died in the flames (1 Kings 16.18). When Ahithophel learned that King David had ignored his advice, he returned home to his own city, where, "having left orders concerning his family, he hanged himself. And so he died and was buried in his father's tomb" (2 Sam. 17.23). Ptolemy Macron poisoned himself when he was accused of treachery (2 Macc. 10.13). Sarah, the daughter of Raguel, contemplated hanging herself when she was the victim of slander (Tobit 3.10).

Most of these suicides are presented as acts of heroism. This tradition continued into the Jewish Wars of the first and second centuries, when it provided many examples of suicide, both individual and collective. Flavius Josephus relates some of these heroic gestures: Phasael, in chains and a prisoner of the Parthians, "bravely dashed his head against a rock, as he was not free to use sword or hand." Josephus remarks, "Thus he showed himself a true brother of Herod, and Hyrcanus a cowardly poltroon."[25] When the Roman army attacked one of the towers of Jerusalem and set fire to it, the trapped Jews rushed to their deaths: "The men on top were suddenly hemmed in by the flames: many of them were burnt to death; many others jumped down among the enemy and were destroyed by them; some turned about and flung themselves from the wall; a few, seeing no way of escape, fell on their own swords and cheated the flames" (118). When he was surrounded near Scythopolis, Simon, son of Saul, killed his entire family. "Then Simon, having gone through all his family, stood over the bodies in view of everyone, and raising his right hand aloft for all to see plunged the whole length of the blade into his own throat" (157). The Romans were not to be outdone: Longus "held up his sword in the sight of the opposing lines and plunged it in his heart" (317–18).

Josephus gives many similar examples, but the culmination of such "heroic acts," as he calls them, was at Masada. In A.D. 73, after a determined resistance, a thousand Jews, who had crowded onto that rocky spur of land, were on the point of succumbing to the Roman attacks. In an extremely long discourse that ranged far beyond the circumstances at hand, their leader, Eleazar, harangued them and asked them to commit collective suicide. His discourse, a closely reasoned argument that injects Stoic, Neoplatonic, and Hindu elements into the Old Testament context, forms a true apologia for suicide. Eleazar put forth the classic arguments of philosophical suicide: Death is like sleep and delivers us from a brief and unhappy existence; it is unreasonable to continue to live when all that can be foreseen is further woes; since we all must die one day, why not decide the best moment to do so? Our soul aspires to leave the prison of the body and to enjoy a blessed immortality after this miserable terrestrial life; suicide is the supreme mark of human liberty and permits us to triumph over all ills; God wants to punish us. Certain passages in Eleazar's harangue have a resonance unfamiliar in Jewish thought:

I think it is God who has given us this privilege, that we can die nobly and as free men, unlike others who were unexpectedly defeated. In our case it is evident that daybreak will end our resistance, but we are free to choose an honourable death with our loved ones. . . . For those wrongs let us pay the penalty not to our bitterest enemies, the Romans, but to God—by our own hands. It will be easier to bear. Let our wives die unabused, our children without knowledge of slavery: after that, let us do each other an ungrudging kindness, preserving our freedom as a glorious winding-sheet. But first let our possessions and the whole fortress go up in flames. . . . Which of us, realizing these facts, could bear to see the light of day, even if he could live free from danger? Who is such an enemy to his country, who so unmanly and so wedded to life as not to be sorry he is alive today? If only we had all died before seeing the Sacred City utterly destroyed by enemy hands, the Holy Sanctuary so impiously uprooted! But since an honourable ambition deluded us into thinking that perhaps we should succeed in avenging her of her enemies, and now all hope has fled, abandoning us to our fate, let us at once choose death with honour and do the kindest thing we can for ourselves, our wives and children, while it is still possible to show ourselves any kindness. After all we were born to die, we and those we brought into the world: this even the luckiest must face. But outrage, slavery, and the sight of our wives led away to shame with our children—these are not evils to which man is subject by the laws of nature; men undergo them through their own cowardice if they have a chance to forestall them by death and will not take it. (360, 361, 364)

As a result, 960 Jews committed suicide that day.

After the poison comes the antidote: Josephus' *Jewish War* also contains a counter-argument to Eleazar's discourse. It comes from the author himself. The situation at Jotapata was delicate: Flavius Josephus and his companions were about to be taken by the Romans, who had promised to spare their lives. He attempted to persuade his companions not to commit suicide. Once again, the discourse reaches beyond the immediate context to take on a more general philosophical and religious dimension. It includes all the arguments reiterated by adversaries of suicide from that day to our own: Suicide is a cowardly act akin to desertion; it is an act counter to nature, which has endowed humankind with an instinct for survival; it is an affront to God, since He gave us life and is the master of our lives; we do not have the right to deprive God of one of his creatures; those who kill themselves go straight to hell and their bodies will be exposed:

The man who doesn't want to die when he ought is no more cowardly than the man who does want to when he ought not. What keeps us from going up to the Romans? Isn't it fear of death? Well, then, shall we, because we fear possible death at the hands of our foes, inflict certain death on ourselves? "No, it is fear of slavery," someone will say. As if we were free men now! "It is a brave act to kill oneself," another will suggest. Not at all! It is a most craven act. *I* think a pilot would be a most arrant coward, if through fear of bad weather he did not wait for the storm to break but sank his ship on purpose. Again, self-murder is contrary to the instincts shared by all living things, and towards the God who made us it is sheer impiety. Of all living things there is not one that dies on purpose or by its own act; it is an irresistible natural law that all should wish to live. For that reason if men openly attempt to rob us of life we treat them as enemies; if they lay a trap for us we punish them. And do you suppose God isn't angry when a man treats His gift with contempt? It is from Him we have received our being, and it is to Him we must leave the right to take it away. . . . If a man throws away what God has entrusted to his personal keeping, does he think the One he has wronged is unaware? To punish runaway slaves is considered right, even if the masters they are leaving are rogues; if we ourselves run away from the best of masters, God, shan't we be judged impious? . . . But if men go mad and lay hands on themselves, Hades receives their souls into the shadows. . . . The wisest of lawgivers has declared it a punishable offence. Those who destroy themselves must by our rules be exposed unburied till sundown, though even our enemies are thought to be entitled to burial. In other lands it is laid down that the right hands of those who die thus should be cut off, since they have made war on themselves, on the ground that as the body has been divorced from the soul, so the hand must be divorced from the body. . . . *I* shall not go over to the Roman side in order to be a traitor to myself. (200–201)

These arguments failed to persuade Flavius Josephus' companions. They drew lots and killed one another, until only Josephus himself and one companion remained. He then won over the other man, and the two of them surrendered to the Romans.

Which version are we to believe, Josephus arguing against suicide when he himself faces death or Josephus pleading in favor of suicide through Eleazar, whose discourse is obviously written by the author? The problem is secondary: What matters is to note that the Jewish world, the direct heir of the Old Testament, had no set position on suicide in the late first century A.D., when Judaism and Christianity parted company. Josephus presents all the arguments for and against suicide, and up to the twentieth century, moralists, theologians, and philosophers had little to add to them. Historical circumstances tilted the balance to the side of indulgence or rigor because no peremptory argument for or against suicide could be drawn from the biblical texts.

Among the Ten Commandments, Mosaic law obviously prohibits killing, but it does not specify whether that prohibition applies also to taking one's own life. As we have seen, mentions of suicide in the Old Testament are never accompanied by the explicit disapproval that pertains to murder. Moreover, the commandment against killing admits exceptions, such as killing enemies in wartime, killing in legitimate defense, or executing criminals. Thus medieval Christendom found little to draw on in the inspired texts, a fact that might go far toward explaining the broad variety of interpretations of suicide during the Middle Ages.

The Legacy of the Middle Ages

Between Madness and Despair

At first, medieval writers seem to have hesitated to take a position on voluntary death: The founding Christian texts were not explicit on the question, and the Church only gradually elaborated a coherent position.

"For These Sheep I Will Give My Life"

In the New Testament, where Christians began to portray themselves as different from the Jewish world, there is no direct discussion of suicide. Was Christ's death a suicide? Put as bluntly as this, the question seems shocking, but John quotes Jesus as saying, "For these sheep I will give my life" and "No one takes it from me; I lay it down freely myself" (John 10.15 and 10.18). Is this a clear statement of voluntary death, a choice that we call suicide? Medieval theologians found the passages in John an embarrassment. Origen, for instance, declares, "If we are not afraid of words and pay attention to things, we might say, finding no other expression that fits the facts, that divinely (in a manner of speaking) Jesus killed himself."[1]

Jesus knew what awaited him when he entered Jerusalem for Passover; he deliberately moved toward his death, and during his trial he did nothing to avoid it. In the context of the Man-God and of redemption, Jesus' suicide has a totally different significance and a totally other dimension from ordinary suicide, but the ambiguity remains. Christians, moreover, who are enjoined to imitate the Master in all things, are invited to sacrifice their own lives: "Whoever would save his life will lose it, but whoever loses his life for my sake will find it" (Matt. 16.25); "If anyone comes to me without turning his back on his father and mother, his wife and his children, his brothers and sisters, indeed his very self, he cannot be my follower" (Luke 14.26); "The man who loves his life loses it, while the man who hates his life in this world preserves it to life eternal" (John 12.25); "There is no greater love than this; to lay down one's life for one's friends" (John 15.13).

The list of New Testament passages in which Paul, James, Peter, Luke, and John invite the faithful to detest terrestrial life seems interminable. They constantly reiterate the notion that this life is to be scorned as an exile that we should hope will be as brief as possible. "I put no value on my life," St. Paul tells us in Acts 20.24, echoing several Old Testament texts.

The first generations of Christians understood this injunction, and during the period of the persecutions they took it literally, willingly giving themselves over to martyrdom. "Love for life did not deter them from death" (Rev. 12.11), John tells us, writing in the late first century, and he places in heaven "the spirits of those who had been beheaded for their witness to Jesus and the word of God" (Rev. 20.4). In his *Apology,* written in the second century, St. Justin (Justin Martyr) praised Christians who seek death, and in the early third century Tertullian and the Montanists advocated voluntary martyrdom. The Acts of the Christian martyrs abound in examples of Christians who turned themselves over to the civil authorities or who, by their responses to interrogation, deliberately chose death.

Christianity emerged and spread in an ambiguous atmosphere, asserting that earthly life—life in "the world"—is to be hated and that the Christian must aspire to death in order to attain God's presence and eternal life. This tendency became predominant in the early Church. St. John reports that Christ's teachings seemed to the Jews so ambiguous that at times they thought he was announcing his intention to commit suicide: "Again he said to them, 'I am going away. You will look for me but you will die in your sins. Where I am going you cannot come.' At this some of the Jews began to ask, 'Does he mean he will kill himself when he claims, "Where I am going you cannot come?"'" (John 8.20–21).

Christian death must testify to faith in God, however; it is not to be sought for itself or out of despair. The joyful death of the martyr was contrasted to the death of the despairing sinner. Hence Judas' presumed suicide soon became the archetype for a shameful, damnable death, not so much for the act itself as for the despair that prompted it. St. Matthew alone states that Judas hanged himself; the other evangelists say nothing about his death, and the Book of Acts reports that he died of a fall: "That individual bought a piece of land with his unjust gains, and fell headlong upon it. His body burst wide open, all his entrails spilling out" (Acts 1.18). Medieval miniaturists reconciled the two accounts by depicting Judas hanged with his belly split open. When Paul and his companions were miraculously delivered from prison, the jailer, who knew he deserved to be punished for his negligence, "drew his sword to kill himself" (Acts 16.27). When Paul stopped him from doing so, the jailer was instantly converted. Killing oneself for a purely human reason or out of despair is a wicked act, St. Paul states.

Life is detestable, but it must be put up with; death is desirable, but it must not be self-inflicted. Christian life was based on that difficult duality. The essential teachings, as they are found in the New Testament and as they were elaborated by the currents of spirituality, created a context predisposing the faithful to voluntary death. It took all the theological skill of Christian thinkers, backed by dissuasive canonical measures, to create instead a moral climate favorable to the prohibition of suicide.

Voluntary Martyrdom

Christianity's founding event was a suicide, and the writings of Jesus' disciples glorified voluntary self-sacrifice. The example of Christ was followed by many willing martyrs, to the point that the Church fathers became concerned and debated the question of suicide for three centuries.

Although as a matter of principle St. Athanasius condemns Christians who commit suicide, in view of the example of Christ he cannot bring himself to condemn them totally. St. Gregory of Nazianzus praises the suicide of the mother of the Maccabees but condemns suicide in general. St. Gregory of Nyssa applauds the voluntary deaths of the martyr Theodore, St. Basil, and St. Julia. St. Jerome is inconsistent, condemning Christians who commit suicide but praising pagan widows who preferred death to remarriage.[2] Peter of Alexandria condemns suicide but congratulates those who refuse to give in under persecution. Although Origen and Dionysius of Alexandria both assert that Jesus killed himself, they advise Christians to flee danger rather than expose themselves to it unnecessarily. St. Cyprian also recommends prudent retreat. St. Ambrose condemns suicide, yet he praises Samson, stating, "When the occasion for a praiseworthy death arises, it should be seized immediately" and "Let us not flee death: The Son of God did not scorn it."[3] St. Clement of Alexandria is nearly unique among the Church fathers in his unambiguous condemnation of Christian suicide: Christians who kill themselves have a false view of martyrdom; they take it on themselves to interpret divine will. On the other hand, Christian texts like the *Didascalia apostolorum* and the *Apostolic Constitutions* are imbued with indecision, torn between admiration for the beauty of the gesture and repudiation of a shameful display of weakness. The historian Eusebius relates, without disapproval, many cases of deliberate martyrdom, some of which inspired spontaneous cults, as in the cases of three Christian women, Domniana, Berenice, and Prosdocia.

Martyrdom was not the only occasion for indecision. Canon 25 of the Council of Ancyra in 314 mentions the case of a pregnant woman who committed suicide in despair after being seduced and abandoned by her lover (he was punished for his crime). Christian moralists of the times usually followed the Neoplatonic stand on suicide, condemning it in principle but admitting certain exceptions, such as killing oneself to carry out an order of the civil authorities (like Socrates), to escape shame, or to avoid an overly cruel fate. In practice, however, doctrine was far from clear: At a time when many sins were subject to strict discipline and required public reconciliation with the Church, canon law contained no sanctions against those who attempted to take their own lives.

As in many other domains, the struggle against heretical currents tightened doctrinal positions and brought stricter disciplinary measures. In 348 the Council of Carthage condemned voluntary death, in reaction to Donatism, which praised the practice. In 381 Timothy, bishop of Alexandria, decreed that henceforth prayers could no longer be said for suicides except in instances of certified insanity, a move that implied that self-homicides were damned.

St. Augustine and the Prohibition of Suicide

The hardening of the Church's position on suicide is even clearer in St. Augustine, whose *City of God* proclaims the rigorous doctrine that became the official Church position:

This we declare and affirm and emphatically accept as true: No man may inflict death upon himself at will merely to escape from temporal difficulties—for this is but to plunge into those which are everlasting; no man may do so even on account of another's sins, fearing they may lead to a sin of one's own—for we are not sullied by others' sins; no man may do so on account of past sins—for to expiate them by penance we need life all the more; no one may end his own life out of a desire to attain a better life which he hopes for after death, because a better life after death is not for those who perish by their own hand.[4]

Prohibition of all types of suicide was based on the Mosaic commandment against killing, which brooked no exceptions. Augustine reinforces his sweeping condemnation with arguments: Those who kill themselves are cowards incapable of withstanding trials; it is vanity that induces suicides to lend importance to what others think of them (both vices were combined in

Cato). No circumstance excuses suicide, not even rape. If Lucretia's soul remained innocent, she had no reason to kill herself; if she drew even involuntary pleasure from the episode, it would have been better for her to live on to do penance for that sin. Nor is a desire to flee temptation a valid reason, Augustine continues, for one commits a sure crime in order to escape a possible sin, and death removes all chance for repentance. Dying to flee suffering and pain is pure cowardice; death from despair caused by a contemplation of one's sins is no better. As with Judas, killing oneself adds a second crime to the first. In no circumstance have we the right to open the gates to eternal life ourselves.

Augustine's uncompromising prohibition of suicide reflects both Platonic influences and an excessively strong reaction to Donatism. Although Platonic philosophers admitted certain exceptions, they held suicide to be an offense against God's rights, an idea reiterated by Plotinus, Porphyry, Macrobius, and Apuleius. Augustine simply takes the notion one step further, recasting it in the light of "Thou shalt not kill." He states that life is a sacred gift from God that God alone can take away. The Donatist heretics were criminals when they defended voluntary martyrdom.

Augustine squarely tackles embarrassing examples and contradictions. Was Samson a criminal? Or St. Pelagia, honored by the Church for killing herself to preserve her virginity? In these exceptional cases that do not fit his scheme, Augustine allows that such people must have received a special call from God. As for Jesus, his death was undeniably voluntary. What is more, Augustine states, the Mosaic commandment not to kill is far from absolute, given that condemned criminals can be put to death and enemies can be killed in times of war. For centuries civil and religious authorities were to continue to wrestle with the paradox that unfortunate individuals who kill themselves to put an end to their own suffering and that of their dear ones are criminals, whereas the slaughter on the battlefield of millions of healthy young men who have no desire to die is a meritorious act. Augustine himself states that "it is better to die of hunger than eat food sacrificed to idols" and that bishops should not flee persecution.[5]

The Sociopolitical Context of Hostility to Suicide, Fifth to Tenth Centuries

How can we explain the hardening of the Christian moral position on suicide after the early fifth century? Albert Bayet sees it as the result of social pressure: Public opinion was deeply hostile to suicide, and it influenced the cultivated elite, which favored a more flexible stance. This hypothesis seems to me hardly credible, since it makes suicide the only moral domain in which the leaders of the Church allowed themselves to be influenced by popular sentiment. Admittedly, there were many examples of contamination, and many superstitions found a lasting niche in Christian practices, but none involved such an essential point. Moreover, nothing proves that the common people were in fact more hostile to the practice of voluntary death than the elite.

There is a link, however, between the emphasis on the preservation of human life in both civil and canon law and the evolution of the Roman Empire in the late fourth and early fifth centuries. Beginning in the reigns of Diocletian and Constantine, the Roman state was undergoing a serious economic and demographic crisis and was becoming transformed into a totalitarian system in which individuals lost all right to dispose of their own persons. The system of agricultural exploitation by *coloni* spread throughout rural areas: The *colonus* was free but attached to the land and was dependent on the *dominus,* or "master." He could not marry, become a priest, or join the army without his master's permission. In 332 Constantine decreed that a runaway *colonus* must be returned to his master. In cities and towns members of corporations were fixed within their social and professional conditions. An acute shortage of manpower dictated the requisitioning of all human lives for the service of the economy and the defense of the empire. One result was harsher civil legislation, which replaced the Roman world's traditional indulgence toward suicide. Henceforth the possessions of anyone who committed suicide in an attempt to avoid trial were confiscated by the state, gradually establishing a connection between confiscation and culpability in suicide.

As for the Church, it launched a campaign to enhance marriage, condemning as deviant any view of sexual abstinence as an obligation for all Christians or of virginity as something to be glorified. All forms of contraception and abortion were prohibited, and an imperial edict of 374 prohibited infanticide. The abandonment of infants was discouraged. All these complementary measures were aimed at promoting and protecting human life; they were a defense mechanism put into play by a society that felt its existence threatened by a declining birthrate. It is useless to ask which power, civil or religious, influenced the other, because after Constantine the two worked in close collaboration.

The Church, whose landholdings had grown considerably, had no reason to seek the emancipation of *coloni* or slaves. Their lives belonged to their masters, and in 452 the Council of Arles condemned the suicide of all *famuli* (slaves and domestic servants). The servant who kills himself robs his master and owner; his suicide is an act of revolt, and he himself is "filled with diabolical fury." In 533 the Council of Orléans, confirming Roman law, prohibited oblations in the name of suspected criminals who had killed themselves before coming to trial. Thus the repressive and dissuasive arsenal against suicide was slowly being put into place. Social, economic, and political conditions put pressure on morality, criminalizing suicide as an offense against God, nature, and society. For the Church the fact that voluntary martyrdom, the only honorable form of suicide, disappeared with the conversion of the Roman Empire to Christianity meant that no religious motivation remained to excuse suicide. In civil society and religious thought alike, the master had the power of life and death over his dependents, who in turn owed everything to him.

This attitude was reinforced during the age of the barbarian kingdoms, when civil and religious authorities continued to act in concert. In the early sixth century the Lex Romana Visigothorum introduced distinctions: The possessions of a suicide would be confiscated if the act had been motivated by remorse for having committed a crime, but not if it had been inspired by a distaste for life, by shame caused by debts, or by illness. Damnation was by no means an automatic consequence: In the Life of St. Martin of Tours, the saint is shown resuscitating a slave who has killed himself and men who have thrown themselves into a well. Such distinctions disappeared during the late sixth century. The Council of Braga in 563 and the Council of Auxerre in 578 condemned all types of suicide and forbade commemorative offerings and masses for suicides. This meant that suicide was now punished more severely than murder, which entailed only the payment of a fine.

In the Anglo-Saxon penitentials of the eighth and ninth centuries, only the insane or the possessed are excused from punishment for suicide, and then only if they had lived honorably before falling into the clutches of the devil. Killing oneself out of despair was considered the most culpable type of suicide. The Church was beginning to insist on individual confession of sins, a practice that reinforced its hold on souls. Persons afflicted with *desperatio* committed suicide because they believed their sins beyond all pardon; like Judas, they sinned against God by doubting his mercy, and they sinned against the Church by doubting its powers of intercession. Despair was among the gravest sins precisely because it contested the role of the Church in pardoning faults through absolution just when the Church was beginning to assert its role as a universal and obligatory intermediary between God and humankind.

The penitentials paralleled civil justice when they forbade prayers in favor of persons who committed suicide out of fear of criminal justice, or even persons who killed themselves for reasons unknown, suspected of having something on their conscience. The Frankish synods were particularly severe: In Châlons in 813, Paris in 829, and Valence in 855 the bishops defined death in a duel as suicide and forbade prayers and Christian burial for the victims. In the mid-ninth century Pope Nicholas I decreed, in response to questions raised by the newly converted Bulgarians, that all types of suicide were forbidden and that suicides were beyond help and irremediably condemned. The hunt to ferret out suicides began. In the early tenth century Reginon of Prüm directed bishops to inform themselves regarding all cases of suicide in the parishes in their dioceses. In the period before the Crusades, when anti-Muslim feeling began to run high and some Christians revived the practice of voluntary martyrdom, the ecclesiastical authorities proclaimed their opposition to it.

After a long period of indecision during the first four centuries of Christianity, barbarian rule brought total prohibition of suicide to Western Europe. The severity of both the civil and the religious authorities regarding self-murder might strike us as odd in the general climate of bloodthirsty violence and scorn for human life that reigned from the fifth to the tenth century. The seeming contradiction needs to be set within the context of an age of changing relations between God and humankind that reflected other changing relations between masters and dependents. Ties of dependency multiplied in the late Roman Empire, and God's interests reflected those of the property owners: Taking one's own life was an offense against the rights of both God and the master. Civil and religious authorities carried on a parallel combat against suicide using complementary dissuasive measures—confiscation of earthly possessions and promise of eternal damnation. In both domains the prohibition of suicide entailed a loss of human freedom. Stripping people of their essential right to dispose of their own persons worked to the benefit of the Church, which directed all aspects of their lives and drew its strength from the numbers of the faithful, and to the benefit of the lords (some of whom were churchmen), who needed to maintain and increase their labor supply in an underpopulated world where exploitation of the domain was regularly compromised by famine and epidemic disease.

The Theological Bases of the Prohibition of Suicide

From the eleventh to fourteenth century the civil and religious opposition to suicide gradually became a system. Existing notions concerning suicide were given a rational and juridical framework in the great scholastic syntheses and in treatises on canon and civil law, thus helping to turn what had been a transitory adaptation to a specific historical situation into an absolute with an intangible value of its own. The result was the extremely durable notion that suicide brought infamy. From the Renaissance to the Enlightenment, the "wall of shame" that medieval theologians, jurists, and moralists had erected around suicide made challenge difficult.

The theologians were unanimous. In the late eleventh and early twelfth century, Abelard used Platonic arguments to condemn all suicides in his *Sic et non,* while St. Bruno called suicides "Satan's martyrs." St. Bonaventura saw an immoderate self-love in suicide, a notion with which John of Salisbury and Jean Buridan agreed. Duns Scotus wrote in the fourteenth century, "No one can be a homicide of himself without a special command from God."[6]

Two thirteenth-century doctors of the Church subjected the question of suicide to the scholastic method, giving arguments for and against and offering their own *resolutio.* Alexander of Hales cites five passages from Scripture as arguments in favor of suicide: two statements of St. Paul's ("For me, it is a boon to die" and "Who can free me from this body under the power of death?" [Rom. 24]); one phrase from Job ("All that a man has he will give for his life" [Job 2.4]); a phrase from the Psalms ("The body is like a prison"); and a statement of Jesus ("Whoever loses his life for my sake will find it" [Matt. 16.25]). Alexander also recalls the glorious suicides of Samson and Razis. He then presents eight arguments against suicide taken from both Scripture and pagan writers: St. Paul's statement (Rom. 3.8) that one should not commit an evil deed in view of a good end; the argument that a virgin who has been raped is not guilty of any crime, hence she kills an innocent person when she kills herself; the Mosaic commandment that prohibits all murder; Plato's statement that our life belongs to God; Plotinus' statement that only a blameworthy passion can effect a violent rupture of the ties that bind the soul and the body; the argument that personal improvement is only possible in life; the argument that sinners must live in order to repent and do penance; and the argument that it is passion that urges us to put a premature end to our days in order to enjoy eternal bliss, and passion is sinful.

Alexander then offers his own opinion. Scripture requires interpretation: Man can only give what does not involve sin; even if the body is a prison, that does not give us the right to leave it; losing one's life means only renouncing bodily pleasures; to desire death refers only to death to the world; man is duty-bound to love himself; "thou shalt not kill" is an inviolable law. His conclusion: "In no case, under no pretext, is it legitimate to kill oneself."

In his *Summa theologica* (part II-II, q. 64, art. 5, "Whether it is lawful to kill oneself?"), St. Thomas Aquinas treats the problem more philosophically. His solution provided arguments against suicide for centuries to come. As arguments in favor of suicide he states the following: Killing oneself commits no infraction of justice; public authorities can kill malefactors, hence a person holding public power who has broken the law can kill himself; killing oneself permits avoidance of worse ills; the Bible praises the suicides of Samson and Razis. Thomas offers only one argument against suicide: that the Mosaic commandment prohibits killing. He states in his *resolutio* that all the arguments in favor of suicide are fallacious: Suicide does an offense to both God and society; no one has the power to pass judgment on himself; killing oneself does not avoid greater evils because the act itself is the greatest evil since it prevents repentance and penance. Suicide, he concludes, is absolutely forbidden. He offers three basic reasons: first, it is an offense against nature and against charity because it contradicts both a natural inclination to live and our duty to love ourselves; second, it is an attack on society because we belong to a community in which we have a role to play; third, it is an offense against God, who is the proprietor of our lives. Thomas offers an enlightening comparison: "Whoever takes his own life, sins against God, even as he who kills another's slave, sins against that slave's master." As for Samson and Razis, Thomas declares that they had special commands from God. Aristotle and Plato, human reason, St. Augustine, and Scripture all concurred to forbid suicide.

Diabolic Despair the Culprit

Moralists and poets threw the weight of their talents onto the balance. Vincent de Beauvais condemned "distaste for life," and in Canto 13 of the *Inferno* Dante reserved a special place for suicides among the violent in the seventh circle of hell. Because they are guilty of injury to themselves, suicides in Dante lose all human form and become trees bearing faded leaves in an immense, dark forest. Because they have refused life, they are eternally fixed in place, twisting in the wind and moaning. Their spokesman is Pietro Della Vigna, the minister to Frederick II who committed suicide in a fit of despair. Despair is not a psychic state here, but rather a sin prompted by the devil, who persuades the sinner that damnation is certain and leads him to doubt divine mercy.

To turn Christians away from killing themselves, the Church made use of a large body of pious literature that circulated in the form of tales, exempla in sermons, and episodes in mystery plays. The moral of these tales is that one must not despair, since miracles are always possible. One of them tells of the misadventures of a pilgrim making his way to the shrine of St. James at

Compostela. Deceived by the devil, who has taken on the form of St. James himself, the pilgrim slits his throat, but he is resuscitated by the Virgin Mary, who snatches his soul away from Satan.[7] In other tales the desperate sinner is saved at the last minute by the intervention of a saint or the Virgin, by making the sign of the cross, or by a timely sprinkling of holy water. *The Cloud of Unknowing,* a fourteenth-century English mystical text, warns against a diabolic seduction that pushes minds inclined to melancholy toward "nonbeing." In *Piers Plowman,* an allegorical work written between 1360 and 1370, William Langland shows Avarice sinking into despair, attempting to commit suicide, and being saved by Repentance. Similarly, John Skelton shows Magnificence persuaded by Despair that his sins are beyond pardon and choosing to stab himself, only to be saved by Good Hope.[8]

The best cure for despair, and thus for suicidal urges, was confession, which brought pardon for one's sins and reconciliation with God. The eleventh and twelfth centuries were the decisive moment of the elaboration of a theology of penitence. In the twelfth century St. Bernard exhorted the faithful to confess without delay and to hold fast against despair should they feel themselves falling back into sin. In 1215 the Fourth Lateran Council decreed, "All the faithful, of either sex, when they arrive at the age of discretion, must personally and loyally confess all their sins to their parish priest at least once a year." The procedures of the "tribunal of penitence" were accordingly simplified and made more flexible. Until around 1000, confession of sins had been separate from reconciliation (where grievous sins were concerned, an event that occurred only once a year, on Holy Thursday). Beginning in the eleventh century, however, confession of sins, penitence, and pardon were brought together. Thus repentant sinners were reconciled with God even before fulfilling a penance because the priest, who held "the power of the keys," could give absolution, thus offering the faithful immediate reassurance and removing all cause for despair. Given this, it seemed impossible that anyone in his right mind would kill himself, which meant that should a suicide occur, the church would presume insanity.[9]

Penalties for Suicide in Canon and Civil Law

The faithful now had infallible recourse against suicide, so those who were not insane and yet killed themselves could expect no mercy. Canon law, fixed in the twelfth century in the works of Burchard of Worms, Yves de Chartres, Gratian, and Gregory IX, was extremely severe. From then on we find indications that Christian burial was refused to suicides, although the first incontrovertible written proof of this severity appears only in 1284, at the Synod of Nîmes. The synod confirmed the refusal of Christian burial to the excommunicated, to heretics, to men killed in tournaments, and to those who took their own lives; exceptions were to be made only in the presence of signs of repentance in extremis. Raymond of Peñafort states as much in his *Summa,* and in his *Speculum juris,* written in the late 1300s, Guillaume Durand, bishop of Mende, offers a model letter requesting the exhumation of the cadaver of a suicide erroneously buried in the cemetery.

Civil law added its rigors to those of canon law.[10] The medieval customals are an invaluable source of information on local practices concerning suicide. In France the question was more likely to arise in the north of the kingdom, where the law clearly assimilated very old superstitious practices aimed at preventing suicides from returning to haunt the living. One of the oldest texts, an ordinance of the municipal government of Lille in the thirteenth century, stipulates that the body of a male suicide is to be dragged to the gallows, then hanged; a female suicide's body is to be burned. Similar customs pertained in Anjou and Maine. The *Très ancienne coutume de Bretagne,* compiled in the fourteenth century, specifies, "If a man deliberately kills himself he must be hanged by the feet and dragged like a murderer, and his movable goods will be acquired by whoever has claim to them."

The *Loi de Beaumont* went a step further: A suicide's corpse was to be dragged "as cruelly as possible in order to make a show of the experience to others." The stones on which a suicide had walked were to be taken up. In Metz customary law stipulated that the body of a suicide be removed from the house through an opening dug under the threshold. The body should then be thrown into the river, nailed up in a barrel bearing a sign commanding that it be left to drift: "Throw it downstream; let it go; it is by justice." The accursed body would thus be borne far away, without polluting the local river water. This would avoid the legendary misadventure supposed to have occurred when the body of Pontius Pilate (thought to have killed himself) caused disastrous floods after being thrown into the Tiber. The remains of a suicide were thrown into the Rhine in Strasbourg, where the body of a bishop who had supposedly hanged himself was blamed for causing a similar disaster.

The authorities in Zurich treated the body of a suicide in accordance with the manner of death: Suicides who had stabbed themselves had a wooden wedge driven into their skulls; those who died by drowning were buried in the sand five feet from the water's edge; those who died in a fall were buried under a heap of stones with big stones on their head, stomach, and feet. It may have been in the interest of making the site unrecognizable and preventing the return of a suicide's spirit that in Lille and Abbeville the body of a suicide was thrown out a window or "passed under the threshold of the house through a hole, face down like an animal." In some parts of Germany the body was first dragged on a hurdle, then hanged in chains and left to rot. The corpse was usually dragged and hanged upside down.

In England the body of a suicide was buried under the high road, preferably at a busy crossroads, and it was pinned to the ground by driving a wooden stake through the chest. With the corpse immobilized and trodden upon in this manner, there was less chance that the spirit would emerge to haunt the living. Suicide was a form of malefic death and an illustration of the work of the powers of evil, identified in pagan times as evil spirits and in the Christian age as the devil. The execution of the corpse was both a rite of exorcism and an example intended to dissuade imitation. It was also a dreadful trial for the suicide's nearest kin, who were forced to watch a public spectacle that brought dishonor to the entire family group.

Another trial awaited the survivors. Confiscation of the suicide's estate appears in France as early as 1205 in the report of an inquiry conducted by royal commissioners who "assigned to the king or the baron the movable goods of those who have killed themselves or drowned themselves voluntarily."[11] In 1270 the *Établissements de Saint Louis* stated, "If it should happen that any man hang himself, drown, or kill himself in any manner, the goods will be for the baron, and also those of his wife." Suicide fell under high justice, and confiscation might take various forms: confiscation of movable goods in the customary law of Anjou, Maine, Normandy, Poitou, Brittany, and the Beauvaisis; confiscation of both movable and immovable goods in Bordeaux and elsewhere; confiscation of a portion of the estate, as in a decree of the treasurer of Rouen in 1397 that gave one-third of a suicide's possessions to the king and two-thirds to the widow and the children (a clement division that seems an exception to the rule of severity). In some provinces of France—Maine and Anjou, for example—a further custom, called *ravaire* or *ravoyre,* called for removing the roof of the house in which a suicide had taken place and dismantling the walls on either side of the hearth. In addition, the fields that had belonged to a suicide were to be burned and his vines and woods cut down to the height of a man.

Legislation in England is better known, thanks to the jurists who wrote on English common law beginning in the mid-thirteenth century. In the seventh century the Council of Hertford prohibited Christian funeral rites for suicides, and in the mid-tenth century a law of King Edgar confirmed the provision. Acts from the 1230s bear witness to the confiscation of goods in

Surrey, and Henry de Bracton shows in his *De legibus et consuetudinibus Angliae,* a systematic treatise on English law compiled between 1250 and 1260, that the courts differentiated between suicides who were *non compos mentis* and those who were *felo de se.* In the latter case the lands and goods of the deceased were confiscated.[12] In the late fourteenth century King Richard II distributed the estates of several suicides to his courtiers.

The Practice of Suicide in the Middle Ages

The study of actual events is a more delicate matter than the study of medieval law because the documentation is scant and uninformative. Nonetheless the evidence suggests a decidedly more indulgent attitude in practice than the severity of the juridical texts would lead us to suppose.

Jean-Claude Schmitt draws several conclusions based on a sampling of fifty-four cases of suicide in the Middle Ages.[13] Men were three times more likely to kill themselves than women were; hanging was the means most often used (34 cases out of 54), followed by drowning (12), stabbing (5), and leaping to death from high places (4)—proportions that are strangely similar to those for suicides in the twentieth century. The same is true of the seasonal distribution of suicides: March and April were the peak months, followed by July. Leaving aside biological rhythms, the role of which is as yet unclear, bodily weakness from Lenten fasting in March and April, and heavy agricultural labors in July may have played an important role in rural Christian societies.

A seeming preference for Fridays and Mondays is more difficult to explain. Was there an atmosphere of penitence and remorse on Fridays and, on Mondays, a sense of discouragement at having to face a new work week? Medieval suicide seems to have been largely nocturnal: Two-thirds of the instances studied took place between midnight and dawn. Here a connection between darkness and despair may have provided an added inducement, along with the absence of a better occupation for the mind, left to solitary thoughts in the darkness. The available data are too few to allow us to draw definite conclusions. To end the list, people usually committed suicide at home.

People of all social categories took their own lives, but proportions are falsified by the nature of the evidence, which consists for the most part of court records from an urban setting. The great majority of the townspeople who committed suicide were craftsmen. The absence of nobles can be quite easily accounted for by their lifestyle, which offered many opportunities to exercise violence freely and to risk one's life, as we have seen, but it can also be explained by the fact that nobles controlled justice. It was an easy matter to camouflage a suicide as an accidental or natural death, given the complicity of both the kinship group and the civil and religious authorities.

Clergy had access to the same methods of dissimulation, which makes the rather high proportion of priests who took their own lives (19 percent of all cases) all the more troubling. The clergy's greater vulnerability to despair might also explain the particularly strong insistence on this point in pastoral letters. A more acute sense of guilt and an awareness that some sins were irremissible might have had something to do with a relatively high suicide rate for clergy.

Insanity: A Frequent Excuse

Most suicides probably originated in the tribulations and unbearable sufferings of life: hunger, illness, destitution, the death of loved ones, extreme poverty, imprisonment and fear of judicial torture, and jealousy. Honor, a sentiment reserved to the nobility in literature, is conspicuously absent from this list. All cases of deliberate suicide were attributed to a precise cause that brought an excess of physical and moral suffering. It is interesting to note that simple distaste for life is categorized among forms of madness, as Bracton's treatise explicitly states. The medieval mind could not even imagine that anyone might doubt the goodness of existence. What the eighteenth century later called "philosophic suicide" was not among the possibilities in the Middle Ages. It was inconceivable that someone in his or her right mind might come to the objective conclusion that life was not worth living. Simply entertaining such a thought for no precise reason was in itself a symptom of madness, of the mental imbalance that was beginning to be called *melancholia*. That term, derived from Greek and meaning "black humor," designated a physical affliction, an excess of black bile that clouded the brain and prompted somber thoughts. Brunetto Latini, writing around 1265, was among the first to use it.

This first type of madness manifested itself in depression and gloom. A second type, called *frenesy* or *furor*, gave rise to violent fits. Often brought on by alcohol, it was manifest in hallucinations, delirium, violent or brutal acts, and a tendency to complain of everything and everyone. The least sign of strange or unaccustomed behavior might be interpreted as proof of alienated reason, and it was often accepted as evidence by the investigators. The criminal records of Saint-Martin-des-Champs mention five cases of suicide, four of which are excused with the notations, "furious and out of his senses," "mad and out of his senses," or "raving and out of his senses."[14] Sixteen (30 percent) of the fifty-four cases studied by Jean-Claude Schmitt were attributed to insanity, at times seemingly with good reason, but at other times somewhat more dubiously.

When a suspect death occurred, the body was not to be touched until the authorities arrived. In cities and towns these were the *échevins;* in rural areas, the proper authority was the representative of whoever held high justice in the locality; in England, it was the coroner. A report was drawn up, and it was followed by an inquiry during the course of which the kin and close acquaintances of the deceased would be called as witnesses. It is clear that public opinion played an important role in these proceedings and that the dead person's relations had every reason to pass off the death as the result of an accident, a crime, or an insane act. This was not a difficult task, providing the village community gave moral support to the survivors, as usually seems to have been the case. Barbara Hanawalt demonstrates that this occurred in fourteenth-century England: When jurors drawn from the local communities were charged with conducting the inquiry and arriving at a verdict, they produced a high number of acquittals, and the coroner (an unpaid post) was open to bribery by the family of the deceased.[15] Should the jury produce a guilty verdict, the goods of the deceased were appraised at much less than their real worth.

Philippe de Beaumanoir states that in the Beauvaisis in the thirteenth century a suicide's goods could not be confiscated unless the deceased person's full responsibility was clearly established. If the body was found at the bottom of a well, for instance, the site of the well, the reasons the deceased may have had for going there, his or her mental and physical state, and the likelihood of a fainting fit (which would indicate accidental death) all had to be taken into consideration. In one case in Bedfordshire, a jury called in April 1278 concluded that the victim, who had been ill, had been seized by a fit of weakness, but a royal inquiry conducted soon after declared his death to be suicide.[16] Beaumanoir tells us that if the deceased had been heard to say, "Someday I will kill myself," it was sufficient proof of intention, but statements of the sort had to have been reported to the authorities. If in spite of all these loopholes there seem to have been many confiscations, it may be because the courts could also use the fact that someone died intestate as a pretext for confiscating the estate.[17]

Confiscation might be avoided, particularly when the suicide was a married woman. Or the king might issue a pardon, as Charles VI did in 1418 for a man who had killed himself because he had lost his fortune, his children had died, and his wife had fallen ill.[18] In 1278 the Parlement de Paris acquitted

Philippe Testard even though the evidence was not conclusive. Albert Bayet interprets the silence of customals from southern France on the question of suicide as a sign of an absence of condemnation, at least among the more notable citizens, and as a result of the influence of a renaissance of Roman law after the twelfth century.[19]

Signs of Indulgence

In the fourteenth century some jurists called for mitigation of the laws regarding suicide. In his *Somme rural,* for instance, Jean Boutillier (d. 1395) argues for a return to Roman law. When a suicide occurs, he writes, the lord's justice should conduct an inquiry, and no penalty should be applied unless the deceased killed himself to escape a sentence, in which case the corpse should receive the same punishment that would have been meted out to the living person. In all other cases—that is, illness or madness *(forsennerie)*—he should be buried in the normal manner. "If it was out of sickness or madness or for any woeful path, such as the sudden loss of his wife, his children, or his posses-sions (and please note that for these two things anyone would be stricken with despair), even if he loses his life, he should not lose his wealth or his body; nor should he be turned over for criminal execution, such as being hanged, nor put to public justice, for the body has done no offense to justice, but [only] to itself."[20] Once again, suicide out of distaste for life was, by implication, classified among cases of madness.

I might add, finally, that even the theologians and the moralists, usually so severe where self-murder was concerned, recognized the grandeur of such suicides of classical antiquity as Cato, Diogenes, and Zeno. Alain de Lille and Vincent de Beauvais also praised the courage of voluntary martyrs. Other writers, anticipating the works of the casuists of the sixteenth to eighteenth centuries, admitted Christian suicide in extreme cases. Brunetto Latini states that one can die of starvation rather than steal bread; Hugues de Sainte-Marie asserts that death is preferable to aiding a heretic. Jean Buridan and Duns Scotus intimate that war and crusades can serve as substitutes for suicide, Buridan by declaring that on occasion death is preferable to flight, and Duns Scotus by stating that someone who has committed homicide can redeem himself by "exposing his life in a just cause, as, for example, in a struggle against the enemies of the Church." Other writers—Guillaume le Clerc and Philippe de Vitry—reintroduced the notion of Christ's suicide.[21] No medi-eval theologian or moralist called for or justified refusing Christian burial to a suicide or subjecting a suicide's body to criminal punishment.

In the final analysis, medieval attitudes toward suicide offered many more nuances than we might expect from the macabre rites of execution performed on the corpse, the unappealable pronouncements of St. Augustine and St. Thomas, or the global statements in the customals. The age was not tender toward homicides either. Popular beliefs, official religion, and civil authorities all recoiled in horror before murder, an act that simultaneously offended nature, society, and God. Paradoxically, however, suicide—an exclusively human gesture—seemed so inhuman that it could only be explained by the direct intervention of the devil or by insanity. In the first case, a suicide was the victim of a diabolical despair for which the Church offered the remedy of confession. Anyone who succumbed despite that aid was consigned to hell. In the second case, the unfortunate person was not responsible for his or her act, and thus might be saved. The age took a very broad view of madness, and the pity or the fears of the victim's family did much to enlarge its definition even further. Literature recognized the grandeur of suicides for love or honor, and the nobility had their own substitutes for direct suicide.

Ordinary suicide in the Middle Ages concerned the world of laborers *(laboratores)* above all others. It was peasants and craftsmen who died by their own hand, often following a brutal worsening of their condition. The *bellatores* (warriors and nobles) preferred indirect methods for killing themselves. The *oratores* (religious) killed themselves on occasion, but insanity was always offered as the cause of an ecclesiastical suicide and clerics' bodies were not subjected to punishment. The bad sorts of suicide—petty and egotistical suicide, the suicide of the coward seeking to avoid tribulations—were always those of the rustic, the serf, the manual laborer, or the craftsman, a fact that contributed much to the low esteem accorded the act.

By explaining suicide uniquely as the result of the devil's instigation or of insanity, the Middle Ages turned it into a totally irrational act. Suicide after mature reflection or out of a simple distaste for life could only be classed as melancholy, a form of madness. The Middle Ages may have excused suicide on occasion, but only to condemn it more strongly. There was no such thing as sane suicide.

With the fifteenth century, the earliest humanists began to reflect on another heritage that offered a quite different image of voluntary death—that of classical antiquity. The scholastics were acquainted with Lucretius, Cato, and Seneca, but because those ancient philosophers had not received the revelation of Christianity, their conduct could not serve as a moral example. The humanists' greater knowledge of classical antiquity and their growing admiration for its values slowly changed attitudes. We need to recall the classical legacy in order to understand the first timid (but nonetheless audacious) attempts to appreciate suicide that arose during the Renaissance.

THREE

The Classical Heritage

Perfecting the Timely Exit

In the fifteenth century, when the first signs of changes leading toward the modern world began to emerge out of the socioeconomic, political, military, religious, and cultural tumult of the age, the first humanists enthusiastically turned their restless curiosity to deciphering the immense heritage of pagan antiquity. A great challenge to intellectual and moral certitudes had arisen in the fourteenth century with the Ockhamist revolution; it had been amplified by the Nominalist movement, by the religious contestation of John Wycliffe and Jan Hus, by schisms in the church, by the scientific audacity of Nicholas of Cusa and Nicole d'Oresme, by the last struggles of a moribund feudal order, and by demographic crises and the ravages of war. All this brought European intellectuals back to the long neglected treasures of classical philosophy.

Christian thought, of course, had an answer to everything: the fathers of the Church, the councils, and the theologians of the Middle Ages had provided increasingly precise rules for both scholarship and norms of conduct. In the moral sphere, which was the most solid domain, the Ten Commandments formed an unquestioned basis for obligations and prohibitions imposed by those in authority and internalized by the faithful. Deviant behavior met with unanimous reprobation, and it was repressed by the civil and religious powers with the full approval of society. Even in the domain of good and evil, however, the prestige of the authors of classical antiquity led humanist thinkers to raise questions when ancient thought manifestly disagreed with Christian moral teachings: Hadn't the theologians proclaimed that God had endowed all humankind—believers and nonbelievers alike—with universal principles of conduct? Respect for human life seemed the most self-evident of these principles. The prohibition on killing was absolute (certain strictly defined instances aside), and it extended to killing oneself. Classical antiquity, however, offered Christian thinkers illustrious examples of heroic suicide, justified by lofty philosophical thought. Meditation on ancient practice underlay the questions raised during the Renaissance on the right to self-murder. An admiring rediscovery of the Greek and Roman past and its great men led to reflection on a long list of suicides: Aristodemus, Cleomenes, Themistocles, Isocrates, Demosthenes, Pythagoras, Empedocles, Democritus, Diogenes, Hegesias, Zeno, Cleanthes, Socrates, Lucretia, Appius Claudius, Crassus, Caius Gracchus, Marius, Cato, Lucretius, Antony, Cleopatra, Brutus, Cassius, Varus, Piso, Cocceius Nerva, Silanus, Seneca, Calpurnius Piso, Otho, and others. Could one indiscriminately qualify voluntary death as an act inspired by a culpable cowardice that led to damnation, in the cases of persons as worthy of respect as these?

Disagreement among the Greeks

The essential difference between classical and medieval attitudes toward voluntary death lies in the plurality of opinions in ancient times versus the monolithic stance of Christianity. Pagan antiquity was far from unanimous in its acceptance of self-homicide. In the Greek world each philosophical school had its own position on the question, and opinions ranged from the Pythagoreans' categorical opposition to suicide to the welcoming approval of the Epicureans and the Stoics.[1]

This diversity is reflected in law, some cities (Athens, Sparta, Thebes) stipulating punishment of the body of a suicide and others not. Everywhere, however, actual practice seems to have leaned toward indulgence, and Greek history is studded with famous suicides, both historical and semi-legendary. The reasons behind these suicides varied. There were patriotic suicides, such as those of Meneceas, Themistocles, Isocrates, and Demosthenes. Aristodemus killed himself out of remorse; Cleomenes for honor; Pythagoras out of fidelity to a religious ideal; Democritus and Speusippus in order to avoid the decrepitude of old age; Pantheia, Hero, and Sappho for love; Hippo to preserve her chastity; Charondas for civic reasons. Zeno, Cleanthes, Hegesias, Diogenes, and Epicurus committed philosophical suicide to show their scorn for life. The death of Socrates is debatable, but it can be accounted a suicide because of his provocative responses during his trial and his refusal to flee.

From the most remote ages of history, Greek thought posed the fundamental problem of philosophical suicide. The Cyrenaic school, the Cynics, the Epicureans, and the Stoics all recognized the supreme worth of the individual, whose liberty resided in the ability to choose whether to live or die. For these groups only the good life—that is, a life in conformity with reason and human dignity that brought more satisfactions than woes—was worth living. When this was no longer the case, it was foolish to conserve life.

Within this general scheme each philosophical current emphasized one aspect of the question or another. The Cyrenaics, who pushed individualism to an extreme, were pessimists, and one of their masters, Hegesias, is reported to have been expelled from Alexandria for having induced several people to commit suicide. The Cynics professed complete detachment from life if it could not be lived in accordance with reason; Antisthenes was of the opinion that people of insufficient intelligence would be better off hanging themselves. His disciple Diogenes carried that principle to its logical conclusion, arguing that death, which one does not perceive when it comes, is not to be feared, hence people should not hesitate to kill themselves if they cannot live reasonably. To live well, he claimed, one needs right reason or a rope. Diogenes Laertius attributes to him many statements, such as these: "Why then do you live, if you do not care to live well?" (*Lives of Eminent Philosophers* VI.65; Loeb ed., 2:67); "When someone declared that life is an evil, he corrected him: 'Not life itself, but living ill'" (VI.55; Loeb ed., 2:57). He ceaselessly repeated that one must confront life with a healthy mind or hang oneself, and "when Antisthenes cried out, 'Who will release me from these pains?' replied, 'This,' showing him the dagger. 'I said,' quoth the other, 'from my pains, not from life'" (VI.19; Loeb ed., 2:21).

According to the Epicureans, wisdom dictates that when life becomes intolerable one should commit suicide without fuss. After mature reflection and without precipitation, as if leaving a room filled with smoke, one should move quietly out of life. The Stoics also recommended suicide after careful reflection when reason shows it to be the worthiest way to reach conformity with the order of things or when the line of action we have laid out for ourselves proves impossible. Life and death are equally indifferent, as everything will be swept away in a pantheistic universe. "The wise man can with reason give his life for his country and his friends, or he can kill himself if he suffers serious pain, if he has lost a limb, or if he has an incurable illness." This is how Diogenes Laertius summarizes Stoic thought on suicide, giving the death of Zeno as the perfect example. As he was leaving his school, Zeno (who was ninety-eight years old) "tripped and fell, breaking a toe. Striking the ground with his fist, he quoted the line from the *Niobe:* 'I come, I come. Why dost thou call for me?' and died on the spot through holding his breath" (VII.28; Loeb ed., 2:141).

The Pythagoreans gave two reasons for their opposition to suicide. First, because the soul falls into a body as the result of an original profanation, it must pursue its expiation; second, the association of body and soul is regulated by numerical relations whose harmony would be broken by suicide. This did not prevent Pythagoras from deliberately starving himself to death out of weariness with life, as Heracleitus tells us. According to Hermippus, he was killed by the Syracusans as he was fleeing from them. They caught up with him because he stopped in his tracks, refusing to cross a field of broad beans (a sacred legume), which might be considered a form of suicide.

Plato's Distinctions and Aristotle's Rejection

Plato and Aristotle, the two giants of Greek philosophy and the thinkers who had the greatest impact on Western thought (though often in contradictory ways), disagreed with earlier currents of thought. Both men considered humans as essentially social beings operating within a community. Hence individuals should not reason in terms of personal interest but rather should take into account the duties owed to the divinity who placed them in their positions in society (Plato) or the city, where they had a role to play (Aristotle).

Plato's position regarding suicide is at once more supple and more hesitating, as if he himself had not quite made up his mind. Christian thinkers intent on recapturing his thought twisted what he says about voluntary death, which is quite subtle in the original. In a passage of the *Laws* omitted by opponents of suicide, he states that public burial should be refused to "someone who slays himself, violently robbing himself of his Fate-given share of life" (*Laws* IX.873C; Loeb ed., 203). A suicide should be buried anonymously in an isolated site and without a marker. Plato goes on to state, however, that the rule does not apply to one whose death is "legally ordered by the State" or who is "compelled to it by the occurrence of some intolerable and inevitable misfortune" or who has fallen into "some disgrace that is beyond remedy or endurance" (ibid.). Thus Plato's prohibition of suicide has three exceptions: condemnation (Socrates' case), painful and incurable illness, and the miseries of fate, which might cover a broad range of situations from abject poverty to shame. In the same work Plato states (he is addressing temple robbers) that if you are unable to cure yourself of evil penchants and if seeking the company of virtuous men has had no effect, "then deem your death the more noble way, and quit yourself of life" (IX.854C; Loeb ed., 203).

Plato also raises the question of suicide in the *Phaedo,* where Socrates debates with his friends before drinking the hemlock. The least one can say is that Plato's thought is extremely tortuous, the way he expresses it is discouragingly obscure, and Socrates' interlocutors find what he has to say downright disconcerting. Cebes nearly gives up trying to understand him at one point. Socrates, who is about to drink the poison, tries to show them that although suicide is perhaps not acceptable in the city, death is so desirable that a philosopher must necessarily wish for it. He begins by paying lip service to the official attitude: The gods are our masters, we belong to them, and we have no right to quit their company. His "opposition" to suicide is presented with a degree of circumlocution that speaks volumes about his own level of conviction: "Thus perhaps from this point of view it is not unreasonable to say that a man must not kill himself until god sends some necessity upon him, such as has now come upon me" (*Phaedo* 62.D; Loeb ed., 217). This seems a rather reticent condemnation of suicide, particularly in the light of the lyrical evocation of the advantages of death that immediately follows.

Cato is reported to have read the *Phaedo* twice before he committed suicide, which shows that its meaning may not have seemed totally clear to him, and also that Socrates' arguments against voluntary death did not persuade him. If death is so very desirable, and if it opens the way to such bliss, one must have strong reasons for not taking one's own life. In the Christian context, Platonism eventually gave rise to what might be called "mystical suicide"—death to oneself and to the world in an effort to attain, in this life, the felicity of otherworldly life. When physical suicide was not a choice, later mystics practiced spiritual suicide.

Compared to Plato's ambiguous message, Aristotle writes with martial brutality. He condemns suicide because it is an act counter to justice committed against one's own person and against the city, because it is an act of cowardice in face of responsibilities, and because it is counter to virtue. We must remain at our posts and confront the vicissitudes of existence with serenity. Yet he declares in the *Nicomachean Ethics* that magnanimity does not consist in preserving one's life, since "the great-souled man . . . holds that life is not worth having at every price" (*Nicomachean Ethics* IV.3.23; Loeb ed., 221).

Disquietude in Archaic Roman Thought

Of all Western civilizations, Rome is reputed to have been the most favorable to suicide, a reputation founded on the popularity of Stoicism among the Roman elites and the impressive number of famous people who put an end to their days. In a noteworthy study, *Le suicide dans la Rome antique,* Yolande Grisé offers twenty pages of statistics on 314 cases of voluntary death among prominent Romans from the fifth century B.C. to the second century A.D., a higher proportion than one would find for Europe from 1300 to our own day.[2]

The Roman world, like its Greek counterpart, was far from unanimous in its attitude toward suicide. Many shades of opinion appear, varying from one period to another and also according to social category and sociopolitical milieu. From earliest times, Roman society was divided between hostility toward an antisocial act and admiration for a manifestation of individual freedom that permitted a way out from the abuse of the strong and from a tyrannical state power.

The particularly tragic nature of suicide, which seemed to force the hand of fate and nature, engendered worries about the cadaver, which, if it were possessed by evil spirits, might return to harass the living. It has been noted that all primitive societies have rites aimed at immobilizing the dead body or mutilating it to render it powerless. Louis-Vincent Thomas has furnished African examples of this:[3] When someone of the Baganda people of Central Africa hangs himself, the body is burned at a crossroads, using the wood of the tree he used. When the women pass by, they cover the ashes so that the spirit of the dead cannot penetrate them and be reborn. The Ewe of Togo leave the body of a hanged man attached to the branch from which he did the deed and drag it through sharp-thorned bushes. They then bury the lacerated corpse in an isolated place. At times a spike is driven through the chest of a suicide's body; elsewhere the body is mutilated (femurs broken, ear torn off, hand cut off) so that the dead person, shamed and powerless, will no longer disturb the living. Still elsewhere the body is buried under the roadway at a crossroads.

Certain of these same rites were practiced in Greece in archaic times: In Athens the right hand of a suicide was cut off so he could commit no crimes. (This did not prevent the Athenians from holding differing opinions on suicide itself, as we have seen.) All these practices—rites of purification, mutilation of the corpse, expulsion of the corpse from the community, erasure of all trace of its passage to avoid its return—can be found in the Middle Ages and can be attributed to a common fund of superstitious fear of uncommon, hence supernatural, acts.

Although there is no mention of such practices in early Rome (the Law of the Twelve Tables, for instance, says nothing on the subject), we can see similar beliefs reflected in the decrees of Tarquin in Rome under the kings, as related by Pliny the Elder. Tarquin commanded that the bodies of people who had committed suicide in protest against his tyranny be crucified. His aim was to prevent the dead from wreaking vengeance on him. When the bodies were nailed to wooden crosses (which gave them no contact with the ground) in an out-of-the-way spot, the evil spirits would be paralyzed and the birds who feasted on the cadavers would absorb the evil.[4]

This is the only mention of legal prohibition of suicide in early Rome. Grisé parts company with previous interpretations to show that the Law of the Twelve Tables did not prohibit voluntary death and that suicides' funerals were conducted in the normal manner. Among the various ways to take one's own life, however, hanging was reputed to exert a particularly malignant influence. The reasons for this belief are unclear: Was it because of the horrible aspect of the hanged corpse, with eyes bulging from their sockets, tongue hanging out, gaze fixed, and limbs twisted? More probably, this form of death was considered sacrilegious because in ancient Roman religious practice the victims sacrificed to the telluric gods were suffocated, so that they displayed no flow of blood. Until the early modern age, suicide by hanging continued to have pejorative connotations in comparison to the more "noble" suicide by the sword.

For obvious economic and patriotic reasons, suicide was forbidden to two categories of ancient Romans, slaves and soldiers. The suicide of slaves was considered an affront to private property (a notion that was later essential in medieval serfdom); the army had specific penalties for soldiers who survived an attempted suicide.

Suicide and the Free Citizen

There was no legal or religious prohibition of suicide for free men in Rome. Life was not considered a gift of the gods, a sacred breath, or a right, and Romans could dispose of it at will. For Cicero suicide was neither good nor bad in itself; instead, it lay somewhere between the two and was to be judged above all by its motivation. Cato's suicide, for example, was a model of total liberty because in killing himself when his life was not threatened he placed himself on a higher plane than fate. Cicero criticized other suicides, however, judging them in the light of his (rather debatable) interpretation of Platonism. He cites the *Phaedo* to state that Plato forbade killing oneself unless the gods made it necessary, and he cites the *Republic* on our not having a right to abandon the post the gods have assigned to us. Most Roman historians presented the same nuanced opinion, condemning some suicides and praising others. They tended to praise wives who chose death rather than outlive their husbands, women who had been raped, and men who wanted to escape a shameful punishment, who refused to die at an enemy's hand, who preferred death to dishonor, or who wanted to flee the decrepitude of old age.

Virgil also distributes the shades of suicides to the underworld or to the Elysian Fields, according to their motivations. Suicides who kill themselves for patriotic reasons, in an act of courage, or in affirmation of their liberty are among the blessed spirits; those who died out of sheer distaste for life and who want to return to their miserable existences on earth are elsewhere, lodged in the neutral zone of hell along with stillborn infants, those who were condemned to death by false accusations, women who were victims of love, warriors killed in battle, and the mass of the unfortunate—all of whom more closely resemble victims than criminals.

Roman history offers many examples of famous suicides, and there must have been many anonymous ones as well. Seneca writes to Lucilius of "men of all grades of rank and fortune, and every time of life, who have cut short their sufferings by death."[5] The suicide rate does not seem to have been any higher in Rome than in other ancient civilization, and any notion of a wave or "epidemic" of suicides in Rome is more legend than fact. Voluntary deaths did indeed reach a record level of frequency during the troubled years between 100 B.C. and A.D. 100, but this was a circumscribed phenomenon whose causes—for the most part political—are well known. We shall return to them.

Grisé lists reasons for self-homicide based on her scrutiny of historical sources: suicide by ordeal in archaic times, when a criminal was turned over to the judgment of the gods by being put in a situation of mortal danger; suicide in the games among gladiators who had volunteered to compete; "criminal" suicide committed by persons who had murdered someone; suicide as a means of vengeance or a result of blackmail; altruistic suicide to save the life of another or others; suicide out of mourning; suicide as self-punishment; suicide as an escape from an intolerable situation, such as physical suffering, military defeat, or the threat of criminal pursuit; and suicide out of shame after being raped. The archetype of the last motive is Lucretia: Livy relates how the wife of Tarquinius Collatinus killed herself with a knife after being raped by Sextus, the son of Tarquinius Superbus. The episode became a standard reference in debates on suicide, and it has provided a subject for painters from Lucas Cranach to Rembrandt, including Joos van Cleve, Titian, Cagnacci, and many others.

Taedium Vitae

Another type of voluntary death, distaste for or weariness with life, was unknown during the Middle Ages but was rediscovered in the Renaissance. Humanist commentary often focused on one of the most famous of these suicides, the death of Cleombrotus, a handsome, wealthy, and well-loved young man who killed himself, after reading the *Phaedo,* so as to go to a better world. His story is an additional indication that this particular Platonic dialogue was not read as opposing suicide.

We find suicide out of weariness for life in Rome above all during the civil wars and in the early empire. In fact, this form of suicide seems in general to be linked to crises of civilization, moments when broadly shared attitudes are overturned and traditional values, moral certitudes, and established verities in the religious, scientific, and intellectual domains are challenged. Typically, suicide out of weariness for life appears in transitional phases—times of a radical shift in the collective mentality—that occur between long periods of equilibrium in civilization. It is, so to speak, the suicide of cultural revolutions. It was the suicide of the Renaissance, the first all-European crisis of conscience from 1580 to 1620, of the second crisis from 1680 to 1720, and of the age of revolutions. It is also the suicide of the late twentieth century.

Suicide from weariness with life affects an intellectual minority whose reflection on human destiny leads to a radical pessimism about human nature. Rome in the first century B.C., a society in just such a state of flux, was particularly afflicted with *taedium vitae.* As Grisé states: "Before the apocalyptic vision of a world threatening to collapse amid the ruins of Rome and the massacre of its most eminent citizens, a boundless discouragement seized the most enlightened souls and minds. Disappointed and nauseated by the horrors of the first civil wars, and worried that what was to come would be still more terrible, citizens in search of escape, oblivion, and repose free of any bitter awakening or dreadful tomorrow sank into a sort of morbid and anxious boredom."[6]

The poet Lucretius perhaps best represents a generation of disillusioned intellectuals beset by an ancient version of existential anxiety. A solitary and tranquilly pessimistic man, Lucretius expresses immense pity for a humanity tormented by fear—fear of death, fear of the gods, fear of punishment, fear of illness, suffering, and the pangs of conscience: "Thus each man tries to flee from himself, but to that self, from which of course he can never escape, he clings against his will, and hates it" (*De rerum natura* III.1066–70; Loeb ed., 2:67). Such strong anxiety can only dissipate when we ourselves disappear. Lucretius committed suicide in 55 B.C. at about forty-five years of age.

One hundred twenty years later, another writer imbued with a resigned pessimism, Seneca, killed himself. Seneca analyzes the distaste for life of those whose passions or whose desire for personal accomplishment are unsatisfied by participation in public life or solitary studies and who, perennially hesitant, seek in vain to flee themselves:

Hence the boredom, the disgust for oneself, the tumult of a soul fixed on nothing, the somber impatience that our own inaction causes, especially when we blush to admit the reasons and when respect for others retains our anguish: tightly contained in a prison with no exit, our passions are asphyxiated. . . . Hence the voyages that one undertakes with no goal, the wanderings along the coasts, and the mobility, always an enemy of the present state, that tries us from sea and from land. . . . One trip succeeds another; one spectacle replaces another. As Lucretius states, "Thus all continually flee themselves." But to what purpose, if by so doing one cannot escape oneself? We follow ourselves; we cannot get rid of that intolerable company. Thus we persuade ourselves that the sickness we are suffering from comes not from the gods but from ourselves. We lack the strength to bear anything: work, pleasure, ourselves, everything in the world is a burden to us. There are some whom this leads to suicide because their perpetual variations make them turn forever in the same circle and because they have made all novelty impossible for themselves, they lose their taste for life and the universe and feel rising up in themselves the cry of hearts made rotten by pleasure: "What? Always the same thing?"[7]

This spiritual malaise (nineteenth-century France called it *spleen*)—a feeling characteristic of periods of relativism, widespread skepticism, and uncertain opinions and values—was unknown in the Middle Ages, when (as we have seen), it was considered a form of madness. In an age sure of itself, its future, and the meaning of this world, a morbid melancholy was incomprehensible and could exist only in a deranged mind.

Distaste for life does not seem to have led inordinate numbers of Romans to kill themselves. It was a state of mind that intellectuals indulged in but only rarely followed through to its logical conclusion, precisely because those who suffered from it lacked energy and decisiveness. Its most typical manifestation was floating in a perpetual state of indecision between life and death. Seneca himself committed suicide when Nero commanded him to do so, not out of distaste for life. In his works, moreover, he seeks to prepare his readers for death but does not urge them to it hasten it. To the contrary, he advises them to resist a desire to die. Death should not be feared, but neither should it be sought for no good reason. Seneca's own biography illustrates this point. Very few of the known suicides of his time were due to *taedium vitae*. Rather, they all had precise motivations, to which boredom with life was perhaps an added incentive.

Old Age and Suicide

Seneca states that as long as the body and the mind enjoy possession of their full faculties and one can live a worthy life, there is no reason to kill oneself. On the other hand, he sees continuing to live when we are afflicted with the decrepitude and sufferings of advanced old age as the height of folly, when we have it in our power to deliver ourselves from them:

The man who awaits his doom inertly is all but afraid, just as the man who swigs off the bottle and drains even the lees is over-given to his liquor. In this case, however, we shall try to find out whether the last part of life is really lees, or something extraordinarily bright and clear if only the mind's uninjured [and] the senses come unimpaired to the aid of the spirit. . . . If, on the other hand, the body's past its duties, it may be (why not?) the right thing to extricate the suffering spirit. . . . Old age, if it lasts very long, brings few to death unmarred: for many of the aged life collapses into lethargy and impotence. After that do you consider a scrap of life a more poignant loss than the freedom to end it? . . . I shan't cast old age off if old age keeps me whole for myself—whole, I mean, on my better side; but if it begins to unseat my reason and pull it piecemeal, if it leaves me not life but mere animation, I shall be out of my crumbling, tumble-down tenement at a bound. . . . Still, if I'm assured that I can never be free of it, I shall make my exit, not because of the actual pain, but because it's likely to prove a bar to everything that makes life worth while. The man who dies because of pain is weak and craven; the man who lives to suffer is a fool.[8]

In the late first and early second centuries A.D., many aged Roman patricians versed in Stoic philosophy proved they had learned this lesson well. In his letters Pliny the Younger mentioned admiringly several instances of old men riddled with illness who chose to leave this life in a dignified manner. When one of his friends, a man lamed by gout who had suffered "most incredible and highly undeserved pains," took his own life, Pliny noted that the act "prompts my admiration before his greatness of soul." In another letter he spoke of Titius Aristo, who managed to "examine critically the arguments for dying" before killing himself (*Letters* 1:I.22). In another passage he wrote of a seventy-five-year-old man who suffered from an incurable disease: "Weary of life, he put an end to it." Another case he noted was that of Arria, a Roman woman who set an example for her old and ill husband by killing herself before his eyes. Another touching anecdote concerned two elderly ordinary citizens. The man suffered terribly from ulcers; his wife "saw that there was no hope and urged him to take his life; she went with him, even led him to his death herself, and forced him to follow her example by roping herself to him and jumping into the lake" (*Letters* 1:IV.25).

Political Suicides

Although Tacitus' accounts may have given them more notoriety than they deserve, political suicides were frequent in Rome during the years of the civil wars and the early empire.[9] There were suicides prompted by a reversal of fortune or a desire to retain one's liberty (the most famous was Cato in 46 B.C.); senatorial suicides imposed by the imperial power (Julius Marinus in A.D. 32); suicides to avoid a criminal sentence (Calpurnius Piso, A.D. 20); suicides inspired by a disgust with public affairs (Cocceius Nerva, A.D. 33); and suicides of defeated generals (Varus, A.D. 9).

In certain years the number of voluntary deaths among men active in politics was impressive: There were nineteen such deaths in 43 B.C. and sixteen in the following year; sixteen in A.D. 65, twelve in 66. These heroic suicides by falling on one's sword or by slitting one's veins are reported admiringly by Roman historians as illustrations of the supreme freedom of individuals who rose above their fate. Cato, Cassius, Brutus, Casca, Antony, and Cleopatra all became legendary models; even emperors like Nero or Otho partially made up for their wretched deeds by their suicides. Literature furnished its quota of martyrs in Petronius, Lucan, and Seneca. The heroic anecdotes written about such personages and the memorable statements the historians attributed to them helped to glorify their act in the eyes of posterity. Such legends include Arria's "Paete, non dolet" ("It does not hurt, Paetus" [Pliny, *Letters* 1:III.16]); Brutus' "Virtue, you are nothing but a word"; Scipio's response, "Safe!" to the soldier who asked where was the commander when Scipio had just run himself through with his sword;[10] and Nero's "Qualis artifex pereo!" ("What an artist the world is losing with me!" [Suetonius, *The Twelve Caesars,* Nero 49; Loeb ed., 2:177]). Comedy and black humor might also be brought into play: When Bonosus, a general known for his excessive drinking, killed himself, some wit exclaimed, "That isn't a hanged man, it's a bottle!"

Humanists and philosophers from the sixteenth to the eighteenth century referred constantly to the famous Roman suicides. Imperial Roman law left citizens free to choose their death. Albert Bayet and Gaston Garrisson list the circumstances in which a suicide's estate would not be confiscated.[11] These included distaste for life; unhappiness caused by the death of a son; a desire to have people speak admiringly of one's fine death; madness, idiocy, or simple-mindedness; escape from illness and suffering; and avoidance of the shame of insolvency. In other words, only people under accusation or awaiting execution of their sentences who killed themselves to prevent confiscation of their estates faced penalties. All other suicides were condoned. Tacitus claims that in the reign of Tiberius the result of this policy was to increase the number of suicides among those threatened with judiciary proceedings: "What made such deaths eagerly sought was dread of the executioner, and the fact too that the condemned, besides forfeiture of their property, were deprived of burial, while those who decided their own fate themselves, had their bodies interred, and their wills remained valid, a recompense for their despatch."[12]

The popularity of Stoicism among the wealthy classes of imperial Rome helped make suicide seem banal: "What does it matter by what road you enter Hades?" Epictetus asks. "They are all the same." Emperor Marcus Aurelius recommended quitting this life the minute it became impossible to lead the sort of life one wanted: "As you intended to live when you depart, so are you able to live in this world; but if they do not allow you to do so, then depart this life, yet so as if you suffered no evil fate. The chimney smokes and I leave the room. Why do you think it a great matter? But while no such reason drives me out, I remain a free tenant and none shall prevent me acting as I will."[13]

Increasing Hostility to Suicide

Stoicism declined during the second century, and at the same time Roman law regarding suicide became more severe. With the Antonines law and philosophical ideas evolved in strikingly similar ways. Both Neoplatonism and the eastern cults condemned suicide. Plotinus declared that it disturbed the soul of the dead person, preventing it from detaching from the body and returning to the celestial spheres, but he admitted self-homicide in face of physical pain, the ravages of old age, or the trials of captivity. Porphyry, who had himself attempted suicide and had been saved by his master's timely intervention, rejected all forms of suicide. Among the mystery religions that were becoming increasingly popular in the empire, Orphism taught that the soul, imprisoned in the body by divine will, could leave it only by divine decree.

The civil authorities began to play an increasingly invasive role in citizens' lives. As barbarian populations put growing pressure on an underpopulated empire, the state tightened its control over suicide, working to put an end to fiscal evasion in the form of suicide to avoid being brought to trial. Suicide attempts among soldiers in the army were more severely punished. One law of the age of the Antonines considered the suicide of suspects to be an admission of guilt and a justification for confiscating their estate. With the third century, suicide for no valid reason was a crime, and if a suicide's widow should remarry, her new husband was vilified.

Even before the triumph of Christianity (and for reasons independent of Christian doctrine), condemnation of suicide gradually became the rule in the Roman Empire. When the Church was the only remaining power, the situation that it inherited was unclear. As we have seen, intellectuals within the Church continued the debate on suicide, which by then was complicated by the question of voluntary martyrdom. The systematic opposition to suicide that began with St. Augustine and later became the rule arose more from the historical context than from any clear basic tenet of early doctrine. The proof that such an attitude did not automatically derive from doctrine is that it took theology at least five centuries to consolidate the Church's opposition to suicide.

The absolute prohibition on taking one's own life became firmly established in the Roman Empire under barbarian rule. Formalized by the scholastics during the Middle Ages, prohibition eventually became an integral part of the basic structures of Christian thought. As a cultural phenomenon, the prohibition of suicide owed much to medieval Christian thinkers' mistrust of ancient paganism. The Greco-Roman heritage—which had been in part lost, in part forgotten, and in part distorted—continued to furnish models in scientific and philosophic contexts, but it was denied all value as a moral reference. Medieval scholars adopted Aristotle and Ptolemy when they spoke of astronomy, but after the Christological revelation, moral authority was exclusively invested in Scripture, as developed by tradition—that is, by the Church fathers, the theologians, the councils, and the popes. The science of classical antiquity was believed willingly, but not its moral teachings: Morality was the business of the scholastics and of canon law.

The fourteenth and fifteenth centuries launched a cultural revolution in all domains. The sixteenth century—age of Copernicus—was also the age of Luther and Montaigne, three men who shook the pillars of truth, even if they did not succeed in bringing down the entire edifice. After them that edifice was still standing, but irreparable cracks had begun to appear in science, dogma, and morality. Heliocentrism was at first only a supposition, Lutheranism just a schism, and skepticism only a habit of raising questions, but the age of certitudes had passed.

All domains were not equally affected by a return to classical antiquity. There was even a marked contrast between the realms of science and morality: Ancient science received blows from which it never recovered, but pagan moral teachings aroused an increasing interest that eventually weakened traditional Christian values. Although no one continued to borrow classical antiquity's explanations of the physical universe, its writers were used as sources for models of noble and heroic conduct. References to the great men of Greece and Rome crowd the pages of authors from Machiavelli to Castiglione to Montaigne. Perspectives changed: For the Renaissance, the grandeur of classical antiquity lay in the moral wisdom of its thinkers and the nobility of soul of its politicians rather than in the knowledge (which had been proven erroneous) of its scholars. One particular model of behavior—ancient suicide—prompted more and more open admiration. One highly symbolic illustration of this change is the popularity of the theme of Lucretia's suicide in Renaissance art. The combination of the beauty of the female body and the fatal outcome of her act is one of the many paradoxes of the new age.

PART II

The Renaissance

A Question Raised,
Then Stifled

FOUR

The Early Renaissance

Rediscovery of the Enigma of Suicide

The Problem of Figures

Some writers of the Renaissance had the decided impression that the number of suicides had risen in their age. Giovanni Boccaccio, writing in the late fourteenth century, was struck by the number of self-hangings in Florence. Much later Erasmus, seeing people's haste to kill themselves, wondered in his *Colloquia* how much worse the situation might be if humanity did not fear death. Luther spoke in 1542 of an epidemic of suicides in Germany, and in 1548 the archbishop of Mainz spoke in similar terms, while in Nuremberg in 1569 fourteen suicides were recorded. Henri Estienne declared, "As for our century, our ears are assaulted with examples [of suicides] of both men and women," and Montaigne repeated his father's claim that twenty-five suicides had occurred within one week in Milan.[1]

A few nineteenth-century historians, overly impressed by such statements (which are actually infrequent and extremely vague), credited the Renaissance with suicidal tendencies. In 1841, for example, Félix Bourquelot wrote, "Voluntary death added its victims to the victims of many furors. We then see a sort of reaction operating in its favor. . . . It becomes more frequent."[2] William Lecky, writing in 1877, stated, "We find many facts exhibiting a startling increase of deliberate suicide, and a no less startling modification of the sentiments with which it was regarded."[3] In 1882 James O'Dea took these statements as established fact and offered an explanation for them: "The growing sensuousness of life, its moral and intellectual paganism, together with the political and social disorders of the period, caused a marked increase in the number of suicides, and soon there arose a literature in its defence based on the notions of ancient times."[4] The following year (1883), Gaston Garrisson wrote, "The sixteenth century, enamored of antiquity, returned suicide to honor. There were illustrious examples."[5] As late as 1928, Ruth Cavan repeated these notions in her book *Suicide*.[6]

Since then other historians have judged differently. Albert Desjardins in 1887, Émile Durkheim in 1897, Henry Fedden in 1938, and Samuel Ernest Sprott in 1961 all saw no serious reason for stating that the suicide rate rose during the Renaissance.[7] More recent studies influenced by the school of the *Annales* and its emphasis on quantification are extremely cautious. Robert Mandrou, writing in 1961, states that "since the necessary evidence has not been collected, we must abandon any attempt to measure or even suggest approximate numbers of suicides,"[8] and Jean Delumeau writes of the earlier assertions that "historical research will have to verify that point."[9]

Such verification is unlikely, given the disparity of the sources and their fragmentary, often subjective nature. Personal journals and memoirs are disappointing as sources because they select the suicide cases they mention in function of the scandal they created and the author's own interests. The anonymous "bourgeois of Paris" who kept a journal in the time of Francis I noted only two suicides, both of prominent persons: In 1525 one Poncet, a young lawyer at the Châtelet and a married man with children, threw himself into the well beside his house "out of great annoyance and anger over some suit he had or out of some jealousy"; in 1534 a canon in Rouen named d'Oyneville hanged himself "in despair and because of a suit he had lost, for which he owed fourteen or sixteen hundred livres."[10]

The journal that Pierre de L'Estoile kept during the last quarter of the sixteenth century is somewhat more prolix, but it can by no means be used as a basis for statistical data. It is interesting, though, for L'Estoile's analysis of suicide cases and his opinions on them, which reflect attitudes typical of a man of some social prominence. Nothing in the motivation for suicide, the means employed, or the social categories involved seems to have changed since the Middle Ages. Despair, at times with no further explanation, is usually the principal reason for the suicide of citizens of a certain social status. In 1576, for example, L'Estoile reports that a Protestant doctor of law from Toulouse named Custos, "a man of high culture and integrity and much esteemed by those of that religion, of which he made wholehearted and public profession, killed himself in the village of Lardi out of a form of despair." In 1584 a physician slit his throat because he was deeply in debt, and L'Estoile remarks disapprovingly that it was "a type of death unworthy of a Christian man who was very learned, a doctor and philosopher."[11]

A third suicide mentioned by L'Estoile is that of François de Saignes, seigneur de La Garde and a *conseiller* of the high court of the Parlement de

Paris, who drowned himself because of illness at the age of forty-five, "afflicted with a fever and a retention of urine, and feeling himself vexed with constant pain and nearing the end of his life." L'Estoile indignantly disapproves of the indulgence of the authorities, who declared Saignes insane to avoid having to confiscate his estate, which he had bequeathed to the son of the *premier président* of the Parlement. L'Estoile reports:

And despite all, [he] was buried with solemnity in the choir of the Cordeliers' [church], with ceremony and in the presence of the *premier président,* de Thou, and a goodly number of *présidents, maîtres des requêtes, conseillers,* and others, thanks to the rumor that was circulated that he had a raging fever and was subject to fits of madness, but also because he had given his estate and benefices to Jacques de Thou, son of the *premier président,* whom he had named sole executor of his will. (*Journal,* 29 September 1578)

It is clear from the examples L'Estoile mentions that social origin had an influence on the treatment reserved for suicides. Some self-inflicted deaths that seem clearly due to insanity nonetheless led to punishments inflicted on the corpse. In Montfaucon in 1584, for example, Sister Tiennette Petit drowned herself after slitting the throat of an aged nun; her corpse was hanged. In 1586 a Piedmontese physician named Sylva, imprisoned in the Conciergerie for sodomy, went mad, killing one fellow prisoner and wounding another. Put into solitary confinement, he strangled himself with his shirt, and his corpse "was dragged by a horse to the high road, where it was hanged by the feet" (25 September 1584; 30 January 1586). L'Estoile also relates the suicide of one Balduin, the leader of a band of Italian ruffians, arrested in Bruges for an assassination attempt against the duc d'Alençon: "Fearing more cruel torture if he waited for the results of the criminal proceedings in view for him, he stabbed himself in the stomach several times with his dagger and died soon after" (Early August 1582).

We cannot possibly gauge the frequency of suicide in the period from the few cases mentioned in such sources. All we have is sporadic mentions when someone commits suicide. A priest named Geoffroy Clouet, for instance, hanged himself in Paris in 1431, rue Saint-Germain-l'Auxerrois, and his case was referred to his ecclesiastical superiors.[12] Henri Estienne claimed that members of the clergy committed suicide as frequently as the laity did.[13]

England

One country—England—does offer exceptional statistical data. This has enabled Michael MacDonald and Terence R. Murphy to produce a book,

Sleepless Souls: Suicide in Early Modern England, that has no equivalent for the Continent.[14] The scarcity of sources for continental Europe makes it imperative to refer frequently to England, but that same wealth of data risks giving the impression that suicide was more widespread there than elsewhere. Montesquieu and the eighteenth-century philosophes fell victim to this illusion and helped to further the myth of suicide as a *mal anglais.*

MacDonald and Murphy have rightly pointed out that figures for the Renaissance (which show a steep increase in suicides between 1510 and 1580) need to be handled with caution. The records of the King's Bench, which ruled on cases of suspect death, show 61 suicides for the period 1500–1509; 108 in 1510–19; 216 in 1520–29; 343 in 1530–39; 499 in 1540–49; 714 in 1550–59; 798 in 1560–69; and 940 in 1570–79.[15] In more than 95 percent of these cases the suicides were judged responsible for their act *(felo de se),* and their possessions were forfeit. This spectacular rise in the suicide rate can be attributed to laws passed in 1487, 1509, and 1510, which reformed the procedures to be followed in cases of suspect deaths and provided means for applying such procedures. From that time on, the coroners were charged with organizing an inquiry, receiving 1 mark (13s.4d.) for every verdict of homicide or self-homicide rendered. The goods of suicides judged guilty were recovered by the king's almoner, thus providing the crown with revenues of several hundred pounds a year. The suicides of wealthy merchants were a particularly lucrative source of revenue: Between 1570 and 1600 ten merchants who killed themselves left estates of over £100 apiece. This means that an entire branch of the royal administration, from the local coroner to the king's almoner, had an interest in a strict application of the laws on suicide. Moreover, after 1540 a climate of religious rivalry accentuated the tendency (of all parties) to diabolize voluntary homicide.

Examination of the trial records shows that a *felo de se* verdict was frequently rendered when no decisive proof of suicide was present. This is particularly true of deaths by drowning without witnesses, which make up nearly one-fifth of the total number of suicides in this period.[16] At times it is even clear that the coroner's jury acted in bad faith, as with the inquest regarding Thomas Spryngold of King's Lynn: Ten witnesses testified to his longstanding insanity, but he was nonetheless declared *felo de se* after committing suicide in 1560.[17] The extraordinarily low proportion of cases of insanity—less than 5 percent of the total number of cases—is in itself a clear indication of partiality in the verdicts. Such considerations make these quantitative sources an unreliable indication of actual suicide rates during the Renaissance; moreover, the example of England is not necessarily valid for the rest of Europe, given that local conditions contributed greatly to perpetuating sizable differences.

Repressive laws are easier to trace. The Calvinist regions of Switzerland (Geneva and Zurich in particular) seem to have been the only places besides England that adopted stricter attitudes toward suicide, but in Switzerland the shift came only in the seventeenth century, and practice often remained more indulgent.[18]

The Return of Ancient Suicide in Literature

There were nevertheless signs of slow but sure change. One leading indication lay in a literature that expressed the dreams, aspirations, fears, and most highly respected values of the intellectual elite. During the Renaissance, that group broadened with the invention of printing. Works were no longer confined to a public of clerics (Latin treatises) and knights (chansons de geste and courtly romances); written culture opened its doors to a new stratum of burghers and minor nobility, both as readers and as writers. Books, now much more numerous, reflected the sentiments of a larger part of the population. Above all, drama reached an even broader public and worked to circulate the ideals of the elite among the illiterate.

One of the most characteristic aspects of this change was a return to classical authors. Thanks to new editions and translations of Plutarch, Livy, Tacitus, and Pliny, the reading public regained contact with the heroic suicides of Greek and Roman history, and Stoic and Epicurean philosophical works and adaptations of Seneca's tragedies revealed a morality, parallel to Christian morality but untouched by it, that was all the more attractive for its brilliant historical and mythological examples. The idea of suicide penetrated surreptitiously into people's minds, and as the image of Lucretius, Cato, Brutus, and Seneca became more respectable, the shame and fear surrounding suicide began to dissipate.

Conflicting values are apparent as early as the first generation of humanists in the late fourteenth century. In his *De remediis* Petrarch makes use of classical culture to oppose suicide. In that allegorical dialogue (a form typical of the Middle Ages) between Dolor and Ratio, he rehearses the classical arguments against voluntary death: We have no right to desert our assigned posts; we must look tribulation in the face; life is a gift of God; killing oneself is against human nature; distaste for life is unworthy; Cato lacked courage. It is interesting to compare this Latin work, written in 1366 for a restricted circle of literati, with Chaucer's great poem, *The Legend of Good Women,* written only ten years later, which glorifies the suicides for love of Dido, Cleopatra, and Pyramus and Thisbe. The tradition of suicide for love is one of the themes of the courtly romances (Boccaccio also uses it in several of the tales in the *Decameron*), but henceforth love-deaths gained added moral value from the historical examples that were beginning to replace the legends of romance.

Chaucer showed that women were just as capable of demonstrating supreme courage as men. In 1528 Baldassare Castiglione recalled the suicide of the women of Saguntum, along with other suicides, ancient and contemporary. In Castiglione, suicide is admired for the beauty of the gesture and the sentiment, which means that he gave a positive moral charge to suicide prompted by noble motives. *The Courtier,* a veritable manual of conduct for the Renaissance noble, sealed the passage of suicide from the domain of fiction to that of real life among the aristocracy.

Another work in praise of female courage, Thomas Elyot's *Defence of Good Women* (1530), speaks favorably of the suicides of Porcia (Brutus' wife), Pauline (Seneca's wife), and several other wives faithful to their husbands unto death. In 1562 Arthur Brooke's *Romeus and Juliet* hesitated between condemnation and pity in its treatment of the suicides of the two famous lovers. William Painter's *Palace of Pleasure* (1566) also displays mixed sentiments, but as he recounts the deaths of Lucretius, Mucius Scaevola, Appius Claudius, Pantheia, Theoxena, and Poris, Painter displays no condemnation of their suicides. Although the horror of death was a specialty of French poetry,[19] English poetry more frequently took up the theme of suicide, and always on the basis of suicides from classical antiquity. One example of this is *The Mirrour for Magistrates,* an anthology published in 1559 that uses the Virgilian theme of a visit to the underworld and judges suicides with severity.

It was above all in the theater that the theme of suicide gained prominence and reached a broad public. Bernard Paulin's exhaustive study of suicide in English literature offers some interesting conclusions.[20] The first concerns the frequency of the theme of suicide. Paulin notes that between 1500 and 1580 thirty or more plays include one or more cases of voluntary death. The second concerns the way the theme was handled. The atmosphere in such plays is still largely medieval, particularly in the morality plays, which firmly condemn self-murder. Suicide is usually portrayed as the result of an immoral life, and it opens the gates of hell. Its direct cause is despair. Judgments on suicide are more varied in plays with a classical subject matter: Appius Claudius' suicide is condemned in *Appius and Virginia* (1560) but approved in *The Wars of Cyrus* (c. 1570) and in *Calisto et Meliboeia* (c. 1520), which all stress honor and love as motivations for suicide. Death by hanging always brings shame; suicide by the sword is noble. Although these early Renaissance dramas by no means advocate suicide, the large number of instances they contain and the presence of some admirable ancient examples helped to inject a degree of doubt into people's minds.

Prose authors were equally torn between standards of morality, and they too were unable to avoid contradiction. Pierre Boaistuau, for example, in his *Histoires prodigieuses* (1560) speaks of Mark Antony's suicide as a well-deserved punishment, but in his *Histoire de Chelidonius* (1578) he speaks with approval of followers of Plato who kill themselves to hasten the liberation of their souls from their bodies. Pierre de La Primauday, who was Protestant, displays obvious discomfort with the topic in his *Académie française* (1580). He praises the heroic behavior of Curtius and Otho (such men were "testimonies of an excellent Magnanimity"), of Cato, Brutus, and Cassius (whom he praises for committing a "noble act, worthy the greatness of their invincible courage"), of Themistocles, and many others. Still, he feels obliged to interpret praise of these figures from classical antiquity, recalling in passing the demands of Christian morality: "Yet notwithstanding, no man that feareth God, and is willing to obey him, ought to forget himselfe so much, as to hasten forward the end of his daies for any occasion whatsoever." Elsewhere La Primaudaye stresses that in this life the soul is prisoner of the body, "and yet whilest we desire to see the end of [this earthly life], we must not be carelesse to keep our selves in it to the good pleasure of God, that our longing may be farre from all murmuring and impatiencie." The example of the ancients was of an "excellent magnanimity . . . though it is true that anyone who fears God and wants to obey him must not forget himself to such an extent that on the slightest occasion he anticipates the end of his days."[21] This was all well and good, but the parallel had been established, and along with it came the danger of a contamination that was pointed out more often than it was exorcised.

One of the scholars who involuntarily contributed to undermining the traditional morality by presenting praiseworthy classical examples was Johannes Ravisius Textor (Jean Texier, seigneur de Ravisy), whose *Officina*, published in Paris in 1520, gives a catalogue of ancient suicides. Not content with reporting some hundred and fifty cases of illustrious voluntary deaths, Textor occasionally adds admiring commentary, notably when he speaks of Lucretia, Thrasea, Atticus, Cato, and Cleopatra (though he speaks disapprovingly of Nero and Pontius Pilate). In much the same spirit but a half-century later, the erudite antiquarian Theodor Zwinger repeated and completed Textor's list in his own *Theatrum humanae vitae.*

French fiction of the mid-sixteenth century was much influenced by such biographical works. Thus in Théodose Valentinian's *L'amant ressuscité de la mort d'amour* (1555), the heroine recalls Cato, Lucretius, and Decius to ask, "Who is there among you who would not prefer to die—even a thousand deaths—should the possibility arise that your reputation might be even slightly tarnished?"

Around 1570 mentions of suicide in literature increase, and suicide is presented in a more and more favorable light. Bernard Paulin refers to one anonymous English manuscript of 1578 that asks "Whether it be Dampnation for a man to kill himself."[22] The work puts Saul on trial. Samuel, his accuser, offers the traditional arguments to state that Saul will burn in hell; Saul defends himself by evoking the examples of Samson, the Christian martyrs, Socrates, and Cato, and he reminds his accuser that we have no right to stand in judgment of our fellow men. Solomon, the trial judge, acquits Saul. In the following year the moral philosopher Pierre de Lostal expressed an unhesitating admiration for the suicides of antiquity in his *Discours philosophiques* (1579). These opinions remained limited to a small fraction of the intellectual elite, but the fact that anyone could express such thoughts in the 1570s shows how much attitudes in that milieu had changed during the early Renaissance.

Suicide, a Utopian Solution to Human Woes

Another literary gauge of evolving attitudes was the elaboration of perfect imaginary worlds, or utopias—a convenient way to expose audacious ideas but avoid censorship. As it happens, these great sixteenth-century fables suggest that a rational organization of society should include the right to kill oneself. Thomas More is an excellent illustration of the contradictions inherent in an author who does not dare counter the moral prohibitions of his upbringing and his training, but who has the audacity to use fiction to shape intellectual creation and express his aspirations. Writing in 1515, More states that when the natives of the ideal island realm of Utopia are stricken by a painful and incurable illness, they can take their own lives. There is a Stoic cast to his remarks:

If a disease is not only incurable but also distressing and agonizing without any cessation, then the priests and the public officials exhort the man, since he is now unequal to all life's duties, a burden to himself, and a trouble to others, and is living beyond the time of his death, to make up his mind not to foster the pest and plague any longer nor to hesitate to die now that life is torture to him but, relying on good hope, to free himself from this bitter life as from prison and the rack, or else voluntarily to permit others to free him. In this course he will act wisely since by death he will put an end not to enjoyment but to torture. . . . It will be a pious and holy action.[23]

This might be Seneca speaking: "If I am assured that I can never be free of [pain], I shall make my exit."

The passage on "deliberate death" in More's *Utopia* is unambiguous, and it was sufficiently embarrassing to the compilers of hagiographic editions of More's works to induce them to omit it. The precautions More takes to set strict limits to the right to die show the seriousness of his intent. In his Utopia all suicides not authorized by the priests and the senate are subject to punishment, and the body is "cast ignominiously into a marsh without proper burial."[24] Self-killing is a decision to be made cautiously, with religion and sanctity in mind. Suicide is a reasonable measure, decided upon in extreme cases as a way to put an end to incurable suffering. The Utopians practice euthanasia, and there is no reason to believe that More was not speaking seriously when he treats the topic. As Bernard Paulin remarks, More (who was chancellor to Henry VIII) nonetheless has his spokesman, Hythlodaeus, state that God has taken away man's right to take life, not only that of others, but also his own.

Thomas More lived in a Christian kingdom, and his personal morality conformed to the Christian ideal of his times. In 1534, when he was a prisoner in the Tower of London, he rejected the idea of suicide for himself, and he wrote *A Dialogue of Comfort against Tribulation,* a work in which he states that all thought of self-murder is necessarily of diabolical origin and (following St. Augustine) that Samson must have received a personal command from God. His eminently reasonable demonstration of euthanasia in the *Utopia* is all the more striking in the light of this statement. Because More himself never had to confront unbearable suffering from an incurable illness, we will never know what choice he might have made between reason and traditional moral teaching.

Later in the sixteenth century, the bishop of Guadix, Antonio de Guevara, had even more astonishing things to say. He praises Cato and Eleazar in his *Libro áureo de Marco Aurelio,* but he goes much further in his *Horologium principum,* where he creates a sort of utopia and states that barbarians from India who had joined Pompey's army observed the custom of systematically committing suicide when they reached the age of fifty rather than being exposed to the miseries of old age: "And these barbarians had the custom of not wanting to live past fifty years, and for that reason when they reached that age they made a great heap of firewood, set it aflame, and burned themselves alive on it, willingly sacrificing themselves to the gods." Guevara expresses ecstatic approval of a custom that revealed such total scorn of the life of this world:

May all feel what they wish in this case and condemn these barbarians if it pleases them; I will not fail to say what I feel about it. O golden age that had such men! O happy people whose memory will live on perpetually through all the centuries! What scorn of the world! What forgetfulness of oneself! What a low blow to fortune! What a scourge to the flesh! What low esteem for life! O what a restraint for the wicked! O what spurs for the virtuous! O what confusion for those who love life! O what a grand example it leaves us for not fearing death![25]

Despair Again; the Catholic Response

Guevara's effusions reveal a tension (which already existed in the *devotio moderna* of the fifteenth century but was intensified in the mystical climate of the Catholic Reformation) between scorn for this world, which ought to inspire a desire for death and for the beatitude of life after death, and the prohibition on putting an end to one's life. The germs of this tension are present in the basic texts of Christianity, the four Gospels and the Epistles of St. Paul in particular, so that it is hardly surprising that Protestant spirituality reflected it as well. Philippe de Mornay devoted his *Excellent discours de la vie et de la mort* (1576) to persuading his readers that life is no more than "a continual death" and that death is desirable because it puts an end to the torments of this miserable existence. Aware of the logical conclusions to be drawn from this argument, Mornay adds, "At that rate, you may say, death is something to be wished for, and in order to leave so many woes, it seems one should hasten [the end of] one's life." Not so, Mornay responds, we have no right to do so: "The Christian must leave this life willingly but he must not flee from it like a coward." The only consistent way out of the dilemma is "to make the flesh die in us and uproot the world from it"—that is, to die to the world and to the self through total detachment, in a sort of spiritual suicide that in many respects substitutes for the physical suicide that has been ruled out.

The religious troubles of the early Renaissance by no means softened the condemnation of voluntary death. If anything, attitudes hardened. For Catholics, Lutherans, Calvinists, and Anglicans alike, suicide was a diabolical act. Hence it was a weapon in the religious wars: When a large number of suicides occurred in the rival camp, they were proof that its cause was satanic and its partisans were in the grip of the devil, who pushed them to despair. Each religious group thus attempted to repress suicide among its own and was quick to exploit any word of suicides among the enemy.

In the Catholic world the medieval explanation of voluntary death by despair was reinforced, with despair becoming one of the gravest sins. Well before the Reformation, suicide continued to occupy a prominent place in literature. In the fifteenth century Despair, an allegorical character in Alain Chartier's *Espérance, ou, Consolation des trois vertus,* depicts the woes of France, ravaged by the Hundred Years' War, and advises suicide as an escape from troubles:

Your age is already turning toward decline, and the woes of your nation are just beginning. What do you think you will see if you live longer, if not the death of friends, the pillage of wealth, fields laid waste, cities destroyed, lordship overturned, the land desolated, and servitude become commonplace? . . . You should regret remaining alive when your country perishes before your eyes and Fortune removes the hope and solace of your life.

At this point Hope (Espérance) arrives and persuades the author that he has no right to kill himself, as to do so would undo the work of God.

François Villon, too, was familiar with the ravages of despair. In his *Grand Testament* he has La Belle Heaumière, grown old, exclaim:

> Qui me tient, qui, que ne me fiere,
> Et qu'a ce coup je ne me tue?

(Who would prevent me, if now I swore to kill myself with a single blow?)[26]

Elsewhere in his *Grand Testament,* Villon states that at times only the fear of God has held his hand:

> Tristesse son cueur si estraint.
> Se, souvent, n'estoit Dieu qu'il craint,
> Il feroit ung orrible fait;
> Et advient qu'en ce Dieu enffrainct
> Et que lui mesmes se deffait

(His heart constricted by wretchedness. Only fear of God and holiness prevent him from some dreadful deed. For else God's law would he transgress, and destroy himself in his dire need!)[27]

Despair was one of the favorite themes of French Renaissance poets from Joachim Du Bellay's *Complainte du désespéré,* where the poet wishes he had been stillborn, to Pierre de Ronsard's *Hymnes.* Ronsard states in the "Hymne de la mort: A Louis des Masures":

> . . . Nous ne sommes rien
> Qu'une terre animée, et qu'une vivante ombre,
> Le sujet de douleur, de misère et d'encombre,
> . . .
> Tant nous sommes chétifs et pauvres journaliers,
> Recevant sans repos maux sur maux à milliers

(We are nothing but animated earth and a living shadow, subject to pain, misery, and burdens . . . so weak are we, poor day laborers with no respite, receiving woes on woes by the thousand.)

In *Les simulacres de la mort* (1538) the author has an old peasant woman from Trechsel state:

> En grand peine ay vescu longuement
> Tant que n'ay plus de vivre envie
> Mais bien je croy certainement
> Meillure la mort que la vie

(In great toil have I lived long, so much that I no longer care to live, but firmly and certainly do I believe death is better than life.)

The annals and chronicles of the period attribute most ordinary suicides to despair. Even the great mystics felt its temptations. On several occasions St. Ignatius of Loyola stated that, overwhelmed by an acute awareness of his sins and feeling sure he could never be forgiven for them, he felt like throwing himself out of the window. Juan de Avila (d. 1569) explained how the devil kindles a despair that urges us to suicide:

The demon, by an artifice quite contrary to the one that inspires pride . . . shows us all the sins we have committed and exaggerates them as much as he can in order to baffle us and discourage us so that, no longer able to bear such a great burden, we fall into despair. This was what he did to Judas. He concealed the enormity of his sin from him while he was urging him to commit it, and after he had committed it, he showed him how horrible it indeed was; at the same time, he prevented him from recalling the infinite mercy of God. This made [Judas] fall into despair, and from despair into hell.[28]

To combat this type of despair, the church still offered confession, and manuals on the art of dying (which flourished during the sixteenth century) paid particular attention to the danger of despair. A 1470 German edition of the *Ars moriendi* that speaks of the temptation to despair depicts six devils surrounding a dying man, showing him all the sins he committed during his life and suggesting, "Go ahead: kill yourself." An angel arrives, however, to reassure the dying man with extraordinarily soft words: "Why are you in despair? Have you committed so many acts of highway robbery, thefts, and homicides as there are drops of water in the sea and grains of sand on the shore? If you had committed all the sins of the world by yourself, never made any.penance for them until now, never confessed them, and had no opportunity to confess them until now, still, you must not despair, for in such a case inner contrition is enough."[29]

One can hardly imagine a better statement on suicide as the worst of all sins. Preachers and theologians repeated this message, without any concession, in an insistence that in its own way reveals a mounting anxiety. In the fifteenth century the topic of suicide appears only infrequently in sermons. In the many texts he studied, Hervé Martin found only one occurrence between 1350 and 1520.[30] Simon Cupersi, an Augustinian friar in Bayeux, based his forty-fourth sermon on the topic "Is Suicide Legitimate?" He responds in scholastic fashion, first by citing St. Matthew for the affirmative ("He who loses his life for my sake will save it"), then by reiterating all the traditional arguments against suicide. He concludes that suicide is a mortal sin.

Sixteenth-century Catholic theologians were unanimous in their intransigence. In his *De justitia et jure* Domingo de Soto developed the three traditional arguments against suicide, which he borrowed from St. Thomas: Suicide is an offense to nature; it is an affront to love of oneself, the state, and society; it offends the God who has given us life. The biblical cases of suicide can be explained by special messages from God. In 1554 Bartholomaeus Fumus stated in his *Summa aurea* that despair, suicide, dueling, and mutilation were mortal sins. In 1557 Francisco de Vitoria repeated the condemnation of suicide in his *De homicidio,* but in his casuistic arguments, which are more refined and more intelligent than those of most of his contemporaries, he admitted that this principle involved delicate questions: "If it were not permitted to expose our lives for the life of others, the physician could not exercise his art in times of plague, nor could the wife brave the danger of contagion to care for her husband stricken by the plague, nor could a shipwrecked man cede to another the plank that is his salvation, which is nonetheless a praiseworthy gesture."[31]

The Council of Trent did little more than reiterate the absolute prohibition on killing, as stated in the Mosaic commandment. The catechism promoted by the council states: "No man possesses such power over his own life as to be at liberty to put himself to death. Hence we find that the Commandment does not say: *Thou shalt not kill another,* but simply: Thou shalt not kill."[32]

The casuist Navarrus (Martín de Azpilcueta) went a good deal further, and his confession manual, published in Antwerp in 1581, reflects the harsher tone of the late 1570s. According to him, it is a mortal sin not only to commit suicide, but also to wish never to have been born, to wish for death in a fit of anger, to expose oneself to danger, to fight a duel, to mutilate oneself, or to expose oneself to martyrdom for personal reasons.[33]

The Diabolization of Suicide in the Protestant World

The Protestant world was no less severe regarding suicide. Martin Luther considered suicide to be a murder committed by the devil: "He breaks the neck of many or makes them lose their wits; he drowns some in the water, pushes many to suicide and many others he leads into atrocious misfortune." For Luther, anyone who commits suicide is possessed by the devil—which also removes personal responsibility for the act. On 1 December 1544, writing about a women who had been possessed by the devil and who had killed herself, Luther declared that the minister who buried her must not be criticized, for the woman might be considered the victim of an assassination committed by Satan. He added that severity was called for, as the devil was growing more and more audacious:

I have known many cases of this kind, and I have had reason to think in most of them, that the parties were killed, directly and immediately killed, by the devil, in the same way that a traveller is killed by a brigand. For when it is evident that the suicide has not taken place naturally, when all you find is a rope, a girdle, or . . . a veil hanging without any knot whatever, wherein you could suspend a fly . . . according to my view of the matter, the only solution of the affair is, that the devil has been deceiving the parties, and making them believe that they were doing something else, and so has killed them. Yet, still the civil magistrate is quite right in punishing this offence without exception, least the devil should make more and more way in this respect. The world merits such warnings, now that it has taken to epicurising, and setting down the devil as nothing.[34]

John Calvin did little more than reiterate the prohibition of suicide, as did all Protestant theologians and moralists from Henry Bulinger, who preached in Zurich, to Agrippa d'Aubigné, writing in his autobiography.[35] Henri Estienne, writing in 1566, deplored the bad example of the pagans of classical antiquity and stated that a suicide cannot be considered a Christian or even a human being: "For though Pagans made little or no Conscience to make away themselves, and though most Philosophers approved it by precept, & some also by their practice; yet the Christian world was never so corrupt, but that it hath condemned these felons de se, and razed them not only out of the number of Christians (by denying them Christian burial) but even of men."[36]

In England, Anglicans and Puritans diabolized suicide and use it as a polemical weapon.[37] For some of them, killing oneself was the result of a divine intervention visiting punishment on a life of sin or on an evil act. Thus when an aged Londoner disemboweled himself in 1577, Edmond Bicknoll presented the man's act as the result of remorse for a theft he had committed some years before.[38] Others considered suicide to be the work of the devil. Hugh Latimer wrote that some are so set upon by the demon that "they rid themselves out of this life."[39] Andrew Boorde, physician to Henry VIII, defined demoniacs as madmen whose chief characteristic is to wound or kill themselves, and he declared them to be possessed by the devil or by devils.[40] Exorcism was best for such persons. In the Roman Catholic Church it was usually the Jesuits who performed that rite, but the Protestants soon imitated them. In 1574 John Foxe exorcised a law student who had attempted several times to kill himself; John Darrel, a Puritan, also performed exorcisms. Others provided depressed persons who had attempted suicide with amulets, or else they anointed them with holy oil to protect them from temptation.

The statement that the devil had a personal role in suicides can even be found well into the seventeenth century in official documents, such as the sworn testimony of witnesses or the minutes of coroners' inquests. It is hardly astonishing that theologians unanimously condemned suicide. Thomas Becon, almoner to Thomas Cranmer, archbishop of Canterbury, held that despair lay at the root of self-murder; Cranmer himself had no doubt that suicides were damned. John Hooper, bishop of Gloucester, contrasted the death of a desperate person to the death of a saint, pointing out that a suicide commits an offense against divine mercy and against the natural law that commands us to love one another. In 1536 John Foxe condemned suicide in his *Acts and Monuments,* but noted that God alone can judge such an act. In 1577 John Byshop wrote in his *Beautiful Blossomes* that human beings have no excuse for committing suicide.

These authors also used the voluntary death of others as a proof of divine approbation of their own form of religion. Foxe, for instance, spoke of the suicides of "papists and apostates," concluding that the Church of England was blessed by God. When Henry Smith, a barrister, hanged himself in 1559 after having abjured Protestantism, Foxe declared that papist idolatry contributed to despair. He added, somewhat rashly, "No man is able to bring forth any one example . . . of any . . . true gospeller, that either killed himself or showed forth any signification or appearance of despair."[41]

While Foxe was writing, something like a propaganda war was taking place in England regarding suicide. The famous jurist Sir James Hales provided a focus for the controversy. An ardent Calvinist, Hales had been one of the principal propagators of Protestantism under Edward VI. When the determined Mary Tudor ascended to the throne in 1553, Hales was arrested and persecuted until he abjured. Stricken with remorse (and still unsure what fate awaited him), he attempted suicide. His major adversary, Stephen Gardiner, took advantage of this suicide attempt to declare that it proved that Protestantism was a "doctrine of despair." John Hooper, an Anglican, disagreed, stating in a manuscript treatise that it was after his abjuration that Hales gave in to Satan, which meant that it was Catholicism that had led him into satanic despair. The affair took on even greater proportions when Hales, freed from prison, drowned himself in another (and successful) suicide attempt. Protestant authors did their best to rescue his reputation. John Foxe suggested that perhaps Hales had killed himself to escape "the pollution of the mass," but Foxe was ill at ease with suicide. Other writers made Hales a Protestant martyr.

Several years later, under the reign of Elizabeth, another famous suicide gave the Protestants an opportunity to strike back. Henry Percy, earl of Northumberland and a Catholic, was imprisoned in the Tower of London for his part in Throgmorton's Plot, an attempt to free Mary Stuart. In 1585, after six months in the Tower, Percy killed himself with a pistol. The Catholics loudly claimed he had been murdered; the Protestants published *A True and Summarie Reporte* on the affair, which concluded that Percy's suicide was a divine punishment: "God by his judgement had for his sinnes and ingratitude taken from him his Spirit of grace and deliuered him ouer to the enemie of his soule, who brought him to that most dreadful and horrible end whereunto he is come."[42]

The Immutability of the Law

The mysterious rites to which, from time immemorial, the cadaver of a suicide had been subjected struck the popular imagination by their terrifying evocation of the forces of evil, and this made people all the more inclined to accept the notion of the satanic origin of suicide. Popular belief and the pastoral role of the clergy supported one another and worked toward the same result. Although the ecclesiastical authorities deplored the superstitious nature of such practices, they tolerated them as a reinforcement of their own teachings. Rites of reversal, for example, made it clear that the body of the suicide, inhabited by Satan, had upset the order of creation. Thus the cadaver was often placed in the ground face down, lying north-south rather than in the usual east-west orientation considered favorable for resurrection, the signal for which would come from the east. Driving a stake through the body was intended to circumvent resurrection, but pinning down the body also kept it from disturbing the living. Burying a suicide at a crossroads had the dual role of confusing the spirit of the dead and impressing passers-by who might be tempted to kill themselves. In 1590 the coroner of London even ordered that the end of the stake pinning down the cadaver of Amy Stokes be left exposed to reinforce the example. On other occasions a suicide was buried in the northernmost part of the cemetery with the excommunicated, the unbaptized, and all others who were excluded from eternal salvation.

In France the medieval punishments were still applied, perhaps with even greater severity. Bodies were dragged head down or hanged by their feet (again, we see inversion rites). In 1524 the body of Guillaume le Conte, a canon of Rouen Cathedral, was dug up, and his heraldic crest was removed from the façade of his house. In several cases a sizable fine was levied on the portion of the estate that had not been confiscated, the proceeds going to whoever held powers of high justice and to the poor.

The law itself was unbudging. Major decrees on criminal matters did not mention suicide, and when local customary law was compiled the jurists promised to point out anything in the ancient customs that "would be found harsh, difficult, rigorous, unreasonable, and thus subject to being tempered or totally corrected, stricken out, or abrogated." As Albert Bayet remarks, no provisions were so noted.[43]

In practice, however, precautions may have been taken to avoid rank injustice. In 1541 a judge, a police lieutenant, and a prosecuting attorney were fined in Toulouse for having hanged the cadaver of a man fleeing from the police who had killed himself. In 1586, again in Toulouse, Du Faur, the presiding judge of the Parlement de Toulouse, reversed a judgment that had given a man who had committed suicide "with no awareness of crime" a sentence calling for the body to be hanged and the estate to be confiscated. The Parlement de Toulouse had a reputation for indulgence, as the *Encyclopédie* recalled in the eighteenth century, when it stated that the court distinguished between "those who killed themselves out of fear of punishment for their crimes and those who kill themselves out of impatience, boredom with life, or an excess of passion or folly." Only those attempting to avoid sentence were punished.[44] Even Paris judges were not totally insensitive: In 1576 the Parlement de Paris permitted La Volpillière's widow to testify to her husband's innocence after he had killed himself in prison because of a calumnious accusation against him. In Burgundy the jurist Job Bouvot, basing his opinion on two decrees of 1502 and 1587, wrote that suicides by drowning would result in confiscation of the estate only when "the proofs are as clear as day."

Inquest procedures seem to have become more rigorous in the sixteenth century. Most jurists specified that a detailed report had to be drawn up regarding the place where the corpse had been found, that the barber-surgeons must examine the cadaver carefully, that the lifestyle and mores of the deceased should be investigated and inquiry made into possible reasons for suicide, and that a "curator of the body" should be named to defend the deceased at the trial and to call witnesses from among the family and the heirs. Unless all these precautions had been met, the sentence would be invalid, and the judges themselves might be liable to sanctions. One jurist, Jean Bacquet, stated that the courts were indulgent toward women who had killed themselves "out of necessity, indigence, and poverty," and another jurist, Anne Robert, declared that "madness is to be presumed" in suicide cases, especially when the deceased was a prominent individual (examples in Pierre de L'Estoile's journal corroborate this point).[45] To end the list, a law of Emperor Charles V, promulgated in 1551, distinguishes between those who kill themselves to escape justice (whose goods are confiscated to the profit of the lord) and those who commit suicide "by the effect of a bodily illness, melancholy, weakness, or some other similar infirmity."

All in all, both the law and judiciary practice concerning suicide changed little until around 1570. With the exception of England, where repression grew in response to laws passed in 1487, 1509, and 1510, prominent persons were always spared, and among the common people madness was quite frequently accepted as an excuse. England was already a special case and a land where a high number of guilty verdicts focused attention on suicide. It is hardly coincidental that systematic reflection on voluntary death developed in England during the years from 1580 to 1620 in writers such as Christopher Marlowe, Shakespeare, John Donne, Robert Burton, and others.

Suicide, Folly or Wisdom? From Brant to Erasmus

Although there was never any real challenge to Christian morality, as examples of suicide from classical antiquity began to penetrate the minds of the intellectual elites, they raised questions or at least elicited an embarrassed comparison between ancient attitudes and Christian positions.

The problem of suicide was also raised indirectly through madness, a topic much in fashion from the late fifteenth to the mid-sixteenth century. From Sebastian Brant's *Narrenschiff (Ship of Fools)* in 1494 through Erasmus' *Encomium moriae (In Praise of Folly)* to the paintings of Hieronymus Bosch and Pieter Brueghel, madness made an impressive entry onto the intellectual and artistic scene. Popular culture had long celebrated madness in the Feast of Fools and Carnival. The intellectual elite (which followed well behind popular wisdom in this regard) discovered this rich theme borrowed from peasant traditions and worked to extract its deeper meanings. We might compare the arrival of madness as an intellectual theme at the end of the fifteenth century to the appearance of surrealism in the 1920s. In both cases, the new movement was a desperate reaction to an existential anxiety. André Breton and his disciples proclaimed their supreme derision in face of an absurd world whose senselessness had just exploded into awareness between 1914 and 1918. Bosch and Brant exorcised the terror born of war and the Black Death, events that had led to the triumph of the macabre throughout Western Europe. Madness was at once a refuge, an escape, and an explanation of a world reduced to nothingness and absurdity. Concerning the broad movement of the 1490s, Michel Foucault, the master of the history of madness, states:

Then in the last years of the century this enormous uneasiness turns on itself; the mockery of madness replaces death and its solemnity. From the discovery of that necessity which inevitably reduces man to nothing, we have shifted to the scornful contemplation of that nothing which is existence itself. Fear in the face of the absolute limit of death turns inward in a continuous irony; man disarms it in advance, making it an object of derision by giving it an everyday, tamed form.[46]

Madness was also one of the masks of death, as amply illustrated in the paintings of Bosch and in Brueghel's *Dulle Griet* (1563). The mad were already dead, to themselves and to the world. Moreover, madness was an excuse and a way of fleeing the wracking problem of sin that so affected Luther's generation. Pursued by poverty, death, and the incubus of sin and hell, humanity set sail on the ship of fools.

But if madness had been an absurd response to the agonizing problems of existence, it soon became a rational critique of absurd human comportment. The perspective changes radically from Sebastian Brant to Erasmus. For Brant, "to seek death is folly, for death will find us soon enough." Erasmus asks, "Who are the people that, merely because of weariness of life, have hastened their fate? Were they not the people who lived next door to wisdom?"[47] Brant thought men mad to kill themselves; Erasmus thought them mad to remain alive. He offers proof:

To how many calamities would he see the life of man subject! How painful, how messy, man's birth! How irksome his rearing—his childhood exposed to so many hurts, his youth beset by so many problems! Then age is a burden; the certainty of death is inexorable. Diseases infest life's every way; accidents threaten, troubles assail without warning; there is nothing that is not tainted with gall. Nor can I recite all those evils which man suffers at the hands of man; poverty is in this class, and imprisonment, infamy, shame, tortures, snares, treachery, slander, litigation, fraud. . . . You will observe, I am sure, what would happen if men generally became wise: there would be need for some fresh clay and for another potter like Prometheus. (41–42)

Why, then, don't people commit suicide? Folly states, "But aided in part by ignorance, and in part by inadvertence, sometimes by forgetfulness of evil, sometimes by hope of good, sprinkling in a few honeyed delights at certain seasons, I bring relief from these ills" (ibid.). What is more, Erasmus adds, haven't the true sages of classical antiquity—Cato, Diogenes, and Brutus— shown us the way? Erasmus' tone is light, and he affects irony, but this statement is audacious to the extreme, and it reveals the surreptitious penetration of a new trend in moral thought. Nor is this simply a witticism: In his *Apophthegmata* Erasmus speaks admiringly of ancient suicides.

The New Suicide: A Yearning for the Absolute (Faust) and for Honor

At the same time, a new reason for despair arose during the Renaissance, and it provided a powerful invitation, unknown in the Middle Ages, to commit suicide. Paradoxically, it emerged out of humanism's excessive optimism. Albrecht Dürer put it this way: "We want to know much and to possess the truth about all things. But our obtuse intelligence cannot attain the perfection of art, truth, and wisdom. Our knowledge is based on lies, and shadows envelop us so mercilessly that even when we cautiously advance we falter at every step." The humanists' immense appetite for knowledge, their Rabelaisian educational program, and their thirst for universal knowledge led the most anxiety-ridden of them to an inevitable awareness of the narrow limits of the human mind. The Middle Ages reserved universal knowledge to God. The Renaissance led some to believe that the humanist man might be able to attain it too. Their disillusionment was all the more bitter: The times were ripe for Faust.

Christopher Marlowe's *Tragicall History of Doctor Faustus* (probably written about 1589 and published in 1604) brought to the stage one of the most significant works of the century. "What Faust finds burdensome," Bernard Paulin writes, "is the very limits of the human condition, within which he feels cramped. Marlowe's Faust does not deny God; he asserts himself in face of God."[48] Of course, Faust fails in his attempt, which leads him to the temptation of suicide. A new Adam, he strives to equal God through knowledge, and the discovery of the vanity of knowledge turns him toward the devil. When the devil disappoints him, there is nothing left but death:

> My hearts so hardned I cannot repent,
> Scarce can I name salvation, faith or heaven,
> But fearful ecchoes thunders in mine eares,
> *Faustus,* thou art damn'd, then swordes and knives,
> Poyson, gunnes, halters, and invenomd steele
> Are layde before me to dispatch my self.[49]

Mephistopheles takes advantage of this despair to offer a dagger to Faust, who cries out in remorse:

> Where art thou *Faustus*? wretch what hast thou done?
> Damnd art thou *Faustus,* damnd, dispair and die.[50]

We see here the medieval theme of despair induced by Satan. The means are new, however: Diabolical trickery takes the form of seduction by knowledge, a typically humanist snare. We have clearly entered into the somber decade of the 1580s.

The sociological and cultural revolutions of the early Renaissance created a context that did much to open the way to reflection on suicide. Admiration for classical antiquity played its part, but so did changes in warfare that gave the noble a new code of conduct. Honor, for an officer in a structured royal or princely army, consisted in successfully upholding the responsibilities entrusted to him. War was no longer the great game it had been in yesteryear, when opposing forces were more interested in capturing knights for ransom than in killing them. Now capture and defeat meant dishonor, to which some, like the heroes of classical antiquity, preferred death. Examples of military suicidal behavior increased during the sixteenth century: In 1523 Guillaume Gouffier, seigneur de Bonnivet and admiral of France, rushed out to meet the enemy forces, braving certain death, after he had made gross tactical errors at the Battle of Pavia. François de Condé, comte d'Enghien, did the same at the battle of Cérisolles (Ceresole d'Alba, in Piedmont) in 1544. Hervé de Portzmoguer, commander of the *Cordelière,* preferred death to surrender in a hard-fought sea battle against the *Regent* in 1513, taking eleven hundred sailors with him to a watery death. In 1591 Richard Grenville did his best to imitate Portzmoguer's example during a naval battle against the Spanish fleet, but the crew of the *Revenge* prevented him from succeeding. In the early sixteenth century Baron d'Allègre (a companion in arms of Pierre Terrail, seigneur de Bayard), whose two sons had just died in combat, voluntarily sought death in the hope of joining them.

A courtier's idea of honor led Filippo Strozzi to commit suicide in 1538. He wrote in his testament: "It is because I found myself obliged to harm my friends, my family, and my honor that I have taken the only course remaining to me, though the cruellest one for my soul: that of taking my own life." John Talbot, earl of Shrewsbury, died with his son in 1453 at the Battle of Castillon, in Gascony, while leading a desperate attack. Brantôme mentions a fencing master who committed suicide after being touched twice by a pupil, and although he recalls pro forma that one should not kill oneself, he states that the man's "courage and generous soul are worthy of all praise." The painter Rosso Fiorentino killed himself in 1541 out of remorse for having falsely accused a friend of robbing him, thus causing the friend to be interrogated by torture.

Women defended their honor as well in the Renaissance. A more dignified role for women in court milieus, where they were increasingly present, was accompanied by new demands, especially for greater autonomy. Men admired Cato; women praised Lucretia. In his manual for courtly behavior, *Il Corteggiano (The Courtier),* Baldassare Castiglione cited several women who followed Lucretia's example, some of them commoners: One Italian peasant girl, for instance, drowned herself after being raped; another did the same to foil the insistent advances of Gascon soldiers. Henri Estienne related how one woman hanged herself because a shoemaker had taken advantage of her, and the Jesuit Juan de Mariana expressed his admiration for a Spanish woman who killed herself to avoid temptation. Brantôme has a store of such stories, but his tone is both moralizing and cynical: "Nor it is permitted to a woman to kill herself out of fear of being raped or after having been raped; if she did she would sin mortally." Still, he reports several cases of such female suicides without disapproval. He remarks that very few women kill themselves following their husband's death; women usually cite the commandment against killing or use the pretext of having children to raise to justify continuing to live. Brantôme speaks critically of Madellena de Soria, who killed herself after assassinating her husband; she would have done better to "give herself a good time afterwards."[51]

The Rise of Individualism and a Challenge to Traditional Values: Cause for Anxiety

During the Renaissance bourgeois individualism invaded the domains of business, religion, and culture. A capitalist in the making required more freedom of choice and began to reject corporative constraints. He also aspired to a more direct, internalized, and deeper contact with God, and he asserted his personality by his tastes, his dwelling, his furnishings, and his reading matter, and by having his portrait painted. But what he gained in autonomy he lost in an increased fragility. Émile Durkheim has shown that the suicide rate is in inverse proportion to social integration. The structured group protects by the ties it creates: Corporation, family, and religious community were ramparts against the temptation to self-homicide. During the Renaissance, the businessman broke his ties with the guilds and corporations, enclosure isolated the rural noble, and communitarian practices declined. At the same time, the influence of Protestantism individualized religious reflection and relaxed horizontal structures in favor of vertical ones that used personal interpretation of Scripture to set up a direct link between the individual believer and God. Admittedly, we have not yet come to the nineteenth century, and lineage, parish, and family still provided a strong framework in this age. Nonetheless, disintegration had begun in the late Middle Ages: The humanist, the man of letters, and the merchant found themselves alone with their problems, worries, and anxieties. Books cannot replace human ties.

A penchant for secrecy further accentuated solitude. Sheltered within his study with his books and his globes, the scholar sought knowledge in isolation, made discoveries alone, and kept his discoveries to himself. Leonardo da Vinci had his secret notebooks and his mirror writing; Jean Fernel insisted on working alone, wishing to owe no debts to others; Niccolò Tartaglia refused to share with Girolamo Cardano his method for resolving third-degree equations; Johannes Kepler could get no information out of Tycho Brahe, who in turn asserted that he had not consulted Nicolaus Copernicus. Copernicus published his conclusion regarding his famous system only after years of hesitation. Perhaps out of a desire to avoid unjust criticism or a fear of condemnation, perhaps because they could not prove their findings, scholars jealously (at times aggressively) cultivated their own individual truths. Dissatisfaction was rampant, beginning with Cardano, Paracelsus, and Cornelius Agrippa. Instability might at times lead such men to suicide, as was the case with Cardano. A temperamental man, part mathematician, part astrologer, Cardano admired the great figures of classical antiquity, and he reflected on ancient suicides on several occasions. He wrote in 1542: "Those who have no hope in a future life die no less valiantly than those who believe the soul to be immortal." His father had killed himself in 1524; in 1577 Cardano followed his father's example after a murky affair involving errors in astrological calculations.

If scholars were solitary beings, cultural incertitude and penury added to their difficulties. Values of all sorts were challenged in the Renaissance: All norms were contested, all hypotheses were tried out. In all fields—geography, cosmology, economics, politics, religion, and the arts—certitudes were questioned, and acquired knowledge was turned upside down. The Americas, heliocentrism, inflation, absolutism, and Protestantism all created a mobile cultural universe whose major trends only the greatest minds could discern. Others doubted, and took refuge in a relativism, even a skepticism, that they had to hide from the authorities, who were quick to discourage any novelty. Intellectuals were often not only isolated and disoriented but also short of money (when they were not frankly poor), which obliged them to seek pensions from wealthy patrons. This was the context that led the humanist Bonaventure Despériers to suicide in 1544. A man with an original mind and a pessimistic bent, Despériers was a freethinker, almost an atheist, who had connections among the disputatious Protestant circles that gravitated around Marguerite de Navarre. An admirer of the ancients, Seneca in particular (whose works he translated), Despériers was already a suspect figure, but he fell into despair when Marguerite, his patroness, abandoned him. He ran himself through with such energy that he was found with his sword sticking out from his back.

Religious anxiety was another cause for suicide. To be sure, both Luther and Calvin opposed voluntary death. Both men had enough intellectual and spiritual resources to protect themselves from the temptations of suicide. But by liberating the faithful from the crushing tutelage of the Roman Catholic Church, they may have placed on the shoulders of the faithful a burden that some were not strong enough to bear. Fragile minds might be led to despair by free examination and free interpretation of Scripture, by an acute awareness of their irrevocable human weakness, by the doctrine of predestination, and by the elimination of confession, a recourse that many had found reassuring. Several cases of suicide were reported, for example, following Presbyterian preaching campaigns in Scotland.[52]

Religious rivalry created situations propitious to suicide, first when abjurations occurred. This was the case, as we have seen, with the English jurist James Hales in 1553 and the barrister Henry Smith in 1559. The climate of religious war led to a recurrence of the mystique of voluntary martyrdom. Denis Crouzet has shown that a rising tide of eschatological anxiety, which had begun in the 1520s, contributed to a liberating but murderous slaughter in which combatants sought death, both for their adversaries and themselves.[53] During the same period there was a wave of astrological predictions in Europe: Henri de Fines predicted a second Universal Deluge in 1524; in 1550 Richard Roussat announced that the end of the world was at hand in his *Livre de l'estat et mutation des temps, prouvant par authoritez de l'Escripture sainct et par raisons astrologales, la fin du monde estre prochaine;* a catastrophic planetary conjunction was predicted for 1564; and Nostradamus put out one woeful prophecy after another. These writings and inflammatory preaching by several monks created a mounting tension that found release in a spurt of violence that associated self-sacrifice with the massacre of heretics. The oath sworn in the Catholic crusade of 1568 in Burgundy stated, "If some of us should die, our blood will be for us a second baptism by which we will go directly to paradise with the other martyrs." The "crusading impulse," as Denis Crouzet calls it, was an impulse for death—for others and for oneself—in a bath of purifying blood.

Admiration for the pagan suicide of classical antiquity, on the one hand, and the Christian sentiment of giving one's life for God and the true faith, on the other, were a curious mixture. Filippo Strozzi said in his testament, written just before he slit his throat: "I recommend my soul to God, and I pray him to accord it (should all other mercy fail) the same sojourn as the souls of Cato and the many other virtuous men who shared his faith."

We find the same inconsistency in Benvenuto Cellini, a man of genius and boundless curiosity, but also an unstable adventurer. Cellini was a murderer and a profligate; he also practiced necromancy. His troubled life is hardly edifying, and his relations with morality were at best incoherent. When he was sentenced to life imprisonment in 1539, reading the Bible led him to attempt suicide. He tells us in his *Autobiography:*

I began the Bible from the beginning, devoutly reading and meditating on it. I was so fascinated that if it had been possible I would have spent all my time reading it. But, as the light failed, all my sufferings immediately flooded back, and I was so tortured that more than once I made up my mind to put out my life with my hand. They had left me without a knife, however, and so I had no easy means of doing such a thing. All the same on one occasion I took a solid wooden beam that was lying there and propped it up in such a way that it would fall like a trap. I wanted to make it crash down on my head, which would have been smashed at the first blow. . . . I had set up the whole contraption, and was resolutely preparing to knock it down.[54]

This seems to Cellini a perfectly natural course of action, and at no point does he mention ecclesiastical prohibitions of suicide. Saved in time by his jailer, he repents:

On reflecting as to what it was that frustrated my attempt I decided that it must have been a divine power, my guardian angel. The following night a wonderful vision in the form of a beautiful young man appeared to me in a dream and started rebuking me. "Do you know who it was who lent you that body that you were ready to wreck before the appointed time?" he said. I seemed to answer that I recognized everything as having come from the God of nature. "So then," he replied, "you despise His works, and you want to destroy them? Leave Him to guide you, and do not abandon hope in His saving power." And he added a great deal else, in very impressive words, of which I don't remember the thousandth part. I began to be convinced that this angelic being had spoken the truth.

This is the bewildering, one might even say infantile behavior of a man who still had a medieval spontaneity but also bore witness to an age in which the great values of classical antiquity were revitalized. Once he has regained his wits, Cellini sets himself to composing a dialogue between his soul and his body on the subject of suicide:

Then I started to write as best I could on some superfluous pages in my Bible, and I rebuked the powers of my intellect for being impatient with life: they replied to my body, excusing themselves on account of their sufferings: and then my body held out the hope of better things. All this I wrote in dialogue, as follows:

> "Powers of my soul, in torment,.
> How cruel it is of you to hate this life!"
> "If you against Heaven are bent,
> Who then will succor us in this our strife?
> Let us depart, to seek a better life."
> "Wait, be not so swift to go:
> Heaven promises you will
> Be yet more happy than you were before."
> "A short while we'll stay below,
> If our great God intends to grant us still
> The grace that we shall never suffer more."

My strength came back to me, and after I had calmed myself by my own efforts I carried on reading my Bible.

Two and a half centuries later, in 1795, another lost child with no moral compass, Cagliostro, committed suicide in prison.

All the ordinary sorts of suicide motivated by suffering, poverty, passion, jealousy, madness, and fear of torture continued during the Renaissance. The suicide rate was probably no higher than in the Middle Ages, but much more was written about the topic than before. Although by far the greater part of expressed opinion remained hostile to suicide, the very fact that many authors thought it necessary to condemn suicide is revealing. Ever since St. Augustine, self-murder, categorized as a form of homicide, had not been open to debate. When suicide was placed within the category of mortal sins suggested by the devil, it could only be excused by insanity, and if in practice madness was often invoked to avoid confiscation and execution of the cadaver, suicide was unanimously and absolutely condemned in principle.

In the early Renaissance, intellectuals discovered the complexity of that apparently aberrant act and its importance as a sign of individual volition. This was not yet a rehabilitation of suicide, but only an incipient interrogation of it. What yesterday had seemed evident became a question. All agreed that Christians do not have the right to kill themselves, but weren't the suicides of the great figures of classical antiquity admirable? And if they were, then on what criteria should the difference between their wisdom and our own be based? These were intellectuals' questions more than moralists'. The moralists sensed danger and loudly reiterated that suicide was satanic. In England repression tightened.

Some authors even began to draw up catalogues, compile lists, and note curious cases. Suicide was at times used to cast aspersions on adversaries: Rumors circulated, for instance, about the hypothetical suicides of Pope Alexander VI and Martin Luther. Voluntary death had come out of oblivion, but until 1580 it remained a topic of purely intellectual debate. The question, "To be or not to be?" was formulated around 1600. It is the only question worth raising, Albert Camus tells us in *The Myth of Sisyphus*. Scholars and writers from Montaigne to John Donne reflected on the problem, but found no clear response to it. For those in positions of civil and religious authority, the question was in and of itself a crime and a sacrilege that threatened the existence of human societies and even creation itself. It was a primordial question, to be stifled because raising it was the first step toward poisoning the self. The Church and the state owed it to themselves to react to it, repress it, and find substitutes for it.

FIVE

To Be or Not to Be

The First Crisis of Conscience in Europe

To be, or not to be: that is the question.
Whether 'tis nobler in the mind to suffer
The slings and arrows of outrageous fortune,
Or to take arms against a sea of troubles,
And by opposing end them. To die; to sleep;
No more; and by a sleep to say we end
The heart-ache and the thousand natural shocks
That flesh is heir to. 'Tis a consummation
Devoutly to be wish'd. To die; to sleep;—
To sleep? Perchance to dream! Aye, there's the rub;
For in that sleep of death what dreams may come,
When we have shuffl'd off this mortal coil,
Must give us pause. There's the respect
That makes calamity of so long life.
For who would bear the whips and scorns of time,
The oppressor's wrong, the proud man's contumely,
The pangs of dispriz'd love, the law's delay,
The insolence of office, and the spurns
That patient merit of the unworthy takes,
When he himself might his quietus make
With a bare bodkin? Who would fardels bear,
To grunt and sweat under a weary life,
But that the dread of something after death,
The undiscover'd country from whose bourn
No traveller returns, puzzles the will
And makes us rather bear those ills we have
Than to fly to others that we know not of?
Thus conscience does make cowards of us all;
And thus the native hue of resolution

Is sicklied o'er with the pale cast of thought,
And enterprises of great pith and moment
With this regard their currents turn awry,
And lose the name of action.
(William Shakespeare, *Hamlet,* act 3, scene 1)

This passage, one of the most famous in world literature, was written in 1600. Shakespeare said it all in these few lines: Given the constraints and limitations of the human condition, how can we justify prolonging our existence? Many things combine to make Hamlet's soliloquy a timeless, universal text: the mystery of the personality of its author, little known behind the façade of his name; the contrast between the simplicity of Hamlet's dilemma and his inability to decide; the internal movement of the text whose ebb and flow so well expresses the interwoven hopes and disappointments of the human condition. Humanity's lot is, precisely, one of intertwined pains and frustrations—humiliations, injustices, emotional distress and physical pain, unmerited defeats, and the scorn and indifference of the great, the proud and the bureaucracies. These accumulated troubles make human life

. . . but a walking shadow, a poor player
That struts and frets his hour upon the stage
And then is heard no more. It is a tale
Told by an idiot, full of sound and fury,
Signifying nothing.
(Shakespeare, *Macbeth,* act 5, scene 5)

Since life is so absurd and so painful, why not put an end to it without delay and slip into eternal sleep? Because we are afraid of the unknown; it is not fear of death that holds us back but fear of what might come after. Our conscience and our imagination keep us from suicide, and we remain suspended between life and death.

The deep-rooted temptation of suicide has never been expressed more tellingly. Is Hamlet Shakespeare? The question is beside the point: What counts is not William Shakespeare the individual, but that the question was formulated and that its echo has continued to resonate to this day. Hamlet is an actor: We are all actors. He is suspended between madness and lucidity: That is our common fate. His question is humankind's question.

Although Hamlet's soliloquy has proven its timelessness and universality, it is nonetheless strongly anchored in a time and a space—England in 1600. For one thing, its expressive sonority defies translation. Its phrases cut like a knife, and anyone who wants to understand them and feel the full impact of their keen analysis, their depressing litany of human frustrations, and the anguish they convey of making impossible choices must read them in English.

The temptation of suicide in *Hamlet* is the most fully worked out expression of an anxiety typical of both English and European thought during the years from 1580 to 1620. During those forty years, more than two hundred suicides appeared on the English stage in a hundred plays,[1] and that figure alone points to the social phenomenon of a public that was attracted by both curiosity and apprehension. Late-sixteenth-century audiences just lapped up voluntary death.

Their interest is confirmed by a series of texts that, for the first time, use suicide as their main topic. These works challenge the traditional prohibitions, examine the motivations of suicide, and judge it in the light of reason and ancient example. In 1580 Sir Philip Sidney's philosophical romance, *The Countess of Pembroke's Arcadia,* presented a discussion between partisans and adversaries of suicide.[2] Between 1580 and 1588 Montaigne discussed the problem of suicide in several of his *Essays,* notably, in "La Coustume de l'isle de Cea" (A Custom of the Island of Cea). Christopher Marlowe's *Tragicall History of Dr. Faustus* was probably written around 1589 (published in 1604). In 1601 Pierre Charron borrowed from Montaigne and from Stoicism to defend the practice of reasonable suicide in his *De la sagesse.* Francesco Piccolomini was organizing debates on the subject in Italy during the same years. In 1604 Justus Lipsius discussed Stoic suicide in his *Manuductio ad stoicam philosophiam.* He also wrote an entire treatise favoring suicide, called *Thraseas,* but he destroyed the work out of fear of the reactions it might provoke. In 1607 Francis Bacon considered the question of suicide, without condemning it, in his essay on death. Around 1610 John Donne devoted an entire book to suicide, the *Biathanatos.* In 1609 Duvergier de Hauranne took on the subject in *La question royale,* where—surprisingly—the future Abbé de Saint-Cyran justified suicide under certain circumstances. In 1621 Robert Burton analyzed suicide as a result of religious despair in *The Anatomy of Melancholy.* A multitude of other works—tragedies, novels, and treatises on moral philosophy—took up the problem as well. It was the first time in Western European history that suicide had prompted such widespread interest.

This does not mean that people were obsessed by voluntary death in the late Renaissance. They killed themselves neither more nor less than in earlier ages, and what was written on the topic makes up an extremely small proportion of everything that was published. Still, it is noteworthy that these works were written at all, because until that time suicide—an act that both morality and the law unhesitatingly condemned and compared to homicide—was simply not discussed. Certain condemnation shifted to question. We are in the same years as Montaigne's "Que sais-je?" (What do I know?). Before examining why this challenge to the condemnation of suicide arose in religious, political, and juridical circles and what reactions it prompted, we need to see what form the challenge took.

The Questions of Sidney and Montaigne

It was philosopher-essayists, moralists, and lay thinkers who displayed the most interest in suicidal behavior. Systematic studies replaced the questioning of the early Renaissance. Rather than defenses of suicide, such works were attempts to understand it—an approach that inevitably led their authors into distinctions, nuances, and excuses. Skepticism was the predominant attitude, but the heirs of humanism had trouble making up their minds: They tirelessly listed arguments pro and con, but drew no conclusions.

Pyrocles, the protagonist of Sir Philip Sidney's pastoral romance, *Arcadia,* contemplates suicide to save his mistress, Philoclea, from unpleasant consequences when the two are discovered in bed together. They engage in a debate on voluntary death in which they rehearse all the known arguments. For Pyrocles, suicide is a lesser evil that would resolve their problems. He puts forth the Stoic argument that benefit to the "general nature" should prevail over that of "private nature." He states that he will die happy and without fear because it will be for her sake; that death will save them from despair; that life is short, and shortening it by a few years will make little difference; and that to die for a good cause is praiseworthy. Philoclea responds, somewhat curiously, with arguments drawn more from Aristotle and Plato than from Christian sources: God has placed us in our bodies like soldiers in a fortress, and we have no right to desert our posts; suicide is an act of cowardice and can camouflage unsavory emotions. Pyrocles does not in fact kill himself, but it is his love of Philoclea that wins him over to life more than her fairly weak arguments. Traditional morality is safeguarded, but not very convincingly.

Montaigne takes a loftier position. He acts as a humanist intent on avoiding prejudices when he turns to the question of suicide. As we know, death was one of Montaigne's constant preoccupations: It is death that makes life precious, but it also makes life an exercise in vanity. We can wait for death or go to meet it, and Montaigne is interested in understanding "those of all sexes and conditions and sects in happier times who have either awaited death resolutely or sought it voluntarily, and sought it not only to flee the ills of this life, but some simply to flee satiety with living, and others for the hope of a better condition elsewhere."[3] The question intrigued Montaigne. He devoted a paragraph to it in his *Journal de voyage,* and he discussed it briefly in some thirty scattered passages in the *Essays* and at length in "A Custom of the Island of Cea," a chapter in the *Essays* that forms a true treatise on suicide. He made nine additions to the chapter in 1588, and another nineteen additions in 1592 (two others appear in the posthumous edition of 1595).

Montaigne's argument, to which he obviously devoted thought and which he structured and polished with care, is a systematic study carried on with total independence of mind, even if he notes at the head of the essay, perhaps as a precaution, that his only guide has been "the authority of the divine will." He first lists statements favorable to suicide taken from authors of classical antiquity, lending them such force of conviction and presenting them in such well-turned phrases that we sense undeniable approval:

> The sage lives as long as he should, not as much as he can.
>
> [Nature has given us a fine gift, for] she has ordained only one entry into life, and a hundred thousand exits.
>
> If you live in pain, your cowardice is the cause, to die all that is needed is the will.
>
> Death is . . . the remedy for all ills.
>
> The most voluntary death is the fairest.
>
> Life depends on the will of others; death, on our own.
>
> For the most violent diseases the most violent remedies.
>
> God give us leave enough, when he puts us in such a state that it is worse to live than to die.
>
> Just as I do not violate the laws against thieves when I carry away my own money and cut my own purse, or those against firebugs when I burn my own wood, so I am not bound by the laws against murderers for having taken my own life.[4]

Montaigne follows these rational arguments (which he borrowed, for the most part, from classical antiquity) with a recapitulation of the arguments against suicide. Religious arguments come first: God is the master of our lives; He has placed us on the earth for his glory and for the service of others; we are not born for ourselves alone, and we have no right to desert our posts. Social arguments come next: The laws prohibit us from disposing of our own lives. Then come moral arguments: Virtue and courage dictate that we con-

front our tribulations. Finally, he gives philosophical arguments: Nature requires of us that we love ourselves; to kill oneself in order to avoid the evils of
this world simply throws us into a greater evil. Taking refuge in nonbeing
cannot improve our situation because we would no longer be able to profit
from the improvement. Nothingness is not a solution; it is the negation of
everything: "When he is no more, who will feel and rejoice in this improvement for him? . . . The security, the freedom from pain and suffering, the
exemption from the ills of this life that we purchase at the price of death bring
us no advantage. To no purpose does the man avoid war who cannot enjoy
peace, and to no purpose does the man flee from trouble who does not have
what it takes to relish repose."[5]

After presenting arguments that resolve nothing, Montaigne offers concrete examples. He is well aware that suicide is not a question of abstract
morality to be discussed in absolute terms in the aim of arriving at universal
conclusions; it is rather a question of situational morality. It is a solution that
occurs to an individual facing a difficult situation that only he or she can
deeply appreciate in its full dimensions. When viewed from the outside, other
people's suicides seem more or less justified according to one's own point of
view. Montaigne reviews famous suicides, pagan and Christian, expressing his
opinion on each one, but he does not generalize from them. The lesson of the
Essays is that such a decision is possible only when one faces it personally.

Although Montaigne is generally admiring in his review of famous suicides, he can at times be critical and even ironic. Brutus and Cassius would
have accomplished more if they had remained alive to defend Roman liberty;
the duc d'Enghien acted too precipitously when he rushed into battle, before
defeat was sure, at Ceresole d'Alba. Montaigne's view of female suicides
following a rape is male to the point of bawdiness. He finds it impossible to
believe that the woman who has been raped has not felt pleasure, and he
suggests that rather than killing herself she would do better to take advantage
of the situation, like one woman who "passed through the hands of some
soldiers" and declared, "God be praised that at least once in my life I have had
my fill without sin!"[6]

Montaigne hastens to add that we should not rush to kill ourselves for
frivolous reasons, and that we should draw all possible pleasure from our lives.
"Not all troubles are worth our wanting to die to avoid them. And then, there
being so many sudden changes in human affairs, it is hard to judge just at what
point we are at the end of our hope." Suicide is justified only at the last
extremity, in cases of intense and incurable physical pain, or to avoid a death
by torture: "Unendurable pain and fear of a worse death seem the most

excusable motives for suicide."[7] This conclusion is both Stoic and Epicurean as well as being based on simple good sense.

Montaigne himself, though riddled with pain from his stone, waited for death. Was he, like Hamlet, afraid of that "undiscover'd country from whose bourn no traveller returns"? We have no way of knowing. Like almost all who wrote about suicide expressing their own doubts, Montaigne did not kill himself. It is as if talking about suicide also exorcised it.

From Charron to Bacon: The Study of Suicide

Montaigne's questions become assertions in the writings of his friend Pierre Charron, whose *De la sagesse* was published in 1601. A priest and a Stoic, Charron borrowed as much from Seneca as he did from Jesus Christ when he reiterated the arguments of Montaigne, whom he had known in Bordeaux in 1589. Thanks to his training as a theologian, however, he treated those arguments systematically: Voluntary death is permissible and rational if it is the result of a mature reflection and the decision is well motivated:

It is first beyond all doubt, that we are not to attempt this last exploit without very great and iust cause (nay I cannot see how any cause should be great and iust enough) to the end that it bee . . . an honest and reasonable departure. . . . It is a great point of wisdome to learne to know the point and period, to chuse a fit houre to die. Every man hath his time and season to die: some prevent it, others prolong it: there is a weaknesse and valour in them both, but there is required discretion. . . . There is a time to gather fruit from the tree, which if it hang too long, it rotteth and growes worse and worse; and the losse is as great too, if it be gathered too soon.[8]

Charron died of apoplexy in 1603, so he did not have time to apply his lessons to himself, but his book caused a scandal among the clergy. What might be tolerated in Montaigne as personal reflection and questioning could hardly be admitted from a well-known preacher and the *grand vicaire* of Cahors. Charron's book was placed on the Index on 9 September 1605, whereas Montaigne's *Essays* had to wait until 28 January 1676 to be accorded that dubious honor.

In 1595 Pierre de Dampmartin reflected on contemporary questions in *La fortune de la cour*. Not bothering with arguments, he simply contradicted himself. On the one hand, he criticized Cato: "I will also say that there are some who consider courageous those who cannot wait for a situation to change but rush to their deaths. . . . I cannot be of that opinion; quite to the contrary, I attribute [such deaths] to a lack of courage and confidence."[9] On the other hand, Dampmartin cited as examples of courage the suicides of Perseus and Otho, who redeemed their ill deeds by a heroic suicide.

Although he steered a careful course between Catholicism and Calvinism, the Flemish humanist Justus Lipsius clearly supported the Stoic position on voluntary death, summarizing it in sympathetic terms in his *Manuductio* in 1604.[10] Applying the old scholastic method of thesis and antithesis, Lipsius warmly developed the arguments in favor of suicide, then refuted them briefly and formally. This trick did not fool the editors of the Index. In his correspondence, however, Lipsius expressed himself more freely, exclaiming, "What cowardice to suffer so many deaths and not die!" Startled by his own audacity, he chose to destroy the manuscript of the *Thraseas,* which might have been the earliest published defense of philosophical suicide.

In 1606 Caspar Scioppius also presented a survey of Stoic philosophy as a pretext for expressing enthusiasm over heroic suicides, Cato's in particular.[11] Only a few years earlier, Honoré d'Urfé, a moralist and novelist, had discriminated between cowardly suicides and heroic suicides in his *Epistres morales* (1598). Cowards, in his view, deserved nothing but scorn: "Since death is sweeter to you than the pain of wounds, go bury yourselves! And since servitude seems to you finer than combat, be slaves!" Heroic suicides, whose prime example was still Cato, showed proof of "courage and magnanimity." Honoré d'Urfé was the incarnation of the aristocratic moral code of the *honnête homme,* the successor to the perfect courtier, whose ruling word was honor. The human condition, d'Urfé stated, involves constraints, but it does not oblige us to bear everything. Men are not "obligated to endure all the indignities that fortune sends them or has in store for them." There are situations where one needs to know how to say no and depart rather than submit to a degrading, dehumanizing humiliation. D'Urfé put this moral stance into action in his long novel, *L'Astrée* (1607), in which several characters commit suicide for love with the blessing of the author.

Elizabethan and Jacobean England seemed quite receptive to such ideas. Debate on suicide had opened in the reign of Henry VIII in the context of Calvinist-Anglican rivalry and a royal campaign to enforce forfeiture of the estate of suicide victims. Although preachers vied with one another to show suicide as the devil's work, one of the effects of their campaign was to draw attention to it and to stimulate intellectual reflection on the subject. In the early seventeenth century translation of French works—Montaigne's *Essays* in 1603, Charron's *De la sagesse* in 1608—were added to the writings of classical antiquity on suicide. In 1607 Francis Bacon, the future chancellor, spoke of suicide (without condemnation) in an essay on death. Somewhat later, in

1623, he studied suicide with scientific neutrality in *The Historie of Life and Death,* where he investigated the impressions felt by a dying man who had hanged himself: "He said he felt no pain. But first he thought he saw before his eyes a great fire, and burning; then he thought he saw all black, and dark; lastly, it turnet to a pale blue, or sea-water green; which colour is also often seen by them which fall into swooning."[12]

John Donne's 'Biathanatos'

The point of arrival in this series of works on suicide, John Donne's *Biathanatos,* is an extraordinary book, especially when we consider that it was written around 1610 by an Anglican, chaplain to the king, who held a doctorate in divinity from Cambridge University and was a reader in divinity at Lincoln's Inn at the Inns of Court, London's great school of law. Donne was a humanist, a preacher, a theologian, a poet, and a man receptive to all the currents of thought of his age. Neither a marginal figure nor an eccentric, he was a responsible clergyman. That fact lends his treatise undeniable gravity.

Donne's somewhat embarrassed subtitle outlines his subject with a double negative: *A Declaration of that Paradoxe, or Thesis, that Selfe-homicide is not so naturally Sinne, that it may never be Otherwise.* In plain terms, in some cases suicide is justified. Donne's treatise was the first work wholly devoted to a rehabilitation of suicide. Donne was aware of his audacity and of his responsibility, and he came close to imitating Justus Lipsius and destroying his manuscript: "I have always gone so near suppressing it as that it is only not burnt," he wrote to Sir Robert Ker in 1619. He absolutely refused to have the work published, limiting himself to circulating copies among friends whom he could trust, and on the copy he left to his son he wrote, "Publish it not, do not print this, but yet burn it not." To Ker he wrote, "It is a book written by Jack Donne and not by Dr. Donne." The book had to wait until 1647, sixteen years after Donne's death, to be published.[13] David Hume showed a like prudence in the eighteenth century when it came to his own treatise on suicide.

Prudence is not quite the right word. Donne was well aware that he was infringing a taboo, and he was afraid of having to take responsibility for suicides that might result from reading his book. It was one thing to profess admiration for Brutus and Cato, figures from so remote a past as to be nearly mythic; it was quite another thing to demonstrate that suicide is an act that does not violate natural or divine law, and thus one that should not be penalized. Donne takes his precautions: He insists that he is not writing a defense of suicide and refuses to specify the precise conditions under which

suicide might be condoned. "I abstained purposely from extending this discourse to particular rules or instances, both because I dare not profess myself a
master in so curious a science, and because the limits are obscure and steepy
and slippery and narrow, and every error deadly, except where, a competent
diligence being foreused, a mistaking in our conscience may prove an excuse." Donne complains earlier in the same work, however, that no one
"brings the metal now to the touch," and he states that we must deliver
"ourselves from the tyranny of this prejudice" (193, 45).

One of the cultural preoccupations of the times and a difficult personal
situation converge in his thought. Donne felt himself a failure in his life, his
marriage, and his career. He became melancholic and contemplated death, a
theme that permeates his entire work. Despite the scholastic form Donne
gave it, *Biathanatos* is not a stylistic exercise. Would he have taken so much
trouble to write this treatise, then hide it, if it had been only an intellectual
game? His book was rooted in both his life and his epoch: In the same years a
young Catholic priest, Duvergier de Hauranne (later better known as Abbé
de Saint-Cyran) also considered cases in which suicide might be an acceptable
course, though with considerable less audacity than Donne.

One of Donne's most daring moves, and a point on which he broke with
all previous interpretations of the question, was to treat suicide within the
framework of Christian thought. Rather than choosing an indirect approach
and reasoning from the examples of Cato, Lucretius, or Seneca, he places
himself, from the outset, within Christian theology and uses only rational and
religious arguments. His attack is frontal: We think it obvious that suicide is
the worst of sins, but if we examine the arguments backing up that seemingly
obvious tenet, we find that suicide might possibly not be a grave sin and
perhaps not be a sin at all. In any event, we have no right to judge whether or
not an individual is damned because he has killed himself, and many actions
that we condemn today were authorized in the Bible.

In the three parts of *Biathanatos* Donne discusses whether suicide is contrary to the law of nature, to the law of reason, and to the law of God. If it is
contrary to nature's law, we would have to condemn all mortification, all
practices that aim at "taming" our nature. The nature that is unique to
humankind is reason, which distinguishes us from the animals. Therefore
reason should enlighten us about what is good or bad for us. It might at times
be more reasonable to kill oneself. Moreover, people have killed themselves in
all places and in all ages, which indicates that such an act is not so contrary to
natural inclination as has been said.

The law of reason is what guides human laws. Certain laws, those of Rome in particular, do not condemn suicide, and canon law itself has not always condemned it. Certain theologians (St. Thomas Aquinas, for one) declare that suicide harms the state and society because it removes a useful member, but could not the same be said of a general who becomes a monk or of an émigré? Excessive mortification can be a kind of suicide in disguise, and no law condemns it. Thus we can renounce life for a higher good.

When he comes to God's law, Donne has no difficulty showing that no passage in the Bible condemns suicide. There is, of course, the Mosaic commandment against killing, but if exceptions are made for capital punishment and for the millions of homicides committed in times of war, why not make an exception for suicides, which are fewer in number? Is not voluntary martyrdom suicide? Was not the death of Christ, on the model of the Good Shepherd, suicide par excellence? St. Augustine's argument that Samson must have received a special command from God is pure supposition.

Donne's reasoning has its weak points; his style is heavy and tiresome; and he overuses syllogism and analogy. Still, his arguments are undeniably forceful.

John Donne, Galileo's Contemporary

In his *Biathanatos* Donne attempted to show that the condemnation of suicide derives from principles falsely considered to be self-evident, and that "self-homicide" is far from being the absolute sin that medieval and early modern theology made of it. Like hellebore, it was medicine "wholesome in desperate diseases, but otherwise poison" (194). Once it was published long after Donne's death, *Biathanatos* met with little success, in part perhaps because its form put off readers, but even more because of its content. Few people were inclined to examine a book with such a sinister reputation: It scorched the hands even of those who shared its ideas but did not want to compromise themselves by citing it. A troublesome ally, *Biathanatos* was used only by a few libertines.

"To be or not to be?" was still the question, however. Any attempt to give too precise a response to it tended to break its spell, which resided in the melancholy and romantic vagueness that spun a mysterious fog over dizzying chasms that the mind sensed but could not clearly imagine. Donne took a step too far, daringly placing himself beyond what his times wanted to hear. His book nonetheless stands as striking testimony to an age that challenged traditional values and sought new guidelines. Like his exact contemporary, Pierre de Bérulle, Donne referred to the new astronomy of Copernicus, Giordano Bruno, and Galileo. The astronomical revolution left its mark on spirituality in the early seventeenth century; it helped to weaken traditional systems and to hasten the emergence of new certitudes in much the way that Einstein's theory of relativity turned culture and morality upside-down in the early twentieth century. During the same decade, from 1610 to 1620, Galileo (b. 1564) gave heliocentrism a scientific foundation; Pierre de Bérulle (b. 1575) elaborated a Christocentric spirituality founded in man's nothingness; Jakob Böhme (b. 1575) perfected a mysticism based on the "abyss" and on an opposition between being and nothingness—and Donne (b. 1572) asserted that human autonomy is sufficiently great to allow free choice between life and death. These events are more than pure coincidence; they indicate a cultural crisis that was to be resolved, temporarily at least, by the generation of Descartes, Pascal, and Hobbes.

Duvergier de Hauranne and the Justification of Certain Suicides

Reflection on suicide was one of the signs of the crisis. To give one illustration: In 1609 Henry IV put before his entourage the question of whether a subject may sacrifice his own life to save the king's. A young cleric from Béarn who was new to the court, Jean Duvergier de Hauranne, took on the task of responding to the king's question in a treatise, *La question royale,* in which he stated that under certain circumstances it is not only legitimate but a duty to give one's life.

The future Abbé de Saint-Cyran began by demonstrating that suicide in and of itself did not deserve condemnation. Like John Donne before him, his first move was to "remove the deformity, so to speak" that had been "insep- arably attached to the act" of suicide. Murder and suicide were evil actions only "if one considers them in themselves, unadorned and stripped of all relations that lend them luster and stamp them with moral rectitude."[14] In other words, suicide should be judged situationally, not absolutely. In certain circumstances, might suicide be legitimate? Since there were so many excep- tions to the prohibition of homicide, why should there be none for suicide? In particular, what if someone went to his death in aid of another who was essential to the state? Such a gesture might not be against nature or reason any more than the act of the soldier who blows up a tower he has the duty to defend. Sacrificing oneself for the king is even a social obligation.

Was Duvergier de Hauranne's treatise simply an occasional work produced by a young and imprudent mind skilled in the casuistics he had learned from his Jesuit teachers? This may be true in part; the author himself later withdrew all copies of the work from libraries. But we also need to take into account the author's troubled psychological makeup. Henri Bremond said of him: "In his case, I find it difficult not to recognize clear signs of morbid tendencies [and] a quite pronounced psychopathic heredity."[15] Bremond in fact believed that Saint-Cyran suffered from a "strikingly obvious mental unbalance." In a further sign of instability, in 1617 Saint-Cyran wrote a treatise to show that ecclesiastics have the right to bear arms. His depressive tendencies, his persecution complex, and his ambiguous attitudes bothered even his friends at Port-Royal. Saint-Cyran transferred (in modern terms, sublimated) his neurotic attraction to morbid topics to a spiritual yearning for personal annihilation and a hatred for life: "You would have to be sick in your soul and possessed by some evil passion to love this mortal life," he wrote. One must "annihilate" oneself in spirit by dying to the world: "For each of us, the aim of the law is to annihilate ourselves and make ourselves enter, through virtue, into the nothingness that pertains to us by nature and out of which we have been drawn by God's overwhelming power."[16] Here we have shifted from physical suicide to spiritual suicide, but the fascination for annihilation remains. Some aspects of French spirituality in the seventeenth century replaced suicide with a refusal to participate in the life of the world. That sort of spirituality arose directly out of the profound crisis of the Christian conscience of the years 1580–1620.

Robert Burton and the Arrival of Melancholy

Another manifestation of the same crisis was the movement to secularize, even normalize, suicide. Although both the Protestant and the Catholic clergy continued to see Satan lurking behind all suicides, urging them to despair, some intellectuals and some physicians began to analyze the psychological process that led to self-murder. They called it melancholia. Despair, they claimed, is a moral notion, a sin; melancholy is a psychological notion, an imbalance in the brain. When suicide became the object of medical study, it became secularized.

We need to guard against exaggerating that distinction, however. In his *Treatise of Melancholie* (1586) Timothy Bright presented suicide as the product of both divine vengeance and diabolical temptation. For a long time melancholia was viewed in moral terms, particularly because its physiological explanations were quite vague, at times whimsical. In 1607 Jean Fernel related the "melancholic humor" to the earth and to autumn, and he defined it as a liquid "thick in consistency, cold and dry in its temperament."[17] An excessive amount of that humor in the brain was responsible for the somber thoughts that afflict melancholiacs and lead them to fix their attention obsessively on an object: "All their senses are depraved by a melancholic humor spread through their brain," Johann Weyer wrote.[18] Some blamed black bile for leading melancholiacs to murder, but Weyer stated that some melancholiacs "fear death, which they yet cause most often to themselves." As early as 1583 the English physician Philip Barrough remarked that persons who suffered from melancholia "desire death, and do verie often behight and determine to kill them selves," while in 1580 Pierre de La Primaudaye wrote in his *Académie française* that black bile drives some people to hate themselves, fall into despair, and kill themselves.[19] In 1609 Felix Plater put melancholy on his list of "functional lesions."[20]

Melancholia, which caused suicide, was indeed a disease.[21] But where did it come from? That was the question that Robert Burton examined in 1621 in his famous treatise, *The Anatomy of Melancholy*. That disease, Burton says, particularly affects studious people, whose meditations can easily turn to morbid rumination. He himself was inclined to it, which is why, he confides, "I write of Melancholy, by being busie to avoid melancholy."[22]

Burton's description of the disease long remained the standard one: Melancholia is both physiological and analogical, thanks to universal correspondences; it involves an excess of black bile, a substance associated with the earth, the most somber of the elements, and Saturn, the most somber of the planets. An inclination to it is innate, hence certain people are predestined to have a somber temperament, but the tendency can be either corrected or aggravated by social environment and the person's own actions. Thus what today is called psychosomatic therapy can attenuate the effects of melancholia or even turn it into a positive quality that confers an exceptional profundity of mind, as was the case with some great men and religious prophets.

Marsilio Ficino's Neoplatonic writings had already suggested music, fresh air and sunshine, fine perfumes, and savory food and wine as cures for melancholy. Burton adds to the list certain herbs recommended by the ancient Greeks and Romans and, above all, psychological treatment to help melancholiacs regain their equilibrium by diversifying their activities, reading fewer books, and developing broader interests. There is no universal remedy; rather, every melancholic must adopt an appropriate personal lifestyle. The solitary person should seek out company and confide in family and friends; the worldly person should seek solitude now and then. It is advisable to frequent beautiful women, the sight of whom makes the heart rejoice, and to have a normal sexual life (sexual frustration is a source of melancholy), but to avoid debauchery. The melancholic should take up mathematics and other sciences that absorb the mind, such as chronology. In short, one should lead a balanced life. Burton also indirectly suggests a socioeconomic cause for melancholia when he states that poverty is a major cause of psychic troubles. His thought is extraordinarily modern in all this, and it is quite unlike the supernatural explanations of the clergy of his times. Burton is indignant at the thought of treating melancholia by exorcism or astrology.

If melancholia is a malady that responds to therapy, however, it can also worsen under certain circumstances, and when that happens, somber thoughts focus on a search for death. Melancholiacs have "a cankered soul macerated with cares and discontents, [and] *taedium vitae,* impatience, agony, inconstancy, irresolution precipitate them unto unspeakable miseries. They cannot endure company, light, or life it selfe. . . . They make away themselves, which is a frequent thing, and familiar amongst them" (1:406). The physiognomy of the sick person "changes suddenly, his heart grows heavy, overwhelming thoughts crucify his soul, and in an instant he is defeated or tired of living; he wants to kill himself." Various things can lead him to this point—poverty, sickness, the death of a loved one, loss of liberty, education, calumny—but amorous jealousy and religious terror are particular dangers. The jealous person is inclined to kill the object of his jealousy and kill himself afterward; the religious melancholic kills himself because he is persuaded he cannot be saved.

Burton blames both Catholics and Protestants for religious despair, the Catholics because of their superstitious and idolatrous beliefs, which aid the devil's work, and the Protestants because they sow terror by preaching apoc-alyptical sermons. As a good Anglican, Burton values equilibrium and mod-eration, believing that "too much of anything is harmful" is a rule that pertains in religion as elsewhere. Atheism is obviously to be avoided, for there the devil reigns supreme. Religious excess is hardly better. Asceticism un-hinges the mind; the free examination of Scripture can lead to despair. Cal-vinist predestination encourages despair by persuading people that they are damned no matter what they do. Unhappy people whose minds are fragile see themselves already in hell: "Some . . . dare not bee alone in the darke, for fear of hobgoblins and divells: hee suspects every thing he heares or sees to be a Divell, or enchanted, and imagineth a thousand Chimeras and visions, which to his thinking he certainly sees, like bugbears, talks with black men, Ghosts, goblins &c" (1:386). Terrified by such visions, some melancholiacs commit suicide.

Burton turns next to the act itself. We feel he is of two minds. How can he condemn the unhappy people who kill themselves, once he has shown they are not responsible for an act that is the result of a mental illness, aggravated by external circumstances and an unfavorable social context? He begins in the traditional manner, recapitulating opinions favorable to suicide and listing authorities ranging from the ancient authors, for whom suicide was an act of liberty and courage, to such contemporaries as Thomas More. He tendentiously places St. Augustine among those who excuse voluntary self-homicide. He then recalls famous cases of suicide in classical antiquity and concludes, though with little conviction, "But these are false and Pagan positions, prophane Stoicall Paradoxes, wicked examples." The retraction is totally pro forma. In reality, Burton is pleading for indulgence and pity. No one knows whether suicides go to hell; that is for God to decide. For our part, we would do better to pity them:

Those hard censures of such as offer violence to their own persons, or in some desperate fit to others, which sometimes they doe . . . are to be mitigated, as in such as are mad, beside themselves for the time, or founde to have beene long melancholy, and that in extremity, they knowe not what they doe, deprived of reason, judgement, all, as a ship that is void of a Pilot, must needs impinge upon the next rocke or sands, and suffer shipwrack. (1:438)

Suicidal tendencies, which result from melancholy, are thus an illness and not a satanic sin: Burton's work marks a turning point in how self-homicide was imagined. His secularized interpretation was obviously not to the taste of the churches of the time, which were intent on reinforcing the moral condemnation of suicide. From then until the nineteenth century, there were two antagonistic conceptions of suicide. In 1620 the religious conception was clearly predominant. Burton himself had not totally renounced the notion of diabolical intervention: Among the remedies for melancholia that he suggests are plants, such as peonies, angelica, and above all St. John's wort, also known as *fuga daemonum,* reputed to chase away the devil, as well as betony, which was used in cemeteries even in classical antiquity to ward off evil apparitions.

Still, the explanation of suicide by melancholy was a first step in the direction of removing suicide from the realms of religion and criminality, and it provided a precedent for later partisans of tolerance. In the seventeenth and eighteenth centuries an entire medical and philosophical current attributed suicidal tendencies to physiological disorders resulting from melancholia. That current included such figures and works as Hippolyte-Jules de La Mesnardière, *Le traité de la mélancolie* (1635); Johannes Jonstonus, *Idea universae medicinae practica* (1644); Murillo, *Novissima hypocondriacae melancholiae curatio* (1672); Thomas Willis, *De anima brutorum* (1672); Richard Blackmore, *A*

Treatise of the Spleen and Vapours (1726); François Bossier de Sauvages, *La nosologie méthodique* (1763); Carolus Linnaeus, *Genera morborum* (1763); Anne-Charles Lorry, *De melancholia et morbis melancholicis* (1765); Faucette, *Über Melancholie* (1785); Charles-Louis François d'Andry, *Recherches sur la mélancolie* (1785); and Weickhard, *Der philosophische Arzt* (1790). For all these writers, as for the author of an entry in the *Encyclopédie,* melancholia was a "particular delirium, returning determinedly to one or two objects, without fever or furor, in which it differs from mania and frenzy. This delirium is usually accompanied by an insurmountable sadness, a somber humor, misanthropy, and a decided penchant for solitude."[23]

If we can believe some of the physicians of the time, on occasion an early form of psychotherapy succeeded in curing religious melancholiacs of their suicidal tendencies. In his *Praxis medica* of 1637 Zacatus Lusitanus described a cure by dramatic representation: A man thought himself damned because of his sins, and no amount of reasoning with him could console him. The physician then entered into his delirium, appearing to him as an "angel" dressed in white and bearing a sword, exhorting him to take courage and declaring that his sins were pardoned.[24]

The Debate on Suicide in Novels and Romances

"To be or not to be?" was a question that invaded literature between 1580 and 1620, as well as philosophical thought and medical and psychological investigation. Characters in novels, poems, and plays, where fiction permitted avoidance of official condemnation, committed suicide with increasing frequency. The deluge of voluntary deaths in works of the imagination teaches us two things: that the theme was popular, and that the authors displayed no reprobation of the act. No reproving moral lesson emerges from these works. The good and the wicked alike commit suicide, and whether their death is an admirable or a cowardly act depends on its motivation and the circumstances.

Suicide is a prime ingredient in the highly precious fiction that flourished throughout Europe under a variety of labels—gongorism in Spain, marinism in Italy, euphuism in England. In the refined intrigues of the *pays du tendre,* it was good form to throw oneself into the nearest body of water, as did Céladon in Honoré d'Urfé's *L'Astrée,* the minute amorous complications arose. Suicide was an elegant and convenient way out; it was a device that authors used, to the accompaniment of heavy sighs, with little consideration for traditional morality or even simple logic. In *Les comptes du monde aventureux,* heroines kill themselves after declaring that suicide is the road to hell. The hero of Ollenix du Mont-Sacré's *Amours de Cléandre et Domiphille* (1597) calls suicide an "execrable crime," but when he makes up his mind to kill himself, he calls it his "glory." Antoine de Nervèze has Marizée, the heroine of his *Amours diverses* (1617), repent of having killed herself, but we note that the lady is in heaven. Albert Bayet declares, after passing in review all the major French novels of the period, "I do not know of a single case in which suicide renders a character odious. Quite to the contrary, those who kill themselves to save their honor, out of remorse, or for love are invariably likable."[25] We will take his word for it, especially as he furnishes a long list of literary suicides caused by unrequited love, remorse, or a desire to defend chastity or honor.

Rather than following the meanders of interminable novels such as these, we would do better to focus on passages in which the protagonists discuss the problem of suicide.[26] One character in Jacques Yver's *Printemps* (1572) airs pagan ideas on suicide, approving it when committed "for some praiseworthy cause," such as preserving chastity, being curious about the next world, rendering service to society, or having grown weary of life. The list leaves few blameworthy motives. Bénigne Poissenot acknowledged two standards of morality in his *Nouvelles histoires tragiques* (1586), one for pagans, for whom suicide might be glorious, the other for Christians, for whom it is prohibited. The novels of Ollenix du Mont-Sacré teem with debates of the sort. In *Les Bergeries de Juliette* (1585), for example, Arcas eloquently argues the case for the grandeur of a suicide that offers an opportunity to end mortal woes. Nature has "put into our hands the proper and salutary remedy for those miseries, which is a fine exit from this world." Since the doors of that exit are at hand, it is dishonorable to beg others for material or moral help: "There is a proper and particular remedy, which is death." Let it not be said, Arcas continues, that killing oneself harms our country or our family, for someone desperate enough to commit suicide is of little use on this earth, where he can "do no good." Furthermore, those who kill themselves are "praised and esteemed by everyone," and the famous suicides of classical antiquity showed by their deaths that they rose above "not only nature, but all the powers of heaven." Arcas's interlocutor, Phillis, "had no idea what to say." She can do no better than offer two weak arguments: We should not destroy the work of the Creator; some people must be left to praise God. Arcas, unpersuaded, makes up his mind to kill himself. In the same novel Juliette praises Bransil, who starved himself to death, even though he had previously called suicide disobedience to God.

In his *Œuvre de la chasteté* (1595) Ollenix presents the problem of suicide through a character stricken with love's despair. His hero wonders whether a man whom suffering renders so much an enemy to himself that he expects no death crueller than life should not try to leave this world, so that in dying he stifles the murmur against God that will not pass his lips and the despair that tempts him to self-homicide. We must take the lesser of two evils, and such a one, it seems to me, would do better to die than to live and cause his soul to die in sin.[27]

Fiction gave authors an opportunity to raise questions freely, and the simple fact of raising them challenged traditional morality, as is evident in *The Unfortunate Traveller, or, The Life of Jacke Wilton* by Thomas Nashe (1594). In this work Heraclide, who is placed in circumstances that recall the death of Lucretia, first discusses the grandeur of suicide and its Christian prohibition (at some length), then stabs herself. A character in *La Marianne du Philomène* (1596) works up the courage to kill herself by praising the "bravery," "constancy," and "magnanimity" of Porcia, Cleopatra, and Sophonisba. The same sort of exhortation appears in *Les amours de Cléandre et Domiphille*. Honoré d'Urfé's *L'Astrée* (first part, 1607) is full of examples of suicide for love, which was by then an automatic response to unrequited passion, to the threat of being forced not to keep faith with a beloved, or simply to the decision that beyond a certain level of indignity life becomes unbearable. In *Le lict d'honneur de Chariclée* (1609) Jean d'Intras reintroduces debate on the acceptability of suicide when Mélisse, the hero, is spurned by Chariclée. He examines the question and concludes that the four reasons that oppose self-inflicted death— divine law, the law of nature, love of oneself, and posterity's opinion—will not hold up against the demand for liberty that is man's grandeur. When, at the end of the book, the heroine also decides to kill herself, the author praises her death, "which, according to the world, I must not praise too highly." In Gilbert Saulnier Du Verdier's *Temple des sacrifices* (1620), the hero comments on the suicide of a lover: "As for me, I cannot condemn these actions when they give proof of a true love. To the contrary, I greatly praise a decision that can only be found in fine souls, since they alone are capable of loving well."[28]

The allegorical poetry that the age showed great fondness for also contains debates on suicide. In Edmund Spenser's *Faerie Queene,* the Redcrosse Knight, who represents holiness, attacks Despair, in particular the religious despair that leads to suicide. The knight, defeated in combat, escapes death only thanks to the intervention of Una (or Truth), and Despair, frustrated, hangs himself. Traditional morality is saved, but as is often the case, it does not come out unscathed. Like Burton, Spenser, a pessimist and himself tempted by death, sought to exorcise his own melancholy by writing of his fears.

Medieval romances and poetry had also presented suicides, without commentary, as heroic acts in the context of chivalric morality. What was new in this later period was that the novelists writing between 1580 and 1620 presented scholastic debates for and against their characters' suicides. This may not be enough to constitute a genuine trend, but it is safe to conclude that both authors and readers now found the question of interest. Suicide was clearly included among the cases of conscience debated at the time, and if the legitimacy of suicide was discussed, it means that despite the massive condemnation of political and religious authorities, doubt had crept into people's minds.

Suicide in Drama

Hamlet's question echoed from stages throughout Europe as tragedy became an increasingly successful genre. In all languages, in all forms, before all sorts of audiences, the great question, "To be or not to be?" rang out.[29] Suicide packed the house in France around 1600; its merits were declaimed everywhere:

> Quand il est interdit de vivre librement
> C'est faire un très beau coup de mourir bravement

(When it is prohibited to live freely, it is a fine gesture to die bravely.)[30]

> Vous vainquez tout d'un coup en ce dernier effort
> Deux pestes qui sur vous emportent la victoire:
> L'envie au cœur malin et la cruelle mort

(You vanquish with one blow in that last effort two plagues that carry off the victory against you: the envy of the wicked heart and cruel death.)[31]

> Craindras-tu de t'ouvrir d'une dague le flanc?

(Do you fear to open your side with a dagger?)[32]

> Il faut, il faut mourir, il faut qu'une mort belle
> Une mort généreuse à mon secours j'appelle

(I must, I must die, a fine death, a generous death, to my aid I call.)[33]

> Ceux-là tant seulement sont chétifs ici-bas
> De qui le cœur poltron redoute le trépas,
> Qui, craignant de mourir et lâches de courage,
> N'osent en se tuant racheter leur servage

(Only those whose cowardly heart dreads death are wretched here below, who, fearing to die and lacking courage, dare not redeem their servitude by killing themselves.)[34]

O que beaucoup auront sur vous envie
Qui finissez vaillamment votre vie,
Qui par vos morts acquerrez un renom
Lequel doit rendre immortel votre nom

(Oh! Many will envy you who end your life valiantly, who by your deaths will acquire a renown that will make your name immortal.)[35]

Suicide was a nearly obligatory ingredient of tragedy in England in the years 1580–1620 (on which, see Bernard Paulin's fine study, *Du couteau à la plume*). It was rampant in works that ranged from Shakespeare's *Romeo and Juliet* to plays on subjects borrowed from classical antiquity: Some tragedies present as many as five self-inflicted deaths. There was even an inflationary tendency in stage suicides, from 43 in the period 1580–1600 to 128 in the period 1600–1625, not counting the 52 suicides in Shakespeare. Motivations show a slight shift. Although love persists as the principal reason for doing away with oneself, honor gradually declines in favor of remorse; despair, so popular during the Middle Ages, sinks to fourth place, while financial ruin—a new socioeconomic reason linked to the rise of capitalism—advances. The sociological explanation that had appeared in Robert Burton timidly begins to rival the psychological explanation, and supernatural explanations recede, lingering only in the last morality dramas with a medieval tone, such as Nathaniel Woodes's *Conflict of Conscience* (1581). In one version of that work the devil urges on Francis Spira (Francesco Spiera, an Italian Protestant), who hangs himself out of remorse for his abjuration.

Playwrights do not pronounce judgment on suicide, but they do present it in a favorable light as an admirable act. There is no reference to traditional morality in these works; they are ruled by aesthetic criteria and speak only of circumstances and motivations. Their overwhelming preference for suicide with bare steel is a sign of nobility. Hangings, drownings, and poison are rare.

In the hundred or so plays studied by Bernard Paulin, tragedies in imitation of Seneca are marked by macabre ritual and a fondness for atrocity, as in Robert Wilmot's *Tragedie of Tancred and Gismund* (1591). Other tragedies (by Mary Sidney, Samuel Daniel, and Thomas Kyd), based on the works of Robert Garnier, offer opportunities to debate suicide; Marlowe is more interested in the viewpoint of the instigator. The thirty-nine suicides in the tragedies on classical subjects of Samuel Daniel, Ben Jonson, John Marston, Thomas Heywood, Francis Beaumont, and John Fletcher are dictated above all by honor and political vicissitudes. There is even one example of a gratuitous suicide, committed for no real reason and out of pure indifference, in William Rowley's *All's Lost by Lust,* where a young woman named Dionisia declares before dying, "I must dye one day, and as good this day as another" (act 5, scene 5).

In Thomas Dekker's Christian tragedies, suicide is reserved for the wicked, as it is in the works of Philip Massinger, who was firmly opposed to voluntary death. On the whole, though, the Jacobean age presented a more confused and gloomier perspective than the age of Elizabeth. Bernard Paulin states, "One wonders more and more whether the playwrights were inviting approval or blame for those who kill themselves: The Jacobeans indisputably display their moral confusion here."[36] Suicide had become more diversified in its motivation, its modes of execution, and its purpose. Suicide as blackmail appears, as do feigned suicide, suicide as a means of vengeance, and suicide as trickery. When suicide is integrated into the interplay of social relations as a way to put pressure on others, it becomes neutralized and gradually loses its urgency in moral debate.

Shakespeare and Suicide: From Question to Ridicule

In the fifty-two cases of suicide in his plays, written between 1589 and 1613, William Shakespeare investigates all facets, circumstances, and motives for the act. His immense oeuvre might even be seen as one long variation on the theme of being and nonbeing, a dilemma he crystallized when he gained full command of his artistic powers.

Shakespeare was not a moralist but rather an observer of the human condition. He offers no formal defense of suicide, and one of his most incisive observations is, precisely, that speech often opposes action. Hamlet, the Shakespearean character who talks the most about committing suicide, does not do so. Those who do kill themselves do so rapidly, with a minimum of talk. Lucrece (the Roman Lucretia) is an exception. In her long monologue she comes to the realization that weighing the reasons for killing herself threatens to keep her from acting: "This helpless smoke of words doth me no right" (*The Rape of Lucrece,* line 1027). Too much talk about suicide weakens resolve: The idea hints at a therapy by demystification of the real and essentially egotistical reasons for suicide.

Shakespeare goes much further than his contemporaries, moving the question of suicide into a timeless dimension. The only lesson he preaches is a modest one that demystifies all knowledge and denounces all certitudes. What do all the works of human wisdom contain? "Words, words, words," Hamlet says (*Hamlet,* act 2, scene 2). Those who claim to possess the truth and impose it on others are odious. And what could be more impenetrable than suicide? As Henry de Montherlant said, "We have to make a pretense of the immense joke that is History when it meddles in other things than an exposé of the facts (as if that were not enough!) and, for instance, motivates suicides." If Shakespeare speaks a good deal about suicide, it is to investigate its mystery.

The diversity of Shakespeare's suicides supports all possible viewpoints, but it also reduces their ability to shock. The glorious suicides of classical antiquity (Brutus, Cassius, Antony and Cleopatra) parade before our eyes, but so do unhappy lovers (Romeo and Juliet), somber suicides going to meet their fate (Macbeth), and piteous suicides stricken with remorse (Othello). All are the playthings of circumstance, urged on to death by merciless external mechanisms. The melancholy Hamlet, who talks to the skulls in the cemetery and deliberates the pro and con of suicide, does not act and is not killed by his own hand. Ophelia kills herself without saying a word to anyone, leaving the spectator with no explanation. In reality, like Romeo and Juliet, she kills herself out of a tragic misunderstanding, and in the final analysis all suicides, even the grandest who die for honor, do the same.

Honor? "What is honour? A word. What is in that word honour? What is that honour? Air; a trim reckoning! Who hath it? He that died o' Wednesday. Doth he feel it? No. Doth he hear it? No. 'Tis insensible, then? Yea, to the dead. But will it not live with the living? No. Why? Detraction will not suffer it. Therefore I'll none of it. Honour is a mere scutcheon: and so ends my catechism" (*Henry the Fourth, Part One,* act 5, scene 1). This is Falstaff speaking—a vulgarian, a coward, and a comic foil for Prince Hal. But aren't this odious buffoon's actions similar to Hamlet's? Each in his own way, the prince of Denmark and the brigand refuse suicide, the first out of fear of what lies beyond death, the second out of fondness for the pleasures of this world. "Why, thou owest God a death," Prince Hal tells Falstaff, who answers, " 'Tis not due yet; I would be loath to pay him before his day" (ibid.). Hamlet asks himself if there is sufficient reason for remaining alive; Falstaff asks whether all reasons for dying are not vain. Should one die for words, for ideas, for honor, for "smoke"? Knowledge of the future would be the only sufficient reason for suicide. If one could read the book of fate, King Henry IV states,

> The happiest youth, viewing his progress through,
> What perils past, what crosses to ensue,
> Would shut the book, and sit him down and die
> (*Henry the Fourth, Part Two,* act 3, scene 1)

In Shakespeare, even the most famous, most glorified suicides of antiquity—Brutus and Cassius in *Julius Caesar*—are prone to illusion and blindness.

As for Romeo and Juliet, they are manipulated by a fatality that excludes all individual judgment. Bernard Paulin writes, "Instead of demonstrating, Shakespeare shows. He gives meaning to suicide through his entire dramatic and poetic production. That is why Shakespeare never offers a defense of suicide, but only of love, or, more accurately, of love as Romeo and Juliet experience it. In that existential viewpoint, suicide does not just end life, it prolongs it."[37]

Critics have long noted the symbolic importance of one suicide that stands out from the rest in Shakespeare's works, that of Gloucester in *King Lear*. Everything is false in the episode: Gloucester is a disillusioned old man, doubtless once an extremely sensual person much attached to the world, but now disappointed with it and disgusted by the universality of evil. Tired of living, he wants to kill himself. But does he really? He chooses the most passive form of suicide, throwing himself off the Dover cliffs, but since he is blind, he needs a guide to lead him there. His guide is his son Edgar pretending to be a fool. A blind man led by a fool: This is how humanity, lamentable and tragic, advances. " 'Tis the time's plague, when madmen lead the blind," Gloucester states (*King Lear*, act 4, scene 2). The very act of suicide is grotesque. Edgar places Gloucester on a minuscule rise, from which he jumps, doing himself no harm, but Edgar persuades him that he has been led by the devil and has miraculously escaped death after a dizzying fall. Gloucester, cured of his desire to kill himself, declares:

> . . . Henceforth I'll bear
> Affliction till it do cry out itself
> "Enough, enough," and die.
> (*King Lear*, act 4, scene 6)

Everything is ridiculous in this episode, and critics have given very different interpretations of it. For Wilson Knight it offers a moral lesson: Humankind must take care not to fall into despair, not to let Satan be its guide, but rather await the hour that God has fixed for death.[38] For Jan Kott the scene presents a very modern nihilism, the notion of which is reinforced by a completely bare stage: Everything is empty, even heaven; everything is illusion, even life and death.[39] We should not discard any interpretation without examining it, but if we compare Gloucester's failed suicide with Hamlet's nonsuicide, the suicides by misunderstanding of Romeo and Juliet, the suicide by misinterpretation of Othello, and the suicides due to failure on the part of the great political figures of antiquity, we see that Shakespeare's real question is, Has suicide any meaning? Gloucester, blind, unaware, and led by a fool toward a failed suicide, decides to live: His tragedy has no meaning. Might not the best response to Hamlet's question, "To be or not to be?" perhaps be "The question makes no sense"?

Literary Suicide: A Symbolic Liberation for a Troubled Society

The heights of Shakespeare's art take us far from ordinary morality. It certainly means something that around 1600 the problem of suicide was presented on stages everywhere and that the public flocked to see and applaud such plays. The pervasiveness of debate on suicide, a topic of conversation even in the courts of kings and the leading salons, reveals a crisis of conscience in the realm of culture. The shift from scholasticism to analytical reason, from a closed world to an infinite universe, from humanism to modern science, from a world described in terms of qualities to a mathematical language, from innate truth to methodical doubt, from certitude to critical questioning, and from Christian unity to a division between rival confessions could not be made without weakening the entire value system. Fractures typical of times of crisis occurred in the years from 1580 to 1620, a time of transition when the modern mind was forming. One part of the elite rushed enthusiastically and noisily toward the new world; another part (which included those in positions of political and religious responsibility) fell back on traditional values and set them up as indefeasible absolutes. The majority, hesitant and anxious, watched the fray and prepared to join the stronger party. At each of these crises, moral relativism at first gained ground, in particular by the technique of questioning norms. This created an even greater gap between the questioners' language and that of the censors, the authorities, and all who took responsibility for public morals, who in turn tended to move to even harsher positions.

The authorities reasoned and legislated in universal terms, according to general principles, whereas literature showed concrete, individual cases of people in situations of conflicting values. Moral conflict was the stuff of dramatic intensity. The tragedies of Pierre Corneille, an art characteristic of an age of transition and crisis, came soon after. Periods of stability produce encounters between good and evil (both unanimously recognized for what they are) in which the good necessarily triumph over the wicked, as they do from medieval mystery plays to the classic westerns of the golden age of American film. Periods of order and civilizations that are sure of themselves produce Manichaean dramas. During periods of doubt, on the other hand, the good are divided among themselves: Everything comes in shades of gray rather than in black and white, and the good are pitted against one another.

One set of values rivals another, which plays into the hands of the wicked. There is no way out in these new confrontations; everyone loses, and death is often the only solution for heroes and ordinary mortals alike—or for heroes *more* than for others. The mediocre and the second-rate generally find a way to compromise and remain alive. The great soul, the soul that has the stuff of a hero and whose struggles with conflicting values we admire, has no alternative to self-induced death precisely because it rejects half-measures and accommodations. Shakespeare's tragedies and Corneille's—works that differ greatly in form but are profoundly alike on a deeper level—are mechanisms of death in which we feel from the start that a fatal outcome is inevitable. The prominence of plays containing suicides is a sign of an age marked by conflicting values.

Authors sublimate the conflicts of their times. Spectators go to the theater to give full vent to their frustrations. Theater-goers of that age—who were disoriented, torn between rival opinions made even more diverse by printed matter that circulated widely in spite of all the censors could do, and obliged to submit to repressive authorities who imposed their own code of values— found in the suicides of tragic drama a way to deny their own existential conflicts. In a stable society spectators find in the theater the triumph of the good over the wicked and a comfortable confirmation of their own values; in an unstable society they find conflicting values and the voluntary death of a tormented hero. That is, they find reassurance when their own doubts are confirmed, and they derive a symbolic liberation from the hero's suicide. The theater-goer, fearing what lies beyond death, does not dare commit that act himself, but he participates in it in spirit and in the company of an extraordinary figure whose conduct he admires and who cannot be deemed totally wrong.

When suicide reaches the frequency and the proportions that it did in literature and drama between 1580 and 1620, it probably plays a therapeutic social role by helping a troubled generation get through difficult times and by limiting the number of real suicides. As we shall see, casuistry, which prospers in times of conflicting values, and a spirituality of annihilation, which is in many respects the contrary of casuistry, had a similar function.

Interest in the Practice of Suicide

Remarkably enough, this first European crisis of conscience was not accompanied by any real rise in the actual number of suicides. Again, reliable figures are lacking, but data that at least indicate tendencies show no cause for alarm. In England the number of cases brought before the King's Bench remained largely stable: Records show that 923 suicides were registered in the decade 1580–89, 801 in 1590–99, 894 in 1600–1609, and 976 in 1610–19.[40]

Obviously, these figures do not come even close to reflecting the total number of actual suicides. Lost or lacking documents, the negligence of coroners and coroners' juries, and inconsistencies in their criteria produced a decided undervaluation of suicide rates, thus permitting historians to arrive at contradictory interpretations. In 1970 P.E.H. Hair estimated the suicide rate of the age at between 3.4 and 4 per 100,000 in sixteenth-century Essex, which in his opinion reflected a sharp upswing from the Middle Ages.[41] Samuel Ernest Sprott went a step further. In a work published in 1961 he analyzed the London bills of mortality (periodic reports on deaths and their causes that were begun during the plague years and that continued to be put out subsequently at regular intervals). He concluded that Puritanism could be held responsible for a sharp rise in the number of suicides.[42] In 1986 Michael Zell estimated the suicide rate in Kent in the late sixteenth century at about 10 per 100,000.[43] Other scholars have suggested much lower rates, on the order of 4–6 per 100,000.[44]

More recent works are more prudent, as scholars have limited themselves to studying changes in the suicide rate on the basis of more fragmentary but reliable sources. Michael MacDonald and Terence R. Murphy present tables based on the suicide cases reported to the King's Bench between 1540 and 1640. Their data show some points of comparison between the suicide rate and years of poor harvests and low salaries—1574, 1587, 1597–1600, and 1640—but they draw no strict correspondence between suicides and harvests, prices, or salary levels. The worst years in those respects (around 1595 and beginning with 1620) show no rise in the suicide rate. From 1580 to 1620 the rate tends to stabilize (in the ten-year averages) at around 2.1 per 100,000— somewhat lower than during the years from 1555 to 1580, when it averages about 2.8.[45]

Thus it seems that the English did not kill themselves more frequently than they had before. What is new is an interest in suicide, which contemporaries remarked on and analyzed much more than they had previously. One London turner, Nehemiah Wallington, carefully noted cases of suicide in his journals. He even kept a special "Memorial of those that laid violent hands on themselves."[46] Wallington was himself obsessed with suicide. He tried to kill himself eleven times, and as a good Puritan, he attributed his attempts to the devil's work: "Then Satan temted me againe and I resisted him again. Then he temted me a third time, and I yielded unto him and I pulled out my knife and put it neere my throte. Then God of his goodness caused me to consider what would follow if I should do so. . . . With that I felle out a weaping and I flong away my knife."[47]

John Dee noted several similar cases in his diary,[48] and the physician and astrologer Richard Napier reported 139 cases of attempted suicide between 1597 and 1643, carefully noting the circumstances on each occasion. The victims mentioned range from the humblest peasant to John Harington, the godson of Queen Elizabeth. Most of them attributed their act to the devil's influence. Some blamed witches, as did a certain Agnes Buttres, whom Richard Napier treated in 1618 and who claimed that a spell cast on her had led her to attempt to drown herself.[49]

The real reasons for the attempted suicides, as Napier describes them, are both varied and familiar. Far from reflecting grandiose metaphysical questions, the most common causes are the day-to-day reasons for despair among the common people.[50] People killed themselves as the result of an unhappy marriage: There were wives who were mistreated or scorned by their husbands, such as Katherine Wells, whose husband had run through her dowry and had brought discredit and shame to the family, and who was tempted to kill herself every time she saw a knife. There were spouses plunged into despair by the death of their consort, such as Marguerite Langton, who resisted the temptation to kill herself for more than five years. There were mothers who grieved for a lost child, as did Marguerite Whippan. Some killed themselves for unrequited love, as did Thomas May, Dorothy Geary, Richard Malins, and Elizabeth Church; others did away with themselves in a fit of amorous melancholy, as did Elizabeth Lawrence and Robert Norman. Still others killed themselves because of a painful illness, a sudden bankruptcy, or a fit of despondency over their poverty.

For Calvinist pastors, a suicide attempt might also be part of a conversion experience when a convert felt strong remorse for past sins. It might also occur if converts felt that the holy life that lay ahead was too arduous, and fell into despair. Nehemiah Wallington and George Trosse, a Presbyterian minister, were of this type.[51] In the 1670s John Bunyan gave literary consecration to the perils of Christian perfection in his *Pilgrim's Progress*. Both Anglicans and Catholics continued to exploit Puritan suicides as proof that Puritanism was a desperate cause. In 1600 the spectacular suicide of William Doddington engendered lively debates: Doddington, a wealthy and widely known Calvinist merchant and a friend of leading government figures, threw himself from the steeple of St. Sepulchre's in London.[52]

Debate gave contemporaries the impression that the number of suicides

had increased. Richard Greenham (d. 1594) expressed alarm at their frequency, and George Abbot wrote (around 1600) that he heard of suicides
"almost daily." In 1637 William Gouge wrote, "I suppose, that scarce an age
since the beginning of the world hath afforded more examples of this desperate inhumanity, than this our present age, and that in all sorts of people,
Clergie, Laity, Learned, unlearned, Noble, meane, Rich, poore, Free, bond,
Male, Female, young and old."[53]

In 1605, after he had survived one of several assassination attempts, King
Henry IV of France remarked that madness seemed to be seizing more and
more people, and he confirmed this statement by citing the case of a seemingly prosperous man who had thrown himself into the Seine the previous
Sunday.[54] Suicide was talked about at court, but nothing allows us to state that
the number of actual cases rose. The most famous suicides of the epoch were
prisoners who killed themselves to avoid torture or to safeguard their honor.
Pierre de L'Estoile's *Journal* notes several of these. In 1595 Nicolas Rémy, a
judge in Nancy, boasted of having pushed sixteen "witches" who feared his
terrible justice into killing themselves.[55]

In England the earl of Northumberland (in 1585) was not the only prominent person who tried to kill himself when he was a prisoner in the Tower of
London. Another celebrity prisoner, Sir Walter Raleigh, voyager and poet,
attempted to stab himself in the Tower in 1603. He explained his motives in a
letter to his wife:

I am nowe made an enemie and traytour by the word of an unworthie man. . . . Oh
intollerable infamie, Oh god I cannot resiste theis thoughts, I cannot live to thincke
howe I am deryded. . . . O death hasten the unto me, that thowe maiste destroye the
memorie of theis, and laye me up in darke forgetfullnes. O death destroye my memorie which is my Tormentour; my thoughts and my life cannot dwell in one body. . . .
Be not dismaide that I dyed in dispaire of gods mercies, strive not to dispute it but
assure thy selfe that god hath not lefte me nor Sathan tempted me. Hope and dispaire
live not together, I knowe it is forbidden to destroye our selves but I trust it is
forbidden in this sorte, that we destroye not ourselves dispairinge of gods mercie.[56]

This letter, written three years after Shakespeare's *Hamlet,* is a man of
action's response to the question "To be or not to be?" Under certain circumstances, it is legitimate to kill oneself if the deed is done in full awareness and
to avoid infamy in this world, and if one one has confidence in divine mercy.
This was a response to the question that had not the slightest chance of being
accepted by the theologians, but it illustrates how profoundly people's minds
had changed. Discussion of voluntary death helped familiarize the elite with

that viewpoint, and although it did not take away all the guilt of suicide, it at least made opinion view it in more relative terms.

The sentiments of the mass of the faithful had not changed. For them, suicide still had a sinister, diabolic reputation, even if they were opposed both to confiscation of a suicide's estate and to corporal punishment of the corpse, and even if juries tried to get around these penalties by claiming insanity for the victim. The crisis of the years 1580–1620 did more to change opinion among the dominant classes, who were more open to the written word—that is, among the intellectual elite, the aristocracy, and the bourgeoisie.

The religious and civil authorities, who took responsibility for the organization of society, were hostile to any legitimation of suicide. They cited two reasons for their opposition. First, suicide threatened the entire structure of society by eliminating some of its members and by spreading doubt, anxiety, and contestation in an already troubled body social. Second, suicide was an indirect accusation of the sociopolitical and religious authorities themselves. It was proof of their failure to provide justice and a decent life for the entire population. Suicides kindled remorse and disturbed the conscience of a body social incapable of assuring the happiness of its members or consoling the unhappy. Suicide was an accusation directed at society and its leaders because those who kill themselves show a preference for nothingness or choose the risks of the afterlife over a world that has become a living hell. Suicide was a reproach, an accusation, even an insult to the living, in particular to those charged with assuring the happiness of the collectivity.

This is why society's leaders cannot tolerate suicide. It is an affront to all political and religious systems. Anyone who chooses death and its unknowns displays a total lack of confidence in the theories, ideologies, beliefs, plans, and promises of all leaders. In turn, those same leaders have no choice but to call the would-be suicide mad, thus refusing any responsibility for those who have killed themselves, as well as, and perhaps especially, any responsibility for the living. Even the most liberal system is reluctant to permit suicide and tolerate free expression where suicide is concerned. It is one of humanity's last great taboos. The religious and political leaders of the early seventeenth century, men deeply engaged in trying to regain cultural control in a Europe torn apart by its crisis of conscience, could not afford free debate on suicide. Life must be accepted as it appeared to be and as society's leaders conceived it to be. Those who were tempted to escape faced repression or could choose a substitute for suicide, such as spiritual death. Submission to the authorities in this world or a spiritual retreat from the world were the only options that the Great Century gave melancholic souls.

SIX

The Seventeenth Century

Reaction and Repression

Hamlet's question, "To be or not to be?" had hardly been raised when it elicited a vigorous reaction from religious, moral, and legal authorities. It set off an opposition between awakening concerns, which took the offensive, and traditional values, which mounted a counteroffensive, that needs to be seen in the context of religious reform. The Protestant Reformation and the Catholic Counter-Reform were fighting the same battle, trying to take back control over culture and establish a stable base for European societies shaken by the doubts, experiments, and hypotheses of the Renaissance. What Henry Daniel-Rops called the "Great Century of souls" was built on the ruins of humanist ideals. Aristotle provided the philosophical foundation for the new century, but his thought was buttressed by a principle of authority, order, clarity, tradition, and faith enlightened by reason. Everything—religion, literature, architecture, painting, music, government, even economics—must be subordinated to a unified, monarchical, and hierarchical ideal that formed a definitive interpretation of "tradition," which it took as a guide.

There were to be no exceptions to the rules, which meant that an immense effort of codification took place in all domains. There was an answer for everything, from rules of grammar and orthography to court etiquette. These included the three unities (space, time, and action) in drama, commercial law codes, and a refined casuistry applied to cases of conscience. Society moved from the Renaissance and its exuberance tinged with anxiety to the immobile but reassuring rigor of the age of classicism. In such a world questions were no longer welcome because the answers had already been worked out. The catechisms of the early years of the century are a good example of this. It was a world of certitude, stability, and immobility. If someone had doubts (as Descartes did), they were only apparent, a method for asserting the evident truths of this world with even greater certitude. Neither were there any mysteries left regarding the next world: Theologians had explained all its secrets. Everything that was to occur after death was as well regulated as the progress of a royal ceremony or a criminal trial, and the faithful could know in advance exactly what punishment awaited them and what faults would automatically lead them to purgatory or hell. Sermons dwelt on the etiquette of the Last Judgment.

Every thing and every person had a place in a static harmony: Perfection lay in immobility. The individual was boxed in, guided, and under surveillance; there was no longer any call either for questions or for anxiety. All was foreseen, including eternity. This should have been reassuring. In this view of things, the proper operation of the whole depended on every individual remaining in his or her preordained place. The worst offense was to want to change one's condition; this was equivalent to contesting monarchical and divine order by rejecting one's assigned role and displaying dissatisfaction with Providence. And was not life itself the first benefit of Providence? To refuse such a gift was thus to commit the supreme offense against God. It was also to desert one's post in family society and human society, thus offending both morality and the state.

All this means that political, religious, and legal authorities worked in common during the seventeenth century to quash any sign of a desire to define suicide as a legitimate option. The most rigid condemnation came from the theologians, both Catholic and Protestant, who left no possible loophole. The moralists were slightly more flexible, admitting a few exceptions in extreme cases. The jurists were more indulgent.

The Casuists and Suicide

The theologians' condemnation of suicide was global and unanimous. Concerning principle they had nothing to add to the doctrine defined by St. Augustine, whose prestige was even greater in this age than before. What was new was the development of casuistry, a technique for argumentation that owed much to the Jesuits and is typical of a civilization that seeks to give the faithful of the Church and the subjects of the king guidelines for existence that require unhesitating compliance. Casuistry was an antidote for doubt, fluctuating "states of the soul," and problems of conscience; it was a remedy for the disquietude brought on when great principles are vague or uncertain, and a barrier against all moral snares. It was also the end of any personal searching and of the believer's autonomy and freedom to follow his own conscience. In this new world every signpost was in place, and every eventuality, even the most anomalous, provided for. This all amounted to an enormous effort to advance secularization and to institute tight control over people's minds. By providing guidelines for proper conduct in all circumstances, casuistry simultaneously reassured and imprisoned. It was indeed a fitting child of the great move to control culture that had begun in the late sixteenth century.

The humanists had opened breaches in the defenses that had long prevented suicide from even being discussed. By playing on conflicting values—suicide and honor, suicide and love, suicide and charity—they had suggested that there might be certain situations in which voluntary death is legitimate. The casuists took over the topic, reviewed all possible situations, and closed the doors to them one by one.[1]

In his *Commentaries on St. Thomas,* Cardinal Cajetan (Tommaso de Vio) reexamined the cases of Christian women who had killed themselves in defense of their honor. Could anyone suggest that they did not intend to kill themselves? Ridiculous! Or that they were unaware of the law? No one can be unaware of that particular law, because it is a natural law.[2] In 1581 Martin de Azpilcueta, known as Doctor Navarrus, did his utmost in his *Enchiridion* to block all ways out: It is forbidden to kill oneself in anger; out of impatience, shame, or poverty; because of any sort of misfortune; in a search for martyrdom; or out of weariness with life. He adds that it is a mortal sin to desire one's own death, to wish never to have been born, to expose oneself to danger (for example, by tightrope walking without appropriate training), to fight a duel, to mutilate oneself, or to practice excessive abstinence.[3] In 1587 Louis Lopez found a few more loopholes and rushed to close them in his *Instructor conscientiae:* Someone sentenced to die by drinking hemlock must not drink it willingly; a prisoner sentenced to death by starvation must seek all possible ways to nourish himself. All the famous suicides of classical antiquity had committed an intrinsically evil act; all the traditional exceptional situations were forbidden. The only risk that Lopez authorized was the case of a wife caring for her plague-stricken husband. He, however, was forbidden to care for her.[4]

Jean Benedicti, writing in 1595, formally condemned "anyone who has himself killed by another, or who urges another with words to that effect, or who knowingly rushes into a danger of being killed," and anyone seeking martyrdom "out of presumption or temerity, or out of vainglory, or out of disinterest in living any longer." Benedicti condemned Saul, Cato, Lucretius, and the other suicides of antiquity; Samson and St. Sabina had perhaps received personal commands from God. He also condemned ill persons who do not follow the advice of their physicians and refuse to "take medicines, bleeding, and other remedies" (here he may have been showing excessive confidence in the medical science of his day). "Complaining about life" was just as blameworthy as tightrope walking without practice. Benedicti was more tolerant of mortification of the flesh by flagellation, which is not dangerous "because the skin grows back again well enough."[5]

Francisco de Toledo, a cardinal and a Jesuit, pursued even the most minute motives for suicide, direct and indirect, in his long *De instructione sacerdotum*. A criminal who has been sentenced to be hanged may, without sin, mount the steps alone and put his head in the noose, but he must wait to be pushed and not throw himself off the ladder, since that would be suicide. A prisoner sentenced to death by starvation or by taking poison must do all he can to avoid death (though Toledo admits that some casuists disagreed on this point). A guilty prisoner awaiting execution has no right to escape (though here again, Toledo states that others disagreed). Possible exceptions are risking one's life to defend the faith or the state or to save another shipwrecked person, or voluntary imprisonment to liberate a friend; in all other cases, "for whatever may occur, either in order to avoid a greater evil or an infamy, because of a sin committed, or because of a sin feared as probable, it is never in any way permitted to take such measures." Francisco de Toledo backs up his prohibitions with the familiar Thomist arguments: Suicide is in all instances an act contrary to divine law, natural law, and human law. We find roughly the same reasoning in the English Benedictine Robert Sayr (1560–1602).[6]

Another Jesuit, Leonardo Lessio, published a treatise on justice in 1606, in which he reexamined all the possible motivations for suicide and noted the divergent responses of his fellow casuists.[7] The casuists were in fact in agreement only on major questions, where their responses seem obvious. Their efficacy was weakened by their disagreement on smaller matters, and on the level of complex, extreme, and particular cases, discrepancies opened the door to incertitude, debate on cases of conscience, and even free choice. Lessio's method was to list various opinions, then add his own. For example, in case of fire it is not a sin to throw oneself from a tower, even though death is nearly certain, for one does so not with the intention of killing oneself, but to escape a more atrocious death. When shipwrecked it is permissible to cede one's place on a raft to someone else, since this involves only exposing oneself to danger, not seeking death. During a severe famine it is not sinful to give one's bread to a companion; one may risk one's life for the sovereign or blow up a ship to avoid its capture. On the negative side, a prisoner sentenced to death does not have a right to kill himself before execution because to kill oneself is contrary to "the inclination of common nature." The saints who killed themselves to preserve their chastity did so out of ignorance or through divine inspiration. Ordinary suicide is a crime against the rights of the state and the rights of God, who alone has powers of life and death over us. Another casuist, Paolo Comitoli (Comitolus), also listed divergent opinions, in particular on criminals sentenced to death.[8]

Francisco Suárez, a Jesuit, took refinement even further in a treatise published in 1613. Returning to the case of shipwrecked people grabbing for a floating object, he distinguishes between two possibilities: If no one is already using the plank or raft, one can, without sin, let someone else take it; a person who is already clinging to it commits a mortal sin by ceding his place. "In that case, ceding one's place to another would be like throwing oneself into the sea and having a positive hand in one's own death, which is never allowable." Situations could be subdivided in this way ad infinitum. Suárez recapitulates his colleagues' opinions on the criminal sentence to death by starvation without giving his own opinion.[9]

In 1615 Michael Rothardus globally condemned all suicides, insanity being the only exception.[10] Vincenzo Filliucci (Filliucius), on the other hand, attempted to cover all possible cases. In his *Moralium quaestionum* (1626) he lists ten situations in which suicide is forbidden, but he admits that some of them are unlikely.[11] They are:

1. As a general principle, it is never permissible to kill oneself, except on divine command.

2. It is forbidden to kill oneself to preserve chastity. The saints who did so acted out of ignorance.

3. It is forbidden to contribute to one's own death. A sentenced criminal may climb the gallows ladder but may not throw himself off. One may, however, risk one's life in defense of the faith, for one's country, for one's friends, and for the sovereign.

4. A criminal sentenced to take poison can without sin open his mouth, but he must not pour the poison into it himself; someone sentenced to death by starvation may refuse to eat; the soldier may remain at his post even if he risks being killed; the shipwrecked man may cede his raft.

5. A person sentenced to death has the right not to escape.

6. One must not commit a sin in order to save one's own life.

7. A person in religious orders must not take a wife, even if his life would be saved by doing so. (Filliucci noted that this dilemma had never arisen; it did, however, come up later under the French Revolution.)

8. One may perhaps have a limb cut off or refrain from fasting to save one's life, but ordinary remedies should be applied first.

9. One may eat meat on a fast day in order to save one's life.

10. One may visit the sick, even those stricken with plague.

Many of these same cases appear in Martino Bonacina, Tomas Hurtado, and Hermann Busenbaum.[12] Juan Caramuel was considered indulgent when he stated that a criminal awaiting execution has the right to kill himself. In a treatise written in 1625 (which contains one of the first uses of the Latin term *suicidio*) Caramuel goes so far as to suggest that self-homicide is perhaps less serious than murder, and he relates the troubling history of a monk who hanged himself after having confessed and received absolution. His abbot had the body thrown into the river, but peasants who found the body had it buried without knowing that it was a suicide. After that time, their fields were spared from hailstorms. Caramuel draws no conclusions, but the story merits reflection.[13]

Some casuists openly disagreed on specific cases. Antonino Diana, for instance, wrote that not only can a person guilty of a crime punishable by death deliver himself to justice without sin, but an innocent person can confess to a crime he has not committed in order to escape death by torture.[14] Valère Regnault (Reginaldus) disagreed: Writing in 1653, he stated that someone guilty of a crime is in no way obligated to risk death by confessing to it, even if his silence leads to the execution of an innocent person—an opinion that goes rather far. He condemned the notion of dying to save a private individual, but added that "Catholics who, in our times, have been constrained by the heretics to drink poison or to throw themselves from a high place may be excused, since without [doing so] they risked having to undergo much graver torture." Finally, a wife is excused for caring for her plague-stricken husband, even if all she can do is offer consolation. Once again, the reverse situation of the husband risking his life for the wife was not taken into consideration.[15]

In 1659 another Jesuit, Antonio Escobar, returned to the case of the prisoner sentenced to take poison, repeating that all he can do without sin is to open his mouth. He imagined another situation: If a woman who is pregnant feels such shame that she is determined to kill herself, can she seek abortion if that is the only way she could be dissuaded from suicide? He answered that she can, because abortion is a lesser evil than suicide.[16] If we remember the Church's bitter opposition to abortion throughout its history, we can appreciate the degree of horror that suicide inspired.

Casuistry had its weaknesses, but it also had one great merit: It judged acts in function of intentions. That was also precisely what obliged it to multiply "cases" to excess (a habit that Pascal fiercely ridiculed). Casuistry was a highly moral system in its principles because it substituted the study of particular cases for global condemnation and took conflicting values into account. Its error was to try to codify everything, a utopian enterprise that proved totally impractical and that contradicted its own basic principle. If distinction is used as a first principle, each human instance must be recognized as unique, and circumstances are never identical, hence all classification is useless. Moreover, when casuists multiplied their distinctions to show that suicide was legitimate only in quite exceptional circumstances, casuistry, far from ending debate, simply prolonged it. For one thing, the casuists themselves could not agree; for another, they offered an opportunity for still further refinement of their criteria. The lesson of casuistry was that everything was open to discussion, and that, given sufficient intellectual agility, many illicit actions could be made to seem licit. The dam that casuistry had built proved unable to hold back the flood.

Hesitation on the Part of Catholic Moralists

The discourse of Catholic moralists, clergy and laity alike, was just as unfavorable to suicide as that of the casuists, even though it admitted slight accommodations to the strict doctrine of St. Augustine. In 1597 François Le Poulchre, seigneur de La Motte-Messené, came out against voluntary death in his *Le Passe-temps,* in which he criticized Cato and stated that "true strength is to contain one's cupidity by the judgment of reason, thus purging one's soul of reproachable passions." The poet Jean Baptiste Chassignet also attacked Cato, the symbol of honorable suicide.[17]

Nicolas Coëffeteau, a Dominican and bishop of Marseilles, was more tolerant of the suicides of pagan antiquity. In his *Tableau des passion humaines* (1620), he declared that "according to the custom of the time when the Christian religion had not yet dissipated the vanity of the errors of paganism or the opprobrium of [its] shame by exercises of forbearance," the conduct of Cleopatra and other famous suicides reflected an undeniable grandeur of soul. As a belated humanist, Coëffeteau went so far as to include Socrates and the Christian martyrs in his praise.[18] A fellow prelate, Cardinal Richelieu, did not share that attitude: The *Catéchisme* that he wrote in 1626 flatly condemned suicide, but he was speaking in the name of both God and the king, to whom every subject should dedicate his life. Richelieu's style is as trenchant as an article in a penal code:

He that willingly and knowingly procures his owne death or desires the same, being wearie of his life: or els while he desires it not, doth yet expose himselfe to eminent danger, is more culpable then though he should kill another, desire his death, or putt him, without any iust cause, in euident perill to loose himselfe: because euery one owes more to himselfe then to his neighbour, and for that noe man is absolute Master of his beeing to dispose of it at his pleasure, but is onely a Depositaire obliged to conserue what is putt in his custodie.[19]

All seventeenth- and eighteenth-century catechisms limit themselves to stating that the Mosaic commandment forbidding homicide applies to self-homicide as well. Only rarely do they add further details. One catechism that did so was written by Father Coissard (1618), who described in verse what happens to the cadavers of suicides:

> Par les pieds on les pend et leur coupe on les mains
> Armées les ayant contre leur propre vie,
> Ennemis de nature et Timons inhumains,
> Faisant plus que ne font les tigres d'Hyrcanie

(They are hanged by the feet and the hands that armed them against their own life are cut off; [they are] enemies of nature and inhuman Timons worse than the tigers of Hyrcania.)[20]

In his moral works Jacques Du Boscq calls Porcia and Brutus "monsters" who committed a "crime" comparable to Lucretia's and Cato's.[21] Their deaths were all blameworthy cases of murder and voluntary self-homicide. "Those who kill themselves," Du Boscq says elsewhere, "are not courageous but desperate." Nonetheless, he credits the same classical suicides with nobility and greatness of soul, and says of Lucretia: "It is difficult to condemn her rationally if one does not first condemn her for not having been Christian, but could she have acted according to our principles? . . . Could she obey Scripture of which she was unaware?" Speaking of the suicide of Theoxena, he states, "Must we not admit that courage and constancy appear here with a marvelous brilliance?" Du Boscq's contradictions can only be explained by his interest in showing that women are fully as heroic as men and capable of the same extreme acts. In principle, suicide continued to be totally prohibited.

Several works were published during the 1640s glorifying female courage. There was not only Du Boscq's *Honneste femme* (1643) and *La femme héroïque,* but also *Le triomphe des dames* by François de Soucy (1646) and Madeleine de Scudéry's *Les femmes illustres et les harangues héroïques* (1642). Somewhat later (in 1663) Pierre Le Moyne published *La gallerie des femmes fortes*. These works to the glory of the *beau sexe* took it as their duty to render homage to all women who had done some extraordinary act. For a certain number of them (given the restricted social role of women in traditional societies), the act that brought them fame was their suicide: These of course included Lucretia and Porcia, as well as Christian women who were martyred for the faith or who died to preserve their chastity. Scudéry leaves judgment to the reader, prefacing Lucretia's speech with a plea: "It has not yet been decided whether Lucretia did well to kill herself after her unhappy experience. . . . Hear her reasons, reader . . . [and] give your vote after many others." Soucy recalls that St. Jerome praised the women and girls who preferred death to dishonor. Father Le Moyne has high praise for Pauline, Porcia, Camma, Pantheia, and Blanche of Pavia. He presents Pauline, Seneca's wife, as a role model and an example of moral strength:

> Sages qui nous ôtez les belles passions,
> Apprenez d'une femme à devenir stoïques

(You wise men who deprive us of the fine passions, learn from a woman how to become Stoics.)

Porcia, the wife of Brutus, earned "eternal light" by swallowing burning coals. Lucretia "deserves our praise. Ancient Rome, the nurse of the high virtues of nature and of the great heroes of paganism, brought nothing higher or grander, nothing stronger or more magnanimous than Lucretia." The "chaste and generous Pantheia" deserves like praise.

All this enthusiasm raised some problems for Father Le Moyne, however, and he attempted to put things right by denying that he was inviting women to commit suicide: "I am not putting a sword in women's hands," he wrote, "nor am I calling them to poison, the cord, or the precipice." Above all, he took care to recall that what might have been admirable in pagan morality was in the Christian system "the most enormous of all homicides," a gesture to be classified among "enormous and furious" acts. Voluntary death, he continued, "would be black and hideous in a Christian woman"; in the Christian religion, widows who kill themselves "sin against conjugal love and violate the fidelity they owe their husbands." This was an uncomfortable position, one that led Le Moyne to criticize St. Augustine for excessive rigor in his opinion of Lucretia:

I have seen this trial and the sentence attached to it in the books of the *City of God*. . . . I admit that, if [Lucretia] is judged by Christian law and according to the laws of Scripture, she will find it difficult to prove her innocence. . . . Nonetheless, if she is withdrawn from that severe tribunal where there is no pagan virtue that is not in danger of being condemned, [and] if she is judged by the law of her own country and that of the religion of her time, she will be found to be among the most chaste of her age and the strongest of her land; noble and virtuous philosophy, which so often accuses her, will absolve her from her woe and be reconciled with her.[22]

These moralists all agreed that suicide was no longer permissible, except perhaps, as René de Cerisiers, almoner to the duc d'Orléans, wrote in 1651, "in certain equitable circumstances" when "one might have many reasonable motives for leaving life indirectly." Direct suicide was still forbidden.[23] In 1656 Urbain Chevreau reiterated the distinction between ancient and modern suicides. The former were admirable, "but that virtue of the pagans is today one of our crimes." Guez de Balzac said much the same in his *Entretiens* (1657). After relating the suicide of Filippo Strozzi, he added, "But the laws of Scripture are contrary to that belief, and the new Rome calls despair what the old one called grandeur and courage. It excommunicates today what formerly it would have deified."[24] It is hard to say whether we should read veiled disapproval into the way Guez de Balzac emphasizes the contrast. Just as mysterious is an inscription found in a temple that contains "all that a proper man [honnête homme] must observe," which figures in a novel by François Hédelin d'Aubignac. There the inscription on the base of a statue of Liberty tearing out her entrails reads "On peut mourir malgré la fortune" (one can die despite fortune).[25]

The Troubled Morality of Jean-Pierre Camus

Condemnation of suicide took even more ambiguous forms in the work of some moralists. Jean-Pierre Camus is a particularly perplexing case. Born in 1584, Camus became a disciple of Francis de Sales. He was made bishop of Belley in 1608 at the age of twenty-six and showed himself to be a zealous prelate—too zealous, in fact, for Richelieu's tastes. He was determined to reform his diocese, and he left a gigantic oeuvre of more than 130 titles. When he stepped down from his episcopacy in 1629 he retired to the Abbey of Aulnay, where he died in 1652. He belonged to the restless generation of the turn of the century, and in his moral works he displayed an immoderate, nearly pathological penchant for morbid topics.[26] In a compilation entitled *Les spectacles d'horreur,* Camus presents no fewer than 126 deaths, each more atrocious than the last. His fascination for the macabre, the bloody, and the terrifying makes tales like "Les morts entassés" (Dead Bodies Piled Up), "L'amphithéâtre sanglant" (The Bloody Amphitheater), or "Les martyrs siciliens" (The Sicilian Martyrs) seem to prefigure the works of Abbé Prévost and the marquis de Sade.

Admittedly, Camus wrote with moral goals in mind. Above all, he wanted to show that no one escapes God's justice. Henri Bremond placed him among pious novelists seeking to teach a rigorous morality by concrete example.[27] Bremond also calls him *aimable,* a term one might dispute. Among the sins Camus skewers is suicide, which he illustrates with several edifying examples: In "La Mère Médée" (The Medea Mother) a wife whose husband has been unfaithful cuts her four children's bodies into pieces before slitting her own throat; in "L'inconsidération désespérée" (Desperate Distraction) a worker kills his son in a fit of rage, and when his wife hears of it, she drops the baby into the fire and goes off to hang herself. In another tale, "La force du regret" (The Strength of Regret), an unhappy lover tells the woman's husband that his wife has been deceiving him. When she is chased from the home, she dies of unhappiness; the lover then admits that he betrayed her and poisons himself; the husband, who has been unjustly accused of a crime, accepts his sentence without protest. In "La jalousie précipitée" (Hasty Jealousy) a woman kills her husband and then commits suicide by stabbing herself in the stomach. In "La pieuse Julie" (Pious Julie), a tale based on a real event, Baron Montange is about to commit suicide because the woman he loves has retired to a convent. In "La sanglante chasteté" (Bloody Chastity) a young man wants to become a monk. His father, who disapproves of this decision, tries to dissuade the son by praising the pleasures of the flesh and by placing a nude prostitute in his bed. The young man stabs himself repeatedly. In other tales, Bishop Camus details the horror of suicides' bodies rotting on the gallows: "Those two desperate men, hanged by the feet according to the law, long served as a horrible example to all who contemplated them, and at the end [when they were rotted through] they had no better burial than an ass's."

Camus's lesson is that vice leads to despair and despair to suicide, a mortal sin. Behind this moral pretext, however, the scenes of butchery contained in *Les spectacles d'horreur* make one downright queasy. Suspicion is reinforced by certain comments that stud this hecatomb. Camus makes no effort to hide his approval of the young man who commits suicide rather than sleep with a prostitute: "Several judgments," he writes, "have been made regarding this action, some blaming it for indiscreet zeal, others accusing it of cruelty and accusing him of self-murder. Still others praise it to the skies. For myself, who incline rather to praise than blame, I give my vote to the latter and confess . . . that the contrary and sinister judgment cannot be [allowed] without some sort of temerity."

Elsewhere Camus admires the conduct of a young woman who commits suicide rather than submitting to rape. In "Le désespoir honorable" (Honorable Despair) he relates the story of a man in a besieged city who kills his wife and his daughters before committing suicide himself. He adds this surprising conclusion:

When despair and infamy are joined with servitude, then a soul jealous of glory will rush into a thousand deaths rather than see the light of day with a continual opprobrium on his brow. . . . I know that the spectacle I am about to represent . . . has an effect that shocks Christian maxims, but if you look at the other side of the coin, you will find that although fear of shame took a courageous soul beyond the limits of nature and duty, this simply came of an honorable despair similar to that of the great Cato who is constantly praised in history even though he murdered himself.[28]

In "Les martyrs siciliens," to end the list, a pagan woman decides to kill herself because she cannot marry the man she loves, Agathon, who is Christian. He states that he is very sorry but cannot imitate her because it is contrary to his religion. The girl responds bitterly, "Die of shame that a girl surpasses you in both generosity and courage!" to which Agathon replies, "Even if worst comes to worst, let us die together."

The lesson of these stories is that death is preferable to all forms of sin, a conclusion confirmed by the excessive zeal with which Bishop Camus pursued heresy and backsliding in his diocese. His unhealthy hatred for sins of the flesh, in particular, led him to approve of suicides to preserve chastity. The troubled atmosphere of his bloody tales is a sign of the imbalance that the anxieties of the baroque age and its insistence on purity produced in some minds.

Protestant Theologians and Moralists

Protestant theologians and moralists seem to have been somewhat firmer in their opposition to suicide than their Catholic counterparts. In England and Scotland, Anglicans, Puritans, and Presbyterians were unanimous in their condemnation of voluntary death, and they did not indulge in the subtleties of the Catholic casuists. The impressive list of theologians and pastors who wrote on the subject of suicide between 1580 and 1680 shows that the problem was acute in the land of Shakespeare, Francis Bacon, and John Donne.

In 1583 William Fulke stated that all suicides go to hell.[29] John Case, a professor at Oxford University, attributed suicide to cowardice, and he included Cato, Brutus, and Antony in his strictures. His condemnation extended to children and to the insane: "I think that age does not entirely excuse the infant from every stain of sin, nor ignorance the idiot, nor suffering of mind the insane."[30] In 1586 Timothy Bright admitted no excuse for suicide, not even melancholia.[31] Henry Smith concurred (1591), but Richard Hooker (1593) was somewhat more flexible.[32] In 1594 John King declared suicide counter to nature, and in 1596 Anthony Copley wrote a long allegorical poem attacking voluntary death.[33] William Whitaker went so far as to find even biblical suicides reprehensible, and in agreement with St. Augustine, he refused to grant the Books of the Maccabees a place among inspired texts because they contain praise for two suicides, Eleazar and Razis.

> Razis deserved no praise for his fortitude. For this was to die cowardly rather than courageously, to put himself voluntarily to death in order to escape from the hands of a tyrant. The Holy Spirit judges not of valour by the same measures as profane men, who extol Cato to the skies for committing suicide lest he should fall into the power and hands of Caesar: for he either feared, or could not bear to see him, or sought to catch renown by an act of such prodigious horror. Thus he was crushed and extinguished either by despair, or grief, or some other perturbation of mind; any of which motives are foreign from true fortitude. Rightly, therefore, did Augustine deny those books to be canonical, in which such a crime is narrated with some commendation by the authors.[34]

In 1600 George Abbot, who was later archbishop of Canterbury, returned to the traditional arguments—we have no right to quit this life without God's permission; God has forbidden us to kill—in his discussion of Jonah.[35] William Vaughan's *Golden Grove* was published in London in the same year (1600). The first edition of this work included only one chapter on suicide, but the second edition (1608) had sixteen chapters on the topic, a further sign of the scope of the debate on suicide in the early seventeenth century. The avalanche of arguments that Vaughan uses against suicide is a measure of his anxiety before the mounting tide of contestation, and it shows how much the act horrified him. Suicide, he tells us, is the fruit of despair born in a weak soul, and it is an insult to God. It deprives the state of one of its members. It is forbidden by Scripture, and if there are biblical passages that seem to approve it, they are apocryphal. The Fathers of the Church, the moralists, and the laws all condemn it. Lucretius and Cato were weak, and the latter would have done better to be tortured in the bronze bull of Phalaris than to kill himself in despair. Samson and Jonah received special commands, but virgins who kill themselves to preserve their chastity are wrong to do so, as are those who put an end to their days because they are afraid of being unable to bear suffering, which belittles divine power. In short, Vaughan finds nothing "more damnable or more impious" than to kill oneself. Finally, only God decides the fate of the soul of a suicide.

In 1608, the year in which the second edition of Vaughan's book appeared, the Puritan casuist William Perkins stated that all suicide out of despair was forbidden because the greatest imaginable sin was to doubt divine mercy.[36] In 1614 Andrew Willet condemned all suicides: Pagan suicides, which were not dictated by faith, were worthless, as was Razis' suicide, because his story is apocryphal; Ahithophel, who killed himself in despair, was merely a precursor of Judas, as was Saul. In short, all those who kill themselves are cowards.[37]

The picture that George Strode gave in 1618 was quite different.[38] He agreed that suicide is to be condemned in all ordinary situations; it is a sign of pride and cruelty if we take this way to punish ourselves by this means or if we are weary of life. Those who do not love themselves love no one, and the biblical suicides of Saul, Ahithophel, Zimri, and Judas prove that those who kill themselves are evil. Pagans who killed themselves in the belief that they were escaping tribulation were victims of an illusion; Christians who do so are beyond pardon. Strode added, however, that there are cases in which one can, if not kill oneself, at least desire death: when God is no longer glorified, when one wishes to leave evil company, when one aims to put an end to offenses to God, when one is overwhelmed by the calamities and woes of this life, and when one craves total unity with Christ. These are motives we will also find among mystics with the doctrine of total annihilation, showing a certain kinship between suicide and forms of spirituality hostile to contact with the world.

We might add to the long list of English writers who condemned suicide John Wing (1620) and George Hakewill (1621), who both rejected suicide even in the most dramatic circumstances (among them, a man married to a waspish wife).[39] John Abernethy condemns people who kill themselves out of religious despair because they believe they have committed unpardonable sins. He declares them weak-minded melancholiacs who, by despairing of divine mercy, make a catastrophic mistake and deprive themselves of an opportunity for repentance. Death, he argues, will catch up with us in any event. Abernethy, who was bishop of Caithness, states that suicides are not infrequent in his diocese.[40] In 1629 Nathaniel Carpenter taxed all suicides, pagans included, with cowardice, stating that we must risk our lives only in defense of the faith, justice, or country.[41] In 1633 Richard Capel recalled that

Satan is the cause of suicides.[42] Peter Barker (in the same year) and William
Gouge (in the following year) focused on indirect suicides that were the result
of excesses—not only excessive eating and drinking and uncontrolled anger,
but excessive asceticism as well, a warning they directed at "papists" in particular. Direct suicide was all the more to be condemned, as its instigator was
the devil.[43] In 1634 John Downame, a Puritan minister, treated suicide in
his *Christian Warfare*.[44] We have been placed in our posts in God's armies,
Downame states, and must remain there until relieved. Our only choice is
between bearing the woes of the present life or spending all eternity in hell.
The saints show us the way. In the Bible all suicides but Samson are reprobates. God, the Church, society, and the family all forbid suicide. In 1638
Richard Younge warned against intemperance, which leads to a fall from
grace, despair, and suicide.[45]

Preachers and theologians tirelessly repeated their litanies against suicide.
These included Lancelot Andrewes in 1642; Henry Hammond in 1645, who
wrote a catechism that was republished fourteen times in fifty years; William
Fenner, a Puritan writing in 1648 who called all mortal sins suicides; Thomas
Fuller in 1653; Edward Phillips, who presented suicide as bestial in his 1659
dictionary; Jeremy Taylor in 1660, who measured charity by the love we bear
ourselves; and Thomas Philipot in 1674, who discussed ways to avoid suicidal
melancholy.[46]

These works all reiterate the familiar arguments with little originality.
Their number is nonetheless a sign that the problem of suicide was felt as real,
as Sir William Denny recalled in 1653 in a work titled *Pelicanicidium*.[47] Denny
expressed his alarm at the frequency of suicides and at John Donne's *Biathanatos,* published not long before. Denny stated that he had written a treatise of
his own "lest the Frequency of such Actions might in time arrogate a Kind of
Legitimation by Custom, or plead Authority from some late publisht Paradoxes, That Self-homicide was Lawfull."[48] He listed the most frequent causes
of suicide: love, jealousy, melancholia, debauchery, financial ruin, remorse,
and (among religious extremists) excessive scruples of conscience. His arguments against suicide are conformist: God, reason, nature, the state, and the
family all forbid suicide; by his death Christ redeemed all sins, so there is no
reason to despair.

Thomas Browne and Suicide as an Existential Problem

Sir Thomas Browne was one of the English authors who devoted the most
thought to the problem of suicide and who wrote on the topic over the

longest span of time, from the composition of the *Religio medici* in the mid-1630s to a letter written in 1670.[49] On the three levels of the personal, the paternal, and the theoretical, Browne's arguments have a human and existential quality not found in his predecessors, who reasoned as pure theologians and abstract moralists. What emerges thanks to Browne's multiple viewpoints is a picture of changes and contradictions within the individual as he confronts life's problems.

Browne was a moderate, a believer in the middle road, and a man who valued common sense and wisdom over heroism. In his *Religio medici* he expresses reservations about suicide, even among pagans. Cato, not his favorite hero, would perhaps have done better to face up to life's trials. The patience of Job is preferable to the impatience of such figures as Scaevola and Codrus. Still, within the framework of their religion, the Stoics were not wrong in preferring death to decline, for instance in cases of incurable illness. It is a way out forbidden to Christians, however, and excitable people who seek martyrdom for their faith are simply fanatics: "There are questionlesse many canonized on earth, that shall never be Saints in Heaven; and have their names in Histories and Martyrologies, who in the eyes of God, are not so perfect Martyrs as was that wise Heathen [Socrates]."[50] Browne counseled wisdom and moderation above all.

In *Urne-Burial,* a work written twenty years later (in 1658), we sense that Browne finds greater attraction in classical antiquity and is perhaps more weary of life. At the age of fifty-three, his fellow-physician Guy Patin tells us, he showed signs of melancholy and was attracted to spiritual and mystical suicide. He speaks of the "martyrdome to live" and evokes the "happinesse of the next world." He reproaches Dante for placing Epicurus in hell when that philosopher "contemned life without encouragement of immortality."[51]

When in 1667 Browne's son Tom, an officer in the Royal Navy, wrote to his father of his admiration for Romans who killed themselves rather than surrender, the elder Browne swept aside his tolerance of classical suicides and forbade his son from seeking to imitate them: "I cannot omitt my earnest prayers unto God to deliver you from such a temptation."[52] He added that Plutarch gives many examples of soldiers and captains who surrendered with honor. After 1667 Sir Thomas Browne returned to a much more orthodox position, abandoning all favorable comments on ancient suicides and taxing the Stoics with cowardice.

Browne's attitude illustrates the large gap that has always existed between suicide as an intellectual, theological, or moral problem and suicide as a concrete, existential problem. As always, it is not those who talk most about suicide or who raise the question publicly who kill themselves. Montaigne, Charron, Shakespeare, Bacon, and Donne opened up a dangerous problem, a bomb that they defused in their own cases thanks to their own hesitations, but one that could prove fatal to others who might be more prone to action than meditation. They pose the problem of responsibility regarding writings on suicide. Sir Thomas Browne, a physician and a philosopher, used his culture and his reflection to see suicide in relative terms; his son Tom, a military man, was seduced by concrete instances of heroic suicides and risked succumbing to their appeal because he could not put them in perspective. At which point the father, alarmed, warned his son of the danger. Thus suicide is a purely personal problem and a strictly individual decision, but at the same time it is a question that must be resolved by exchanging thoughts with someone else, which is the only way to evaluate the real situation.

The Devil Again

Theologians and preachers in seventeenth-century England did not limit themselves to the traditional theological and moral arguments against suicide; they also took up and extended the campaign to diabolize self-murder. "Satan doth make many now adais" end their lives, Richard Greenham wrote.[53] John Mirk, Thomas Beard, George Abbot, Lancelot Andrewes, John Sym, and Richard Gilpin agreed. Gilpin wrote in 1677 that "Satan seeks the ruin of our Bodies, as well as of our Souls, and tempts Men often to Self-Murther," and he listed eight ways the devil tempts people to suicide.[54] Many confessions and autobiographies written by Puritans give witness to diabolic temptations: there was Nehemiah Wallington, of course, and also Hannah Allen, who wrote (in 1683) of "the great Advantage the Devil made of her deep Melancholy" to tempt her to suicide.[55] In 1652 Henry Walker, a Baptist, gathered testimony from his congregation, many of whom stated that they had been tempted by the devil to kill themselves.[56]

Charles Hammond's ballad "The Devil's Cruelty to Mankind" dramatizes the story of George Gibbs, who committed suicide by disemboweling himself. Lying in agony for eight hours, Gibbs relates how he first rejected the devil several times, then succumbed to his blandishments. In 1678 John Bunyan's *Pilgrim's Progress* showed the allegorical figures Christian and Hopeful in the "very dark dungeon" of Doubting Castle, tempted by Giant Despair: "He told them, that since they were never like to come out of that place, their only way would be, forthwith to make an end of themselves, either with Knife, Halter or Poison: For why, said he, should you chuse life, seeing it is attended with so much bitterness?"[57] In 1685 an account of the suicide of Roger Long, imprisoned for his participation in Monmouth's Rebellion, declared that those who kill themselves are victims of "the Enemy of Mankind," who "takes the advantage to push them into Ruin, and heighten the Sence of their Guilt into that of a desperate Despair."[58]

Moreover, it is hard to see how to avoid despair before the scene depicted by seventeenth-century preachers, both Protestant and Catholic. If there was one point they nearly all agreed on, it was how few people were among the elect. Jean-Baptiste Massillon was no more optimistic than the most austere Calvinists: "Who, then, can be saved? Few, my dear listener: not you, unless you change; not those who resemble you; not the multitude," he declared in his sermon "Sur le petit nombre des élus."[59] God saved only 2 Jews, Joshua and Caleb, out of 600,000. Why should there be more today? "My brothers, our loss is almost sure." Malebranche was scarcely more generous: "Out of a thousand, not twenty will actually be saved."[60] Jesuits and Jansenists were equally persuaded of this: "There is no more astonishing truth in the Christian religion than the one indicating the small number of the elect," Pierre Nicole wrote.

It is hardly surprising that religious despair accounted for a large proportion of seventeenth-century suicides. When the religion that emerged from the Protestant Reformation and the Catholic Counter-Reform used fear as a prime motivation, the result was diametrically opposed to expectations: Despairing of obtaining salvation, some of the faithful—people of weaker spiritual stamina or those who were undergoing a life crisis—hastened to their deaths. Since damnation was certain, what did it matter when one departed? Many of the more spiritually minded writers of the century nearly succumbed to despair themselves (as we shall see) before they found a technique for counteracting suicidal impulses in mysticism. How many Christians with weaker spiritual armor simply put an end to their days?

John Sym proposed a much more rational approach to suicide. An Anglican pastor in Essex at Leigh, a small fishing port on the Thames estuary, Sym published a book in 1637 that is considered to be the first published treatise entirely devoted to suicide, *Lifes Preservative against Self-Killing, or, An Useful Treatise Concerning Life and Self-Murder.* It helps to put this work into perspective if we recall that at this time John Donne's *Biathanatos* was still in manuscript and was not printed until ten years later.

Sym's aim was to check the progress of ideas favorable to suicide (which confirms the anxiety discussed above), but his book also offered something new in its attempt to describe the psychology of suicide. People who kill themselves, Sym declares, are not really seeking death but rather looking for a positive good and a remedy. Passion and imagination play a more important role in the determination of suicide than pure reason. Some kill themselves out of vengeance, shifting the responsibility for their death onto the conscience of those who oppress them. One example that Sym gives of suicide as revenge is when it is

intended *against others,* by ones killing of himselfe: *when* he is implacably offended by others, from whom he can neither have satisfaction, nor reformation of his grievances; *and when* his death by his owne hands may redound to the hurt, or disgrace, as he thinks, of those that have wronged him. *Which* practice of *self-murder,* upon this motive, is most incident to persons of the weakest *sexe,* and worst disposition and condition; such as be *women,* and *servants,* and *men sympathizing* with them in qualities.[61]

Many who kill themselves cannot really be held responsible for their act, Sym adds. This is the case not only of madmen, children, and idiots, but also of poor people who have suffered great injustices. In his role as pastor of a fishing village, Sym had seen many pitiful cases, and when he touches on this topic, his discourse takes on a much more humane tone than can be found in the purely theological writers. Before condemning a suicide, one should ascertain the causes and motivations for the act and the mental disposition of the victim, because only those who kill themselves deliberately and in full awareness of what they are doing are guilty. The way to combat suicide effectively was thus to aim at its causes: "*Self-murder* is prevented, not so much by *arguments* against the *fact* . . . as by the discovery and removall of the *motives* and *causes,* whereupon they are tempted to do the same." Sym is not advocating a flexible attitude toward suicides. The theologian in him gains the upper hand of the pastor in a sweeping condemnation: "By *induction* of particular *self-murderers* in *Scripture,* who were all reprobates and damned, we may safely conclude, that no *self-murderer* is, or can be saved."[62]

Behind all the motivations and causes that seemed to excuse voluntary death stood Satan and his instruments, pride, despair, and unbelief. These were the sins that led to suicide. John Sym's arguments against suicide are the traditional ones: It is an act against God, against society, and against the person; one is not permitted to expose one's life to mortal danger except to save another person more useful to the community, such as a magistrate or a prince. Despite a few modern tinges, John Sym's thought was yet another contribution to the theologians' and the moralists' massive barrage against suicide.

Canon law and the synodal statutes show the same harsher tone as theoretical writings. The regional councils of Lyons in 1577, Reims and Bordeaux in 1583, Cambrai in 1586, and Chartres in 1587 all repeat the prohibition of Christian burial for suicides. The Council of Reims even stipulated excommunication for anyone who buried the body of a suicide. Prayers for the dead were not to be said for suicides because their damnation was immediate. Exhumations of the cadavers of suicides continued to take place, as in one case mentioned by Pierre L'Estoile in 1596, in which a man who had committed suicide after losing a lawsuit had been buried in the cemetery of the Saints-Innocents in Paris, thanks to a camouflage operation arranged by his children.

Jurists' Distinctions

Although civil law was always just as strict as canon law with regard to suicide, the growing influence of Roman law inclined jurists of the late sixteenth and seventeenth centuries to draw some distinctions.[63] Some, such as Jean Duret in 1572 and Barthélemy de Chasseneux in 1573, relied completely on Roman law. Chasseneux declared that the goods of a suicide should be forfeit only in cases of those who kill themselves after having committed a crime.[64] Duret and Chasseneux were exceptions to the rule, however. For jurists such as Jean de Coras, writing in 1572, suicide was "extremely low, cowardly, and unworthy of a Christian." He nonetheless expressed revulsion at the execution of suicides' cadavers, "a thing most strange and redolent of I know not what barbarity and inhumanity."[65] Bertrand d'Argentré displayed no such scruples in his commentary on Breton law in *Nouvelle Coutume de Bretagne* (1580). He stated that even pagan writers condemned suicides, and if there had been excuses in those remote times, they were no longer valid in the Christian world, where goods should continue to be confiscated and cadavers punished.

Argentré's Angevin neighbor, Pierre Ayrault, was much less categorical. Although suicide is obviously a reprehensible act, is it legitimate to take revenge on a cadaver? Ayrault posed the question in 1591 in a treatise "on trials of the cadavers, ashes, or the memory of suicides, of animals, of inanimate objects, and of persons charged with crimes who refuse to appear in court." He wondered:

Is it not ridiculous and inept, even cruel, even barbarous, to give battle against shadows? . . . Do we not say that death effaces and extinguishes the crime? What do we want with the dead, who are at rest and with whom we have no more business or commerce? It is with God that they must now deal. . . . And it appears that in calling them to him [God] makes use of a right of sovereignty; that is, He evokes knowledge [of that right] if we had already attempted [suicide] or, if it were yet to come, He forbids it to us. Can a dead person die again? Doesn't he pay his debts, criminal and civil, by ceding not only his goods but life itself to all his creditors? . . . Who will not add that it is too much to make sport of our frail humanity, of our feeble and miserable condition, after it has ended to resuscitate yet another mortality and weakness? . . . If it is impossible to chastise and punish the dead, is there turpitude in pursuing them?[66]

Although another jurist, Charondas (Louis Le Caron), did not challenge the mutilation of suicides' cadavers or the confiscation of their goods in his *Somme rural* (1603), he declared that such treatment should be reserved to cases of suicide because of weariness with life or out of remorse for a crime committed, and should not be extended to suicides due to troubles and illness.[67] Many European jurists—Gomezio de Amescua in 1604 and Erasmus Ungepauer in 1609, for instance—limited themselves to noting that Roman law and canon law contradicted one another regarding self-murder.[68]

Another sign of the timeliness of the debates on voluntary death and the contestation that such debates prompted is a case brought before an Angevin court in 1611. The jurist Anne Robert shows us in his report on this case that the traditional arguments for and against suicide could be used in judiciary procedures.[69] One Arnaud, the lawyer who represented the heirs of a man who had killed himself and whose estate had been confiscated, went beyond the strict framework of the case he was pleading to attempt to rehabilitate suicide, calling on Cato, the Stoics, and Seneca for aid. Killing oneself, he stated, is proof of grandeur and valor "when a man of invincible courage is resolved either to conquer his adversities and woes or to put an end to them." Even Christianity admits certain cases of self-inflicted death, but suicide remains a crime that cannot be tolerated. Returning to the case at hand, he noted that at any event, confiscation did not pertain in Anjou, and he added that this particular suicide was probably mad.

When he comes around to offering his opinion on this case, Robert focuses on establishing the criminal nature of suicide. He uses all the familiar arguments, in particular the one of the soldier duty-bound to stick to his post. He also notes that everyone is the property of God: "Is not someone [like] a fugitive serf if he should attempt, by a premature, hastened death, to dissolve and dismember the beautiful harmony and architectural work of the body and the soul?" Robert cites pagan and Christian authors one after the other to attack suicide and justify the confiscation of a suicide's estate.

Antoine Loisel and Joost Damhouder (1616) also supported the most stringent point of view: The cadavers of suicides should be dragged and hanged, and those who attempt suicide should be punished.[70] In 1629 Claude Lebrun de La Rochette was of the same opinion.[71] Toward the mid-seventeenth century, the jurist Antoine Despeisses described approvingly the procedure followed in most French provinces in cases of suspected suicide. First, a report was drawn up describing the circumstances in which the body had been found; next, a barber-surgeon made a report. Then inquiries were made concerning the life and mores of the deceased and the probable causes of the act that led to death. In due time the relatives of the deceased were notified, and if suicide seemed indicated, a *curateur* was named to defend the victim. During all this time the body was preserved in sand or salt or was sprinkled with quicklime to prevent it from decomposing too much before the sentence could be carried out. Once a guilty verdict had been reached, the cadaver was fetched, then dragged through the streets on a hurdle, face down, with a sergeant-at-arms in the lead proclaiming the reason for the sentence. The body was then hanged by the feet from a gibbet, and after being exposed, was thrown onto the communal dump along with rotting horse carcasses. For Despeisses, these were perfectly appropriate measures to take against those guilty of "such a horrible and scandalous violation." The only suicides who were to be excused from such a fate were madmen, the indigent, and others who had suffered such extreme woes that their reason might have been affected.[72]

All the jurists distinguished between culpable and excusable suicides. In 1662 René Choppin declared that aside from cases of insanity, families of suicides could avoid confiscation of possessions if the deceased had killed himself "because of vexation with his life, or out of shame over debts, or through an inability to withstand the sufferings of a malady." Nonetheless, he stated that suicide was a "much more enormous" crime than murder.[73] For François Des Maisons, writing in 1667, it was even "the most odious crime in nature."[74]

Cardin Le Bret declared that suicides were held "in greater horror than all other criminals," but he too tempered this categorical generalization by applying it humanely and drawing distinctions. One example he gives is taken from a decision of his own in favor of a woman who had killed herself after losing a lawsuit. In general, he states, courts should not order confiscation of the possessions of those who kill themselves because of a misfortune, great suffering, or feeblemindedness. "Also it would surely be an inhumane thing to expose to ignominy and loss of goods anyone whose judgment has been impaired by afflictions and misfortunes and whose inability to withstand suffering has turned to madness. Man is an image not only of misery, but also of impotence and weakness; that is why we must bend all our judgments and our opinions to what is gentlest and most in touch with the human condition."[75]

Medicine and Suicidal Insanity

In 1665 Paul Challine, who drew roughly the same distinctions as Le Bret, exempted from condemnation those who kill themselves "because of illness, madness, or other accident." This was a statement that could lead to exculpating all suicides, since all are the result of one sort of "accident" or another. The same might be said of the *petitio principii* Challine used to define the symptoms of *fureur ou frénésie:* The best proof of madness, he declared, is the fact of having killed oneself. Hence all suicides are by definition insane.[76]

Laurent Bouchel was in favor of restricting penalties for suicide to those who had killed themselves to avoid punishment for their crimes. Even in their case, he suggested, such penalties should be carried out on an effigy of the deceased.[77] In 1665 Guy Coquille, also a jurist, showed just as little enthusiasm for the execution of cadavers. He hinted that such procedures are carried out only because the Church creates the crime by refusing Christian burial to suicides. Where civil justice is concerned, he wrote, "I believe that one should not try them as murderers and confiscate their goods," because suicide "is not among the crimes that require inquiry after death in order to condemn the [criminal's] memory."[78] Scipion Dupérier, to end the list, agreed with Challine: Only those who kill themselves to escape criminal pursuits should be condemned; the others are melancholiacs, and melancholia is a form of madness.[79]

Dupérier's view agreed with the medical theories of the age, and probably justice in the seventeenth century had already been influenced by treatises on psychopathology. The famous physician Thomas Willis (1621–75) described the manic-depressive cycle, showing that melancholia can degenerate into madness and bring on suicidal crises. "After melancholia," he wrote, "we must consider mania, with which it has so many affinities that these complaints often change into one another."[80] Most other physicians limited their remarks to noting the frequent juxtaposition of melancholia and suicidal tendencies, without going so far as to link the two.

Willis's explanation resonated in the scientific world and even in judiciary circles. For Willis, melancholia was "a madness without fever or frenzy, accompanied by fear and sadness"; it was a form of delirium and could be explained by a disordered movement of "animal spirits" in the brain that set up a weak agitation and created pores in the brain rather than following the normal circuits. In that abnormal circulation the "animal spirits" became "obscure, opaque, shadowy," acting as a corrosive vapor that upset the brain's functions, fixing it on one object and filling it with sadness and fear.[81]

Thus the idea that suicidal tendencies might have a medical and somatic explanation slowly began to appear. It moved in the direction of considering people who killed themselves not responsible for their act, and henceforth suicides were viewed more as victims than as murderers. The authors who wrote on the topic differed as to the origin of the affliction, but bit by bit they abandoned supernatural and demoniacal causes for insanity and suicide. The self-murderer began to be taken more for a sick person and less for a pawn of Satan. Attempted suicides tended increasingly to be incarcerated, and the registers of asylums and *maisons d'internement* include such mentions as "attempted to do away with himself." Michel Foucault says of this phenomenon, "Thus the sacrilege of suicide was annexed to the neutral domain of insanity."[82] To prevent new suicide attempts, people who had tried to kill themselves had their hands bound and were locked up in wicker cages.

Other therapies existed for melancholia (hence for the prevention of suicide) that corresponded to the explanations advanced by medical theory. For many physicians, a depressive temperament could be attributed to an overabundance of melancholic black humor in the blood. In 1662 Moritz Hoffman proposed blood transfusions as a treatment for melancholia, an idea that was suggested in London as well and, after a good deal of hesitation, tried on a man suffering from amorous melancholia. Ten ounces of his blood was removed and replaced with calf's blood; the operation appeared to have effected a complete cure.[83] In 1682 Michael Ettmüller was still recommending this treatment, but some physicians soon abandoned it in favor of quinine-based medications, and others preferred to prescribe baths, voyages, and music. Such therapies developed further in the eighteenth century.

For the theologians, jurists, and casuists, the soul remained untouched by insanity, and the madman *(le furieux)* bore no moral responsibility, no matter what act he committed. The Cartesian current of thought reinforced the idea that anxiety, viewed mechanistically, was physiological in origin. Descartes viewed anxiety as coming from an imbalanced agitation of the animal spirits; Malebranche made use of recent discoveries regarding the principle of inertia to state that God has put in us a certain quantity of movement that tends toward the infinite good, but when the soul stops progressing toward that good, the presence of such motion, now unused, prompts anxiety.[84]

The seventeenth-century jurists were not insensitive to these medico-philosophical currents, and their works show a clear interest in eliminating penal sanctions in cases of suicide due to a psycho-physiological affliction. Once they had abandoned the diabolical explanation of suicide, they attempted increasingly to exclude the idea of an ethical and penal responsibility on the part of melancholic suicides, although they continued to condemn self-murder in principle.

Repression Relaxed: The Decree of 1670

A growing gap appeared between religious attitudes, which remained extremely firm, and sentences handed down under civil law, which were much more sensitive to changes in the sciences, philosophy, and mores. One flagrant example that Des Maisons relates occurred in 1664. A peasant woman who lived on land owned by the cathedral chapter of Auxerre committed suicide; her family passed off her death as an accident and obtained the permission of a judge to bury her body in a corner of the cemetery. The canons, suspecting some irregularity, brought the affair before the *official* (the judge of the episcopal court), in the opinion of Des Maisons, "as an excuse for getting their hands on this woman's goods, to the prejudice of the six minor children she left." The *official* declared the cemetery polluted and instituted proceedings against her. The chapter stated that although it felt deeply for the children left in poverty, a suicide was a suicide and must never be tolerated. The family appealed to the Parlement de Paris, which decided in its favor.[85]

The Auxerre affair fits well within the cultural atmosphere instituted by the Catholic Reform. The Church had taken great care, using extreme precision and covering all domains, to redefine fundamental matters of dogma, pastoral care, and ethics after the crisis of the years from 1580 to 1620. It then settled into total immobility. Compared with clerical intransigence, jurisprudence was relatively more supple and more comprehending. Very often the law's rigors regarding confiscations were softened to avoid leaving widows and heirs destitute. In the case of the suicide in Auxerre, Le Bret reminded the Parlement de Paris that indulgence was traditional in custom. That, he stated, was what that court "has practiced until now, having always shown itself to be very indulgent in similar occurrences."[86]

There is no lack of examples. In 1630 near La Fère, in Picardy, a man seventy-four years old strangled himself in despair when he proved incapable of consummating his marriage to a twenty-year-old wife. By a decree dated 16 March of that year, his wealth was confiscated, but his widow was permitted to keep 1,500 livres, and another 1,000 livres was set aside for presumptive heirs.[87] In Toulouse in 1634 the heirs of a woman who had committed suicide avoided having her property confiscated because the local courts followed Roman law. In 1670 the jurist Hyacinthe de Boniface related that the Parlement de Provence had annulled the confiscation of property decreed in the case of a woman who had drowned herself, "impelled by some vexatious event." The case involved a problem of form, but there was also a more basic reason for the court's leniency: Those who "wearied of life because of the loss of some lawsuit or [who], out of madness, cut off their days" deserved "no penalty, with the possible exception of being denied Christian burial, given that they are sufficiently punished by quitting the agreeable things of this world." Boniface added that it is God's task to punish such a crime, and that confiscating property only encourages the heirs to commit suicide as well.[88]

In that same year (1670) a major law was enacted. In the view of most historians, this Ordonnance criminelle clearly aggravated the repression of suicide. In my opinion, however, that interpretation is erroneous. In the first place, suicide appears only incidentally among the many articles of this text, specifically in three words found in article 1 of title 12, "The Manner of Putting on Trial a Cadaver or the Memory of a Deceased Person." The dispositions of title 12 are as follows:

Article 1. The cadaver or the memory of a deceased person cannot be brought to trial except for the crime of lèse-majesté, divine or human, where it is pertinent to try the deceased, [or] duel, homicide of oneself, or rebellion against justice with open force in the process of which [the deceased] was killed.

Article 2. The judge will name ex officio a *curateur* [administrator, trustee] for the body of the deceased, if it is still extant (if not, for his memory), and a relative of the deceased will be preferred, if such is available to fulfill this function.

Article 3. The *curateur* will know how to read and write, will swear an oath, and the trial will be conducted against him in the ordinary form: he will nonetheless simply stand and not be seated in the witness chair during the final interrogation; his name will be used throughout the proceedings, but sentence will be rendered against the cadaver or only against the memory.

Article 4. The *curateur* will have a right to appeal the sentence rendered against the cadaver or the memory of the deceased. He can even be obliged to do so by someone among the kin, who, in this case, will be obliged to advance the costs.

Article 5. Our Courts can elect another *curateur* than the person named by the judges to whom appeal is made.[89]

This law simply gathered together all the cases given in the various customals regarding the trial of cadavers, one of which was trials of suicides. It contains nothing new. Article 1 states, moreover, that in all such cases there may be a trial of the cadaver *or* of the memory of the deceased, which in no way implies—Albert Bayet to the contrary—that after the Ordonnance suicides had to stand trial twice, once as a cadaver and again in "memory."[90]

Bayet was alarmed by the very general terms of the definition of the crime in the Ordonnance, which targets "homicide de soi-même" without specifying any circumstances. "It is the generality of this expression that makes it fearsome," he writes.[91] I disagree. For centuries it had seemed so very evident that suicides caused by insanity (to cite one example) were exempt from pursuit in both divine and human laws that it was useless to recall that fact. It would have been absurd to begin punishing the cadavers of insane suicides in 1670.

Moreover, the decree says nothing about the penalties to be applied. It only indicates the procedure to be followed, and the specific details that it gives are guarantees granted the defense. First, the decree is very restrictive in form ("Le procès ne pourra être fait . . . si ce n'est . . . "); next, it specifies that when possible a relative of the deceased should be chosen as *curateur*—that is, someone who knew the deceased well and who has every interest in exonerating him or her. The *curateur* is given all guarantees concerning the respect of his own honor; he can appeal the sentence or be obliged to do so by another relative. In short, if we consider the situation of both jurisprudence and practice in 1670, this decree, far from innovating or from aggravating anything, merely records the most current customs, defining them more precisely in the aim of restraining abuses and guaranteeing the rights of the defense. The Ordonnance was neither an innovation nor a return to the past; it was simply a codification of current practice. As in canon law, immobility was the rule in civil jurisprudence, despite jurists' tendencies toward indulgence.

Suicide as a Noble and Clerical Privilege

No worsening of the repression of suicide is recorded following the promulgation of the Ordonnance criminelle of 1670. Acquittals and compromises remained just as frequent after as before. In the aristocratic milieu, moreover, the question of recourse to the law never even came up. One year after the 1670 decree, a suicide occurred at the royal court of France that provided fodder for conversation in high social circles. We know of it from several sources. Vatel, a man who had formerly been in the service of Nicolas Fouquet but was currently the *maître d'hôtel* to the prince de Condé, killed himself during a visit of the king to his master's chateau at Chantilly. He did so because he thought himself dishonored. There had not been enough roast to serve all the guests, and two tables had been left without meat; the fish that had been ordered had not arrived in time for dinner. The diarists who record the matter offer no reproach, except perhaps to state that the occurrence perturbed the smooth operation of the festivities.

Madame de Sévigné left a famous account of the event. In this text we see that the high nobility felt a certain admiration when it discovered, to its surprise, that a servant (albeit of high rank) might have such a finely tuned sense of honor. Vatel's death is admired as a handsome gesture, but once the agitation has subsided (after only a few minutes), meals and festivities pick up again as if nothing had happened. If the noble guests do express vague regrets, it is because Vatel's death momentarily disturbed the plans of "Monsieur le Duc." The king expresses regret for having been the unwitting cause of this momentary concern for "Monsieur le Prince." Madame de Sévigné writes:

Vatel . . . went to his apartment, and setting the hilt of his sword against the door, after two ineffectual attempts, succeeded in the third, in forcing the sword through his heart. At that instant the carriers arrived with the fish; Vatel was inquired for to distribute it; they ran to his apartment, knocked at the door, but received no answer; upon which they broke it open, and found him weltering in his blood. A messenger was immediately dispatched to acquaint the Prince with what had happened, who was like a man in despair. The Duc wept, for his Burgundy journey depended upon Vatel. The Prince related the whole affair to His Majesty with an expression of great concern: It was considered as the consequence of too nice a sense of honour; some blamed, others praised him for his courage. The King said he had put off this excursion for more than five years, because he was aware that it would be attended with infinite trouble, and told the Prince that he ought to have had but two tables, and not have been at the expense of so many, and declared he would never suffer him to do so again; but all this was too late for poor Vatel. However, Gourville endeavoured to supply the loss of Vatel; which he did in great measure. The dinner was elegant, the collation was the same. They supped, they walked, they hunted; all was perfumed with jonquils, all was enchantment. Yesterday, which was Saturday, the same entertainments were renewed.[92]

La Gazette devoted several pages to a report of the festivities, but it made no mention of Vatel's death.

Like the nobility, the clergy was a social category that almost always escaped prosecution for suicide. Clerical suicides were systematically declared insane and given Christian burial. In the interest of avoiding scandal, the Church was quite willing to "pollute" cemeteries in full awareness of the facts, which raises a question about the sincerity of its theories on the fate of suicides in the next world.

The question of the proper procedures to follow when a member of the clergy died in suspicious circumstances had already been raised early in the century. Although the Church had courts, the *officialités,* to try its own, only royal justice could try cases of violent death. On occasion that division of responsibilities gave rise to conflicts. Thus in 1635 in Toulouse, the Parlement decreed the confiscation of the estate of a priest who had committed suicide, but the Church authorities had the sentence annulled under the pretext that the affair should have been brought before the ecclesiastical judge. The Parlement protested, complaining that this was "a new and extraordinary thing," and expressing its indignation: "The Church should not take such care to protect the interest of those who have betrayed its own in such cowardly fashion."[93] It did no good.

Nonetheless, compromise became common practice beginning in the mid-seventeenth century, as related by the *Recueil des actes, titres et mémoires concernant les affaires du clergé de France.*[94] Ecclesiastical suicides were camouflaged to "avoid scandalizing the priesthood and doing noteworthy harm to the ecclesiastical state and to religion in the minds of the people." For example, a priest lodged in a religious school had been found dead with a rope around his neck and several self-inflicted knife wounds on his body. Suicide was clearly indicated, and the case was all the more embarrassing because the man had given no indication of insanity. To avoid scandal, the principal of the school sent for the *official* and the prosecutor of the bishop's court. The *official* arrived with the surgeon of the royal court, who wrote up a report and transmitted it to the prosecutor. The latter then called witnesses and launched an inquest regarding "the conduct of the deceased, the situation of his mind during his life, and the circumstances that might have led to this accident." On the basis of one witness's somewhat flimsy testimony, the prosecutor ruled that the man had been insane and authorized his burial in consecrated ground, but with all possible discretion, at night and without bells. The *Recueil* states that there were other similar cases.

Civil and religious authorities in the seventeenth century responded to the questions raised during the years from 1580 to 1620 by condemning and punishing suicide. However, their firm position, which for the most part was aimed at impressing the common people, was undermined, as far as the elite were concerned, by many unspoken notions, by innumerable exceptions, and by a certain number of frank disagreements.

The casuists' distinctions suggested that the culpability of suicide depended on circumstances and intention; the jurists' hesitations highlighted the barbarity of executing cadavers, and their increasingly broad conception of *folie* opened breaches in the wall of penal law; the Church's deliberate dissimulation of ecclesiastical suicides thrust into doubt the seriousness of its statements about eternal damnation for self-homicides. To end the list, the nobility's de facto immunity from prosecution inevitably weakened the prohibition of suicide by making it clear that repression was yet another manifestation of class-defined justice.

Was a right to suicide in fact one more noble privilege? The question is legitimate, given that aristocratic cadavers were not subject to execution in seventeenth-century France. As the Vatel affair shows, the royal court might ignore the 1670 decree. Suicide was forbidden to the Third Estate; it was still excused or permitted for the clergy and the nobility.

The same can be said of England, where generalizations can be backed up by data, thanks to the statistics for the years 1485–1714 gathered by Michael MacDonald and Terence R. Murphy. In a table showing the social status of 6,701 suicides, 67.2 percent of peers and gentlemen were judged guilty of suicide *(felo de se)*, whereas 99 percent of servants and apprentices, 94.1 percent of laborers, 93.5 percent of craftsmen, and 86.6 percent of yeomen were judged guilty. Thus nearly all the apprentices and servants who killed themselves were judged to be aware of what they were doing and responsible for their act, whereas a third of gentlemen suicides were considered mad. Unless we jump to hazardous conclusions about the mental health of the English nobility, we are forced to acknowledge that these verdicts were partial. Injustice is even more obvious during the seventeenth century, since after 1650 only 51.1 percent of gentlemen were convicted of deliberate suicide.[95]

Certain cases display flagrant injustice. On 5 April 1610 the daughter of Henry, Lord Mordaunt threw herself out of a window. Hurt but alive, she tried to drown herself soon after and died five days later, either from her injuries or from an illness contracted during all this. The jury refused to recognize the obvious connection between her suicide attempts and her death, and it ruled that she had died a natural death. In 1622 Thomas Howard, the earl of Berkshire, shot himself with his crossbow, but the royal court put pressure on the coroner to attribute the suicidal gesture to madness, which was done.[96] In 1650 the suicide of Thomas Hoyle, a man who had held several prominent municipal posts in York and was a member of Parliament, went unpunished, thanks to the intervention of influential friends.[97]

Everyone knew that laws on suicide were unequally applied, but not everyone accepted that inequality with equal grace. This meant that extreme discretion was called for. We can see this in the case of Anthony Joyce, a cousin by marriage of Samuel Pepys, the diarist. In January 1668 Joyce tried to drown himself. When he was fished out of the water, "he confessed his doing the thing, being led by the Devil; and doth declare his reason to be his trouble that he found in having forgot to serve God as he ought." He was brought home but fell ill. His friends were "in fear that the goods and estate would be seized on," Pepys writes. The family was panic-stricken: "My cousin [Kate Joyce] did endeavour to remove what she could of plate out of the house, and desired me to take my flagons; which I was glad of, and did take them away with me, in great fear all the way of being seized, though there was no reason for it, he not being dead; but yet so fearful I was." Pepys then went to Whitehall to inform himself as to the law in such cases, where he was told that suicide would entail forfeiture of goods. At that point Joyce died. Pepys acted swiftly:

At their entreaty I presently took coach and to White-hall, and there find W. Coventry and he carried me to the King, the Duke of York being with him, and there told my story which I had told him; and the King without more ado granted that if it was found [self-murder] the estate should be to the widow and children. I presently to each Secretary's office and there left Caveats, and so away back again to my cousin's. . . . And so when I came thither, I found her all in sorrow, but she and the rest mightily pleased with my doing this for them; and endeed, it was a very great courtesy, for people are looking out for the estate, and the Coroner will be sent to and a jury called to examine his death.[98]

In the end everything turned out for the best, thanks to the king's intervention: Joyce was buried in the normal fashion, and there was no forfeiture of property. This affair shows, first, that the suicide's family and friends displayed no moral reprobation and, second, that discretion was needed to avoid hostile or self-interested reactions.

The relative immunity of noble suicides from pursuit was already a familiar tale in 1600, when Shakespeare had one of the gravediggers in *Hamlet* say of Ophelia, "If this had not been a gentlewoman, she should have been buried out o' Christian burial" (act 5, scene 1). A century and a half later, in 1755, the review *Connoisseur* published a satirical article that stated: "A pennyless poor dog . . . may perhaps be excluded from the church yard; but the self-murderer by a pistol genteelly mounted or the Paris-hilted sword qualifies the polite owner for . . . a pompous burial and a monument setting forth his virtues in Westminster Abbey."[99]

Thus the repression of suicide allowed various exceptions. Religious and civil authorities in the seventeenth century reacted to suicide with a combination of severity of principle and selective rigor in application. Behind the façade of an apparently unanimous reprobation, the debate that had been launched in the years from 1580 to 1620 continued. At the same time, however, substitutes for suicide and spiritual antidotes to suicide were being developed.

SEVEN

Substitutes for Suicide in the Seventeenth Century

Despite the prohibition of suicide and beyond the discussions of it as a moral and ethical problem, men and women continued to kill themselves in the seventeenth century at a rate that seems to have been roughly the same as in the previous age. Discourse on suicide has little effect on events. People do not kill themselves in relation to the numbers of treatises of theology, morality, or law that are published, but according to their own sufferings, fears, and frustrations. The seventeenth century—France's "Grand Siècle"—was no more an exception to that rule than other centuries. Still, beginning in the 1580s, there was more talk about self-homicide, which gave contemporaries the impression that the number of suicides had grown. An anonymous tract published in England in 1647 declared that drownings and hangings had become so frequent that no one paid attention to them any more, and a few years later William Denny wrote that his ears "tingled" with all the suicide stories he heard in London.[1]

Suicides: Stable Numbers

London provides an example of how rumors amplified people's impressions of the number of suicides. Beginning in the early seventeenth century the city government, worried about the growing death rate due to epidemics, published a weekly list of deaths on which it also noted the reasons for such "casualties." These were the bills of mortality, which were first produced during epidemics of the plague, but later at regular intervals. This means that we have available weekly listings of suicides, parish by parish, that tell how many of these deaths were attributed to madness and what was the profession of the deceased. They also provide opportunities for syntheses and extrapolation of annual totals. Such lists were printed in the newspapers in London and in the provinces. Even beyond the figures they provide, the simple existence of these lists creates an impression of frequency: People got used to the idea of suicide and were struck by its regularity; it seemed an integral part of Londoners' habits. The phenomenon developed further in the eighteenth century, when it provided a basis for the myth of an "English malady." Such statistics exist nowhere else—which reinforces the impression that suicide was an English specialty. There were, of course, some surveys taken in some Italian cities in the sixteenth century, in France between 1670 and 1684, in Leipzig in 1676, and in Stuttgart in 1692, but they did not show the cause of death.[2]

The bills of mortality were exploited as early as the mid-seventeenth century by the first genuine demographer in England, John Graunt, who, incidentally, grumbled at their inaccuracy.[3] According to Graunt, persons not interred in cemeteries (stillborn infants and suicides) were much under-reported. That notion was confirmed later (in 1726) by Isaac Watts, who extended the underreporting to drowned persons.[4] Of those listed by Graunt, how many of the 827 drowned persons, 243 persons found dead in the street, 14 persons poisoned, 51 persons dead of inanition, and 158 cases of madness were in reality suicides? Certainly many of the drownings must have been suicides. Families' tendencies to dissimulate and parish clerks' failure to report deaths add to the uncertainty, but one fact is sure: The published figures are far lower than the actual numbers.

John Graunt covers the years from 1629 to 1660. During that time London averaged 15 suicides per year, with unexplained high points, as in 1660, a year of 36 voluntary deaths. Is there any connection between these suicides and the change of regime that occurred that year, when the restoration of the monarchy may have put an end to the hopes of some Puritans? There is no way to tell. In terms of the total population of London, the suicide rate was somewhat over 3 per 100,000, a rate that is probably much lower than the real case. Still, in spite of their deficiencies, the bills of mortality at least permit us to draw up averages for each decade, from which we can state that the suicide rate in London remained nearly constant until 1680–90, increasing spectacularly during the second European crisis of conscience.

Other sources are purely anecdotal, which means that they suggest motives for suicide. In England the most reliable source of data, the registers of suicides brought before the King's Bench, peters out, then stops completely in 1660. We can see from these records, however, that the number of cases of suspected suicide reported to that court fluctuated with the vicissitudes of politics: 780 suicides are registered in the decade 1620–29, the last decade of peace, when the monarchy could still put relatively effective pressure on coroners and juries. A total of 532 suicides occurred in 1630–39, and there were 356 in 1640–49, during the Civil War, when the disorganization of the administration is reflected in patchy record keeping. Between 1650 and 1659, during Cromwell's protectorate, 720 suicides are recorded (although a smaller proportion of suspected suicides were judged *felo de se*).[5]

Throughout the seventeenth century coroners' juries that were called for inquests regarding presumed suicide constantly opposed forfeiture of goods to the crown, which they considered an unjust spoliation. Such juries were composed of members of the village and local communities, and they frequently worked in concert to dissimulate the greater part of a suicide's wealth, as we can see in many suits brought by royal justice against the next of kin of the deceased and even against the coroners. The means of dissimulation most frequently used were gross undervaluation of the property of the deceased and attribution to the suicide of debts (which had to be settled before the forfeiture could take place) of greater worth than the holdings. Verdicts of natural death were at times given in the face of clear evidence. In 1598 in Norwich, for instance, John Wilkins, a grocer, slit his throat and died a week later. Three surgeons and a physician testified at the inquest that his wound was not mortal, and the jury sustained the notion that Wilkins had died of an illness contracted before his attempted suicide. Michael MacDonald and Terence R. Murphy give as their personal favorite suicide disguised as an accident that of "a man who allegedly fell on his knife while playing football."[6]

The local community resented it even more when the crown delegated forfeited property to a lord, who often had no scruples about leaving the suicide's family destitute. In 1666 in Essex manorial officials fined the village of Witham £15 because 15s.6d. had been held back from the forfeiture and given to the widow of a suicide.[7]

Under the authoritarian regimes of James I and Charles I, the royal administration became more attentive to details, which meant that fewer suspected voluntary homicides were ruled not guilty. The proportion of more lenient decisions rises sharply with the fall of the monarchy, during the decade 1650–60, when many raised their voices to demand the abolition of forfeiture in suicide cases. John March wrote in 1651, "I think there cannot be a more rigid and tyrannical Law in the world, that the children should thus extremely suffere for the crime and wickedness of the Father; the innocent for the nocent."[8] Reform projects (time was lacking to put them into effect before the Restoration) argued restricting forfeiture to cases of suicides among accused or sentenced criminals.

The seventeenth century saw relatively few celebrity suicides, and when well-known people did away with themselves it was for a broad variety of reasons. In 1641 the painter Domenico Zampieri, known as Domenichino, poisoned himself to escape his enemies. In 1647 Uriel Acosta, a Portuguese Jew settled in Amsterdam and a restless spirit gnawed by religious doubts who had shifted several times between Judaism and Catholicism (and was thus the target of persecution from both sets of coreligionists), shot himself with a pistol. In 1654 Simon Bourne, imprisoned in Worcester Castle and sentenced to being drawn and quartered, poisoned himself. Miles Sindercome, who had attempted to assassinate Cromwell, did the same, explaining in a suicide note, "I take this course, because I would not have all the open shame of the World executed upon my Body."[9] His followers saluted him as a new Càto and a new Brutus. In 1664 the writer Nicolas Perrot d'Ablancourt, a tortured soul who had translated Latin works, starved himself to death in what was perhaps one of the first examples of philosophical suicide motivated by weariness with life.

On 2 August 1667 the great Italian baroque artist Francesco Borromini threw himself on his sword after burning some of his drawings. "A bachelor, a melancholic man of a paranoid pride and sensitivity, Borromini had a high awareness of his art," wrote Claude Mignot, who went on to attribute Borromini's act to "a fit of paranoiac madness."[10] This was the suicide of a tormented artist obsessed by a search for natural harmony and imbued with jealousy of his rivals, Bernini in particular. In 1671 we have the suicide of Vatel, the *maître d'hôtel* who took his honor so to heart (see chapter 6), and of Sir Henry North, a man of a melancholy temperament from an illustrious English family, who never recovered from the death of his wife.

Suicide and Plague

The raw numbers for suicides in England rose sharply during times of poor harvests and higher food prices in 1638 and 1639,[11] but the rise was even steeper during epidemics of plague. Fear, despair, and certainty of contagion unhinged people's minds and pushed many to put an end to their days. This phenomenon was noted in Milan during the plague of 1630 and in Málaga at mid-century, where one physician reported that "unparalleled horrors" had taken place. "There was one woman who buried herself alive to avoid being eaten by animals, and one man who, after burying his daughter, built a coffin for himself and died at her side."[12]

Daniel Defoe analyzed suicidal reactions in a time of plague when an epidemic struck London in 1665. His *Journal of the Plague Year* is not, strictly speaking, a historical chronicle, but rather a study of the behavior of people placed in the mortal ghetto of a large city visited by an epidemic. After only a few days, discouragement and fatalism brought many to abandon all precautions, which amounted to indirect suicide:

The People were brought into a Condition of despair of Life and abandon themselves, so this very Thing had a strange Effect among us for three or four Weeks, that is, it made them bold and venturous, they were no more shy of one another, or restrained within Doors, but went any where and every where, and began to converse; one would say to another, I do not ask you how you are, or say how I am, it is certain we shall all go, so 'tis no Matter who is sick or who is sound, and so they run desperately into any Place or any Company. As it brought the People into publick Company, it was surprizing how it brought them to crowd into the Churches; they inquir'd no more into who they sat next to, or far from . . . but looking upon themselves all as so many dead Corpses, they came to the Churches without the least Caution, and crowded together, as if their Lives were of no Consequence.[13]

Other Londoners preferred direct suicide, by drowning in particular, a death that was not listed on the bills of mortality. Defoe states:

I believe it was never known to this Day how many People in their Diliriums drowned themselves in the *Thames*. . . . As to those which were set down in the Weekly Bill, they were indeed few; nor cou'd it be known of any of those, whether they drowned themselves by Accident or not: But I believe, I might reckon up more who, within the compass of my Knowledge or Observation, really drowned themselves in that Year, than are put down in the Bill of all put together, for many of the Bodies were never found, who, yet were known to be so lost; and the like in other Methods of Self-Destruction. There was also One Man in or about *Whitecross-street,* burned himself to Death in his Bed. (200)

Defoe also reports scenes of collective delirium leading to suicide:

People in the Rage of the Distemper, or in the Torment of their Swelling, which was indeed intollerable, [could be seen] running out of their own Government, raving and distracted, and oftentimes laying violent Hands upon themselves, throwing themselves out at their Windows, shooting themselves, &c. . . . Some broke out into the Streets, perhaps naked, and would run directly down to the River, if they were not stopt by the Watchmen, or other Officers, and plunge themselves into the Water, wherever they found it. . . . It was known to us all, that abundance of poor dispairing Creatures, who had the Distemper upon them, and were grown stupid, or melancholly by their Misery, as many were, wandred away into the Fields, and Woods, and into secret uncouth Places, almost any where to creep into a Bush, or Hedge, and DIE. (100, 122)

The law was as rigorous as always, and forfeiture of property awaited families, especially if the estate was a large one. Defoe says of a rich merchant and deputy alderman who had hanged himself: "I care not to mention the Name, tho' I knew his Name too, but that would be an Hardship to the Family, which is now flourishing again" (99).

Waves of suicide were obviously exceptional and the result of extraordinary circumstances—here, the near certitude of a horrible death. Just as infrequent are instances of collective suicide from fear that the world was coming to an end, such as those noted in certain parts of Russia around 1666.[14]

Dueling as a Substitute for Suicide

One type of suicide that was rare in the seventeenth century—and this might seem to contradict the ethic of the *honnête homme*—was noble suicide for reasons of honor. In practice, the aristocratic code offered dueling as an effective substitute for killing oneself. Theologians and moralists were not fooled, and they included the practice in their anathemas on suicide. Canon 19 of the twenty-fifth session of the Council of Trent forbade dueling and refused burial in Christian soil to duelists; the reasons for the measure were the risks of committing homicide (of oneself or of one's adversary) and of dying unprepared. In 1574 Jean Benedicti, in *La somme des pechez, et le remède d'iceux,* qualified dueling as a "sin against hope." Often the only way to save one's honor was by being killed, as La Châtaigneraie demonstrated in 1547 when he tore off his bandages and died of a hemorrhage after his duel with Jarnac.

The mania for duels culminated in the period from 1600 to 1660, despite all the civil and religious laws prohibiting it. Thirty to forty duels per year took place in France, and as many in England, and these figures are doubtless well under the real ones. "In duelling, which is suicide, the hero eliminates himself," François Billacois remarked.[15] It was also during this period that large numbers of manuals on dueling appeared, and many of their authors compared dueling and suicide for the similarity of the states of mind of the adversaries: In questions of honor only blood, and blood shed voluntarily, could efface a fault. Dueling, like suicide, was a desperate and prideful solution, a refusal to acknowledge responsibility before men for a weakness, an error, or a shortcoming. Pierre Boissat qualified duels as a "sort of despair" in his *Recherches sur les duels* (1610), and in 1618 Charles Bodin in his *Discours contre les duels* spoke of "furious and desperate passion." The 1670 Ordonnance criminelle stipulated that the same procedures applied to those who died in a duel and to suicides. A good many of the thousands of men who died in duels in the sixteenth and seventeenth centuries probably used dueling as a palliative for suicide—a more elegant, more noble way to kill themselves.

Ecclesiastical, political, and judiciary discourses seem, in the final analysis, to have had little effect on people's minds. Nor did theological and moral treatises, legislation, and even penal sanctions have much influence on suicide rates. Although condemnations, repressive measures, and threats of eternal punishment continued to rain down on would-be suicides, people continued to kill themselves in reaction to woes, suffering, frustration, and feelings of remorse or dishonor. What hold could threats of hell have when people thought life worse than hell? Suicide will disappear when its causes disappear—that is, when the earth is a paradise and happiness reigns undivided. Until that day, it is illusory to believe that reasoning or laws can have any effect on desperate people. What arguments are there to persuade someone whose ultimate argument is that he or she would be better off dead? Suicide is an act unlike any other because those who commit it place themselves out of reach of all human power. Divine power remains, but people in the grip of despair who decide to kill themselves either do not reflect, cannot imagine any situation worse than their own, are persuaded that divine pardon will be theirs, think themselves damned in any case, or are insane. Suicide falls outside usual norms. The entire and powerless arsenal of laws and anathemas has no hold on reality; it is like a machine turning in the void, a sword striking a blow in water, a cannonade aimed at a ghost.

Taking Refuge in Literature

The debate that the political and religious authorities thought they had settled nonetheless continued. It was particularly lively in literature, which often presented suicide in a favorable light. French classical tragedies often resolve conflicts of values with the protagonist's voluntary and heroic death. Pierre Corneille uses this device on several occasions: In *Polyeucte* the eponymous hero dies for his faith; Mécénée in *La Thébaïde* and Dricée in *Oedipe* sacrifice themselves for others; Arsinoé in *Nicomède* kills herself to avoid being executed; Antiochus in *Rodogune* prefers "the glory of death" to being put in irons; Mandane in *Agésilas* commits suicide to avoid falling into enemy hands. Othon and his daughter Plautine kill themselves, claiming "that noble despair so worthy of the Romans" (*Othon,* act 1, scene 3). *Le Cid* is the prime example of dueling as a substitute for suicide. Don Diègue tells his son, charging Rodrigue with avenging the paternal honor:

> Ce n'est que dans le sang qu'on lave un tel outrage,
> Meurs ou tue

(Only in blood can one wash away such an outrage: die or kill.)

(*Le Cid*, act 1, scene 5)

Rodrigue, weighing his dilemma, thinks first of suicide:

> Il vaut mieux courir au trépas.
>
> . . .
>
> Allons, mon âme; et puisqu'il faut mourir,
> Mourons au moins sans offenser Chimène

(Better to rush to death. . . . Up, my soul; and since I must die, let me at least die without offending Chimene.)　　　　　　　(*Le Cid*, act 5, scene 5)

Then, changing his mind, Rodrigue decides to die fighting:

> Que je meure au combat, ou meure de tristesse,
> Je rendrai mon sang pur comme je l'ai reçu

(Whether I die in combat or die of sorrow, I will give up my blood as pure as I received it.)　　　　　　　　　　(*Le Cid*, act 5, scene 5)

In Corneille, suicide is also a means for making amends for one's crimes. Cinna, pushed against his will to assassinate Auguste (Augustus), declares:

> Mais ma main, aussitôt contre mon sein tournée,
>
> . . .
>
> A mon crime forcé joindra mon châtiment,
> Et par cette action dans l'autre confondue,
> Recouvrera ma gloire aussitôt que perdue

(But as soon as my hand is turned against my breast, it will join my punishment to my forced crime, and by that act, merged into the other, will immediately restore my honor.)　　　　　　　　　　　　(*Cinna*, act 3, scene 4)

In literature, suicide is also a recourse when love seems impossible. After he has killed the count, Rodrigue decides to let himself be killed by Don Sanche, given that he can no longer hope to win Chimène. In all such cases, voluntary death is presented as a courageous resolution that brings glory to heroes and redeems the wicked. Seventeenth-century French tragedy, which was for the most part aimed at a noble public, confirms that moral principle in complete contradiction to Christian doctrine and law. Albert Bayet presents a large number of examples to illustrate this point, drawn from the plays of Florent

Chrestien, Alexandre Hardy, Antoine de Lafosse, Jean de Mairet, Jean de Rotrou, Isaac de Benserade, Jean de La Chapelle, Joseph Lagrange-Chancel, Jacques Pradon, Tristan L'Hermite, Georges Scudéry, Augustin Nadal, Jean Boissin de Gallardon, Claude Billard, and Jean-Galbert de Campistron.[16] Bayet's accumulation of citations is convincing: On the stage, suicide was a glorious act whose praises are sung in vigorous alexandrines:

> Depuis que le malheur étouffe l'espérance,
> L'homme doit courageux malgré l'inique sort
> Ce qu'il ne peut ici le trouver dans la mort

(Since misfortune stifles hope, man, courageous despite iniquitous fate, must find in death what he cannot find here.)[17]

> Quand l'espérance est morte, il faut cesser de vivre,
> Et vraiment il sied mal aux esprits généreux
> De faire état du jour quand ils sont malheureux

(When hope is dead one must cease living, and truly it ill becomes generous souls to value the light of day when they are unhappy.)[18]

> Les hommes courageux meurent quand il leur plaît

(Courageous men die when it pleases them.)[19]

> La mort se donne à ceux que la crainte rend blêmes,
> Et les plus assurés se la donnent eux-mêmes

(Death is given to those made pale by fear, and the most self-possessed give it to themselves.)[20]

> . . . On doit quitter la vie
> Dès qu'on ne la peut garder sans infamie

(One should leave life as soon as one cannot keep it without infamy.)[21]

> Quand on perd ce qu'on aime, il faut cesser de vivre

(When one loses what one loves one should stop living.)[22]

After dozens of examples of glorious suicides clearly praised by the authors and admired by the public, the few phrases in the plays about "mad designs," "shameful despair," and a "criminal attempt" did not bear much weight.

Suicide reaches its greatest tragic intensity in the works of Jean Racine, where the Jansenist spirit launches an ambiguous dialectic vacillating between extreme religious rigor and absolute despair. Racine's heroines Andromaque, Junie, Bérénice, and Phèdre embody true Jansenist heroism, which refuses all compromise, all half-measures, and all human limitation, and aspires to the absolute. It was an attitude that could lead only to death. Death is the logical point of arrival of religious rigor, and withdrawal from the world is only a palliative and a temporary substitute for it. This means that we will have to return later to the tragic atmosphere of Racine's tragedies, which differed so fundamentally from the dramas of his contemporaries.

Seventeenth-century novels reflect many of the same values as the plays. In these noble tales, suicide is a moral duty for all characters who face an impossible situation. Novels mention the Christian prohibition of suicide more often than plays do, but they often refer to Christianity as an excuse for a character who remains alive when noble conduct would dictate death, or as a notion to be set aside courteously in favor of a heroic resolve to die. At times novels state that divine mercy is sure to pardon an unhappy hero. The world of the novel fully illustrates the conception of the double moral standard that had already been tacitly admitted in ancien régime society. To one side there was ordinary morality, strict, meticulous, and destined for the common people, who need to be guided, controlled, and supervised. Incapable of judging for themselves, the people have to be kept within narrow limits, for fear of uprisings. To the other side there was an aristocratic moral code, on a level above ordinary prohibitions, for well-born souls whose spiritual refinement enabled them to discern the limits of good and evil in a given case. Such people were animated by noble designs; their conduct transcended the ordinary prohibitions, because they acted on the basis of superior motivations incomprehensible to the prosaic mass. Even more than was true in real life, novels discriminated between one sort of suicide and another: The suicide of the peasant who hanged himself to put an end to his misery was an act of reprehensible and vile cowardice; the suicide of the noble who ran himself through with his sword for the beautiful eyes of a marquise was a heroic act worthy of a superior soul and one that God himself would not dream of punishing.

The novels of Mademoiselle de Scudéry illustrate this double standard. Innumerable characters declare their intention to kill themselves. In *Ibrahim* the heroine, Isabelle, is perfectly aware of the Christian prohibition on suicide, but at no moment does she consider obeying it as she proclaims her determination to put an end to her days if she loses her lover. Hers is a typically aristocratic reaction: She is above the usual prohibitions and hence can be punished only by God. She states, "If my despair is a fault, I hope that [heaven] will pardon it for the greatness of my misfortune, the purity of my affection, and my own weakness."[23]

In novel after novel, noble heroes commit suicide with the best conscience in the world and for a wide variety of excellent reasons. Women do so to save their honor. As Florinisse says in Pierre d'Ortigue de Vaumorière's *L'inceste innocent* (1638): "It is a thousand times better to lose one's life without stain than to preserve it after such a shameful disgrace."[24] Persons innocent of a crime of which they have been accused kill themselves to escape the infamy of conviction and punishment; the defeated do so to escape dishonor; victims of guilty passions do so gnawed by remorse; lovers do so when they are rejected or their love is impossible; generous souls do so to save their kin. Here again, the reader is referred to the myriad examples in Albert Bayet's study of suicide and morality.[25]

Some authors went so far as to have their characters give a detailed justification of their act, often a reasoned mini-treatise explaining why suicide was the most noble solution in a specific situation. In *L'Illustre Amalazonthe* (1645), Des Fontaines has the king of Marseilles argue for ten pages that to live would be an act of cowardice. In 1630 Merille, the author of *La Polixène,* has his heroine explain that when all hope is gone, suicide is an act of reason, not of despair: "So that no one may believe that despair had more power over me than reason, I beg of everyone who may hear of my death to reflect whether my life could permit me to prolong it further." In his *Cléopâtre* (1661) La Calprenède puts eloquent words justifying suicide into the mouth of his heroine. She sweeps away objections to an "irreparable offense toward heaven" and a possible display of cruelty "to all nature" to state that the only reason she is being urged to live is "to offend me by thinking me capable of being consoled." Gomberville has Cythérée, the heroine of the novel of the same name (1627), scornfully reject her father's argument that religion prohibits suicide: "It is of no use to try to combat my just despair with arguments that unhappy, timid people have invented as an excuse for their cowardice. I want to die. I must do so, and the gods, who are just, cannot disapprove what justice dictates to me." It would be hard to find a clearer statement that the prohibition of suicide applied only to the mass of ordinary people. The remark recalls Shakespeare:

> For conscience is a word that cowards use,
> Devis'd at first to keep the strong in awe.
> (*Richard III,* act 5, scene 3)

On occasion, the religious argument does manage to keep a fictional character from committing suicide, but it is always without enthusiasm that they resign themselves to living, and they seldom fail to present their apologies to the reader, declaring that if it were up to them they would rush to their deaths without hesitation. These works of fiction present the religious prohibition as a categorical obstacle incompatible with heroism and as a humiliation unknown to pagans. "If only I were not a Christian, I would be happy to kill myself!" is in substance what François Eudes de Mézeray has the chevalier d'Orasie say in a novel published in 1646. "It is because I am Christian that I do not kill myself," Placidie declares after a forced marriage with a man she does not love in La Calprenède's *Faramond* (1651); her lover, Constance, declares that he too would have killed himself a thousand times "if fear of heaven, which he had always revered, had not retained him." These are extraordinary statements, in which the Christian prohibition is presented in a purely negative form, as the moral code of the weak, which heroes can transgress. It was an attitude foreshadowing Nietzsche.

Philosophical and Moral Debate

Novelists and playwrights expressed themselves more as psychologists than as sociologists when they placed their characters in quite specific situations and demanded a superhuman moral system, including a right to suicide, for heroes who rose above the common sort. When we come back down to earth, we see that opinion was much more reserved. Authors, philosophers, essayists, and moralists whose viewpoints were far from those of traditional theology nonetheless shared the churches' hostility to suicide. Their reasons, of course, were quite different from the religious ones, but their conclusions matched those of the religious and civil authorities, and when their arguments required it, they did not hesitate to borrow weapons from the theological arsenal.

Thomas Hobbes, whose situation was more than delicate regarding established religion, was a firm adversary of suicide. It is true that he refers uniquely to natural law and reason when he says in *Leviathan* (1651): "A law of nature, *lex naturalis,* is a precept or a general rule, found out by reason, by which a man is forbidden to do that, which is destructive of his life, or taketh away the means of preserving the same; and to omit that, by which he thinketh it may be best preserved."[26] Hobbes barely scratches the surface of the subject here: For a theoretician of the absolute power of the state, suicide poses no problem. The state cannot tolerate the desertion of members of the civil community since, once admitted, that might well lead to the disorganization and ruin of the whole. Subjects owe total allegiance to the service of the Leviathan.

René Descartes, Hobbes's contemporary and, like him, a man whose relations with authority were delicate, was also an adversary of suicide, but for different reasons. It is in his correspondence between 1645 and 1647 with Elisabeth, princess of Bohemia, that he expresses his thoughts on the matter. Descartes's approach corresponds to what we know of his personality: Throughout his life he was guided by prudence and reason. A philosopher who preferred to remove his treatise, *Du monde,* from among his papers when he learned of Galileo's condemnation, who put his love of tranquility ahead of his scientific opinions, and who spoke of himself as a person "who so passionately loves repose that he wants to avoid even the shadow of anything that might trouble it,"[27] Descartes was certainly not the sort of man to rush headlong into death without having a "clear and evident" idea of what was waiting for him on the other side. In the final analysis, Descartes's position is quite close to Hamlet's. Is it reasonable to risk the voyage toward "the un-discover'd country from whose bourn no traveler returns"? Descartes agreed with Hamlet: "For in that sleep of death what dreams may come, / When we have shuffl'd off this mortal coil, / Must give us pause." To be sure, this life is not always happy, but it has some consolations, and it is even possible that the sum of good things outweighs the bad; above all, we know what we have to deal with here, whereas the next world is shrouded in mystery; to kill oneself in the hope of a better fate is therefore to throw away the prey for the shadow, the certain for the uncertain and dubious. Yes, the Church affirms a certain number of things regarding the next world, but reason tells us nothing about it. In the absence of mathematical proofs, it is wiser to remain in this world and endure our petty miseries. Descartes advised Elisabeth in a letter dated 3 November 1645:

Regarding the state of the soul after this life, I have much less knowledge about the subject than M. d'Igby, for, leaving aside what faith teaches us, I confess that, by natural reason alone, we can make many conjectures to our advantage and have fine hopes but no assurance. And because that same natural reason also teaches us that we always have more good than bad things in this life and that we should not leave off the certain for the uncertain, it seems to me that it teaches us that we must not truly fear death, but that we must also never seek it.

Several weeks earlier, on 6 October of the same year, Descartes had written to the same correspondent:

It is true that knowledge of the immortality of the soul and of the felicities it will be capable of once we are out of this life might provide those who are bored with life with a reason to quit it, if they were assured that afterward they would enjoy all those felicities, but no reason assures them of it, and there is only the false philosophy of

Hegesias . . . that tries to persuade us that this life is bad. Real life, to the contrary, teaches us that even among the saddest accidents and the most pressing sorrows one can always find contentment, providing one knows how to use reason.[28]

With Descartes we are far from grand principles, lyrical flights on the nobility of voluntary death, or acceptance of the trials God sends us. For him, suicide seems to become a shopkeeper's calculation: He answers Hamlet's question by presenting a scales to weigh the terrestrial pleasures that reason, used wisely, can furnish us against our woes. Since we can add nothing to the balance regarding the next world, which is wrapped in total uncertainty, let us remain in this life! That is the decision of reason and good sense. Elisabeth objected that there are nonetheless people who kill themselves. "They do so," Descartes responded in January 1646, "because of an error in their understanding, not out of a carefully reasoned judgment."[29]

Although Descartes does not explicitly say so, by this reasoning he would have considered Lucretius, Cato, Brutus, and the other classical suicides to have been fools. To die for ideas is not smart. Of all the adversaries of suicide whom we have encountered, Descartes is the most modest, the most restful, and the most reassuring. He reasons on the basis of known and verifiable givens rather than by abstract principles always subject to caution, always challenged, and always subject to an act of faith, which is risky. Until Descartes, the debate on suicide was carried on in the name of God, nature, the state, society, and honor—words on whose meaning even specialists failed to agree. Descartes reasons in function of what anyone can see and feel (*les évidences,* he called them), and he concludes that it is more reasonable not to kill oneself. His arguments never take religious doctrine into account; he rejects religion from the start because its tenets cannot be proven. For Descartes, suicide is a problem not of morality but of reason. To kill oneself is to commit an error, not a sin. This obviously makes criminal penalties unnecessary, since those who commit an error punish themselves.

Hobbes was opposed to suicide in the name of the state, Descartes, in the name of reason, but neither man devoted more than a few lines to the topic in their works. Opposition to voluntary self-homicide received unexpected support from circles close to the libertines, who argued in the name of nature. Thus the atomist Pierre Gassendi, disagreeing with his master Epicurus, stated that when nature gave us a love of life, it forbade suicide. Killing oneself is a perverse act that insults nature and nature's author.[30] La Mothe Le Vayer also spoke of an offense to nature, "depraved senses," and "great cowardice," and he considered it legitimate to refuse Christian burial to suicides.[31] The philosophic manuals of Scipion Dupleix, Jacques Du Roure, Théophraste Bouju, Pierre Bardin, René Bary, and Pierre Du Moulin contain the same arguments.

Other writers defended more supple points of view, particularly in England, where even before the Civil War a revival of Stoic philosophy influenced preachers. Sir Thomas Browne deplored this tendency; according to him, they "allow a man to be his owne *Assassine,* and so highly extoll the end and suicide of *Cato.*"[32] During the Civil War and the interregnum, when the decline in censorship permitted a flurry of very daring writings, quite a few works challenged the condemnation of suicide.

In 1656 Walter Charleton, a somewhat unorthodox churchman, formerly physician to Charles I, and a friend of Hobbes, published an edition of Epicurus' *Morals* with a long commentary in which he discussed, but did not resolve, the conflict between the Christian and the Stoic systems of morality. As a Christian, he writes, "I hold [Epicurus' view of suicide] to be a bloody and detestable opinion, because expressly repugnant to the *Law* of *God.*" As a "meere *Philosopher,*" Charleton continues, he recognizes that people are free to commit "Selfe-Homicide in case of intolerable and otherwise inevitable Calamity." The law of nature requires that we seek good and avoid evil; hence when life becomes evil, suicide is "an absolute accomplishment of the Law of Self-praeservation."[33]

In 1665 George Mackenzie published a treatise on the Stoics in which he attacked suicide, but with a highly contradictory argument. God, he states, did not prohibit suicide in the Bible because he knew that men's aversion for death was enough of a deterrent. Mackenzie writes in another passage, however, that if God did not speak of suicide, it was to avoid giving humankind the idea. Finally, he states that no suicide mentioned in the Bible is explicitly condemned.[34]

Hence the debate continued. At times it was even reflected in government publications. The *Questions traitées ès conférences du Bureau d'Adresses* indicates that in 1635 there was official discussion of the legitimacy of suicide. The arguments that the adversaries and partisans of voluntary death put forth are not original, but the speeches were clearly impassioned. Among the adversaries we find the notions of suicide as a sin against nature, of the soldier who must not abandon his post, and of the need for courage to bear all woes. Among the partisans we find the demands of honor, heroic examples from ancient Rome, and references to captains who blow themselves up with their ship (and who are more admirable than cowardly captains who surrender). Those who think their suicide would weaken the state have an overly high opinion of themselves, as no one is indispensable.[35] This discussion, which lasted several hours, arrived at no conclusions. That it even took place none-theless shows that the topic was in the air.

Spiritual "Annihilation" as a Religious Substitute for Suicide

From the beginning of the seventeenth century, even religious life was touched by the temptation to voluntary death. As with dueling for the no-bility, certain forms of spirituality presented a troubling kinship with the desire to commit suicide, to the point that they can be regarded as substitutes for or antidotes to suicide. The very particular forms of spirituality born of the Catholic Reform early in the seventeenth century, at the epicenter of the crisis of Christian conscience and just when the question of voluntary death reached a height, contain ambiguities that cannot be coincidental. Many sensitive souls in those times of cultural disarray rejected the world; for some this took the form of suicide, for others, that of mysticism or total withdrawal from society. The same hatred of the world that underlay these avoidance behaviors emerged with violence in the writings of spiritual authors. Father Jacques Nouet thundered, "What, then, is it that pleases you in this vale of tears? Answer again: Why do you love life?" Saint-Cyran echoed him: "As for this mortal life, one must be sick at soul and possessed by some evil passion to love it." Pasquier Quesnel concluded, quite logically, that death is the greatest good we could desire: "It is easier for a true Christian to love death and make it his delight than to love life and find it his pleasure and his joy. . . . Death is my good, my advantage, and my delight."[36]

Declarations of this sort are legion in seventeenth-century spiritual texts. The ideal Christian life rests on an extremely precarious equilibrium: The spiritual individual detests the world and life, aspires to death and to the next world, but is prohibited from crossing that threshold by himself. Living in the world but refusing all its pleasures, the spiritually inclined are like the living dead and must approach death as closely as possible without inducing it. This spirituality was based on a doctrine of "annihilation," which is in reality a substitute for voluntary death and a genuine spiritual suicide. We find this doctrine in all the great mystics and spiritual writers of the early seventeenth century, but at times their writings have a troubling resonance.

The great Pierre de Bérulle (1575–1629), one of the founders of the French spiritual movement, preached inner death, the destruction of all that is our own being, in particular of our intellectual and spiritual faculties, in order to leave room for God. We must, he wrote, "be disappropriated and annihilated, and appropriated to Jesus, subsisting in Jesus, grafted onto Jesus, living in Jesus, operating in Jesus." We must cease to live in ourselves to enable Jesus to live in us; we must become veritable "cadavers," inert instruments animated by the divine spirit. God wants our life to be destroyed "by his own life; he wants us to come out of [life] in order to enter into his life. . . . [He wants] us to die in ourselves; and, while we wait for death to arrive, he wants us to die in spirit, to be in a spirit of death in our own eyes and in those of the present century."[37]

Bérulle described his own experience of the "annihilation of oneself," as he called it: "I resolved to rid myself of all use of myself, both of the spiritual faculties of the soul and of the senses, and to succeed to such a degree that the soul no longer feels itself, where it has nothing, nor any longer wants anything of the self, and where it does not even take the jurisdiction and authority of disposing of itself for the good." At the end of this process, the individual person is as good as dead: "We are dead, and we have no true life but with Jesus Christ in God."[38]

Spirituality shared with physical suicide a rejection of the world, of personal life, and of individual conscience; a desire to merge with the great all that some call nothingness and others call God; and a total effacement of self. Father Charles de Condren (1588–1641), a disciple of Bérulle, carried the analogy even further. From the age of twelve he was inhabited by a desire to sacrifice himself, to immolate himself as Isaac was nearly immolated by Abraham. All his life he was obsessed by a desire for annihilation. His *Lettres spirituelles* are full of such expressions as these: we must "destroy ourselves"; you must "decide to rid yourself of everything you are," "dispossess yourself of your nature," and "lose for yourself all desire to live and to be"; "such a death . . . lets God live in you. . . . Let nothingness . . . find a place for its being in you." Henri Bremond remarks that in Condren:

These are not simple [rhetorical] figures or stylistic exaggerations. The death that Condren preaches to us is much more real—or, to put it better, the word *death* only very imperfectly expresses the total annihilation that the asceticism of sacrifice logically pursues. . . . It is true that from that very destruction a new life, superior to the one he has lost, will be born to the victim, but, precisely, what does having a new and superior life mean, if not a life different from our present one?[39]

Is not a new and better life totally different from the present one precisely what a person about to commit suicide is seeking?

We are on the razor's edge. All these similarities, analogies, and comparisons between physical and spiritual death lend themselves to all manner of ambiguities and confusion. Mysticism, which lodges at an unusually deep level of consciousness, is beyond the categories of a superficial, ordinary awareness. At that profound level limits blur, the unconscious emerges into the conscious, the concrete blends with the abstract, prohibitions are consumed in the forge of desire, and the spirit levitates somewhere between heaven and earth, above barriers of morality or the intellect. The partitions between reason's categories begin to dissolve. To how great an extent a troubling and ambiguous divine love and human love are mingled in the ecstasy of female mystics is a familiar story. Similarly, Bérulle's doctrine of annihilation exerted a worrisome fascination for certain perturbed or fragile minds in which tendencies to physical suicide and a yearning for spiritual suicide are hard to disentangle.

Jean-Jacques Olier (1608–57), a disciple of Condren, went through a grave moral crisis during which he stopped eating and saw himself as already dead: "I did not know how to eat: I was almost losing the habit of it, and it seems to me that I was giving food as if to a dead body." Considering himself lost, Olier compared himself to Judas and imagined himself already in hell: "When people spoke of God I conceived of nothing but an annoying, rigorous, and very cruel being. . . . I took pleasure in the thought of hell, and the description of it pleased me as of the place destined for me." Olier's neuroticism and his neurasthenic crisis led Bremond to say of him: "These were frankly morbid phenomena with nothing whatsoever of the mystical about them (but nothing infamous either), which God permits, for ends known only to him, as He permits lightning to set fire to a church."[40]

For a period of five years, Father Jean Rigoleuc thought himself damned too. Jean-Joseph Surin, a Jesuit (1600–1663) suffered from bouts of madness and suicidal neuroticism: "For seven or eight years I had to withstand an impulse to kill myself," he wrote, and he even seriously attempted suicide by throwing himself out of a window. The Society of Jesus, highly embarrassed by his behavior, opposed the publication of some of his odder writings. He spent twenty years in despair, sure of being damned.

Although it took a variety of forms, the spirituality of annihilation inspired quasi-suicidal attitudes throughout the seventeenth century. Father Jean-Chrysostome (1594–1646), the apostle of pure love and founder of a Society of the Holy Abjection, practiced extreme mortification of the flesh and proclaimed the duty of death of the self. Another adept of pure love, Father Alexandre Piny, preached sloughing off everything of this world in an attitude of total acceptance, even of damnation, even at the cost of arriving "within two inches of the uttermost despair."[41] In 1647 Father Louis Chardon recommended a *déformante* catharsis in *La Croix de Jésus*. The way to "form" God was by extinguishing all the "intellectual and animal powers" in us—memory, imagination, knowledge, and will—and by that means "reducing oneself to nothingness." The end result was a sort of spiritual coma that permitted acceptance of Jesus.

Marie Guyart Martin, a young widow who entered the Ursuline Order in 1630 as sister (later mother) Marie de l'Incarnation, illustrates how entering into religion after a personal loss served as a substitute for suicide. Marie's desire to have done with the world was so keen that, after struggling with her conscience, she abandoned her son Claude, who was eleven years old at the time. She wrote to him later, "In separating myself from you now I have given myself a living death." When Claude himself later joined a religious order and his austerities were affecting his health, she overcame her maternal instincts to tell him, "I do not doubt that your bodily strength is diminishing: Your great retirement, the labor of studies, the cares of business, and the austere practices of the rule may be the cause of it, but we live only to die."[42]

For Marie de l'Incarnation, the annihilation of the self led to a state of perfect quietude. The soul that abandons itself to God is in a state "where there is no more anxiety," she wrote in 1666. "I mean, no more desire, but [only] a profound peace, which cannot be altered by experience." Those who annihilate themselves in God rest in peace, for they are dead to themselves and have nothing more to fear.

It is clear that the spirituality of annihilation was in part an evasive behavior, a means for escaping the disquietude and despair that lay in wait for a Christian conscience sensitized by a climate of religious reform. When disquietude was raised to the level of anxiety, it led some to suicide. Others chose to lose themselves (Condren uses the term *se détruire,* "to destroy themselves") in the spirituality of annihilation. Certain damnation could place even the greatest minds at a crossroads. At the age of eighteen, St. François de Sales, who was a restless and melancholic youth, sought perfection and underwent a serious crisis.[43] Despairing of his salvation, he went without sleep and lost his appetite, declining rapidly until he was suddenly cured of his depression in the church of Notre-Dame-des-Grès. St. Jeanne de Chantal went through a similar phase of despair. Sister Madeleine de Saint-Joseph, a Carmelite, swooned at the thought of the torments of hell.

Some were even willing to return to voluntary martyrdom, an old substitute for suicide. In 1604, for example, six Spanish Carmelites who had come to France to establish a house of their order behaved in a deliberately provocative manner as they went through the Calvinist regions of southwest France. A contemporary account states: "Our holy nuns, with the idea of confessing Jesus Christ openly and gaining the inestimable happiness of martyrdom . . . held their crucifixes and rosaries out of the coach window for the people to see!"[44]

Religious disquietude could encourage a "natural inclination to the sovereign good," as François de Sales said; used by the devil, it could also lead to despair.[45] Two remedies were recommended against the bad sort of disquietude that led to suicide: a spirituality of abandonment to God, which was the way to quietude, and the spirituality of action, which was the choice of Bossuet and the Jesuits, who held that when the spirit was busy with efforts to promote good it could regain its equilibrium. Some Jansenists agreed. Pierre Nicole, for instance, stated that "regarding either sin or temptation, one must always avoid a troubling disquietude."[46]

Devout Humanism as a Remedy

During the first third of the seventeenth century, one spiritual current of thought, devout humanism, fought disquietude and despair with particular zeal. This current is a rare example of a smiling, optimistic spirituality and a true antidote to the suicidal urges that had emerged from despairing doctrines of hell and predestination. The devout humanists rehabilitated laughter and used it to chase away the devil. They repeated Rabelais's injunction that "le rire est le propre de l'homme" (laughter is the essence of mankind). Laughter was good; it was healthy. Christians ought to laugh, Father François Garasse wrote in 1624: "There are among the people of this world some minds so warped that when they see a religious laughing they think him a lost soul and a reprobate. . . . But good lord, what do those people want of us? That we weep constantly?"[47] Pierre de Besse was impenitently cheerful: "I have to laugh, to poke fun at things, to play the buffoon, and mock everything."[48] But wasn't it possible to die laughing, or at least to die of joy? This was what the Jesuit Étienne Binet claimed, stating that he came close to having a heart attack when anyone mentioned the love of God: "As poignant as a dagger-stroke to my heart is the mere act of naming the words love, paradise, or my good master, Jesus."[49] In his *Consolation et resjouissance pour les malades et personnes affligées* (1620), Binet attempted to chase away melancholy humors by telling some pious funny stories. According to him, God the Father is a gruff old jokester, a big buddy who will lead us to paradise with big claps on the back: "Paradise, remember, keeps up the mode of ancient Gaul, where it was customary to be at the church door when a couple was being married, to force the bridegroom to the high altar with blows and beating of a drum."[50]

Life's woes are thus friendly pummeling that we should take in good heart. Even original sin is a "happy sin," because without it there would never have been the marvel of Redemption. The incurable optimism of devout humanism admired the goodness of nature, the grandeur of ancient wisdom, and the extraordinary discoveries of the new science. This current of thought reacted positively to the crisis of conscience of the years 1580–1620; the human mind should not be afraid, but rather should welcome the discovery of an infinite world with joy and delight in the perspectives it opened.

The new science should lead us to love life: Devout humanism's enthusiasm for the new discoveries of the scientific revolution of the times was a genuine antidote to black humors, despair, and meditations on suicide. It was probably much more effective as a remedy than the prohibitions and condemnations of voluntary death had been. Yves de Paris, a Capuchin, mocked melancholiac and sad Christians and preached good humor, optimism, and laughter. Like Father Marin Mersenne, Yves asserted that it is not through mortification, but by studying the world as a scholar would that one approaches God. In 1639 Binet published his *Essay des merveilles de nature et des plus nobles artifices,* a sort of encyclopedia of the arts and sciences aimed at furnishing preachers with concrete and accurate examples of natural lore. Binet marveled at the "most rich treasures of eloquence" of the scientific vocabulary.[51] Léon de Saint-Jean, a Carmelite, wrote *Portrait de la sagesse universelle, avec l'idée générale des sciences* (1655).[52] Devout humanists continued to put out works of a reassuring piety, such as the *Consolateur des âmes scrupuleuses* of Guillaume Gazet (1610); *Des miséricordes de Dieu en la conduite de l'homme* of Yves de Paris (1645); *Les justes espérances de nostre salut, opposées au désespoir du siècle* of Jacques d'Autun (1649), a Capuchin; and *La dévotion aisée* of the Jesuit Pierre Le Moyne (1652).

The Jesuit Louis Richeome (1544–1625) proclaimed the joy of the devout soul. Piety, he asserted, is a pleasure, and laughter is a gift of God. We should love life and our bodies, which are beautiful and reflect the beauty of the soul. Body and soul are united like lovers. Death, which separates them, is a drama that Richeome depicted in a moving allegorical poem in dialogue, *L'adieu de l'âme dévote laissant le corps.* Death rends asunder; there is nothing joyful about it, even if it does prepare future happiness. In this view, suicide is an act of folly, of temerity, or of pride. Cato, for example:

killed himself, driven to an extreme by that very sin of pride. For having always fed his soul on the flies of vanity and popular favors, which gave him no substance nor solid reputation; foreseeing that if he were to fall into the hands of Caesar, his enemy, his reputation would decline; beside himself with frustration and despair and unable to endure that rival, he ripped life from his body, taking the remedy of a cowardly soul, despite his seeming valiance, when he disemboweled himself.[53]

After surmounting his crisis of despair, the master of devout humanism, François de Sales (1567–1622), displayed a resolute optimism throughout his works. In both the *Treatise on the Love of God* and the *Introduction to a Devout Life* he devoted several passages to disquietude and sadness. He states:

> Disquietude is the greatest evil that can befall the soul, except sin; for just as seditions and internal troubles in a nation ruin it utterly, and prevent it from being able to resist a foreign invasion, so our heart, when troubled and disquieted, loses its power of maintaining the virtues which it has acquired, and also the means of resisting the temptations of the enemy, who then makes every effort to fish, as they say, in troubled waters.[54]

Disquietude, which comes from an unsatisfied desire to be delivered from an evil or acquire a good, can be used by the devil to lead an individual to despair. It is the individual's duty to notify his or her director of conscience about it immediately.

Sorrow is an ambiguous sentiment; it too calls for vigilance. According to François de Sales, there is a good sadness, which is sent by God and leads to penitence out of regret for one's sins: "May the penitent always sorrow, but always rejoice in his sorrow." On the other hand, "worldly sorrow brings death" (2 Cor. 7.10). Citing Ecclesiastes, he writes, "Sadness hath killed many, and there is no profit in it."[55]

François de Sales gives three causes for the sorrow that can at times lead to suicide:

> Sometimes it comes from the infernal enemy, who by a thousand sad, melancholy, gloomy suggestions darkens the understanding, weakens the will, and disturbs the entire soul. . . . The evil spirit . . . puts in [man's mind] extreme dejection in order to lead it into despair and damnation. . . . Sometimes sadness comes from a man's natural disposition, when the melancholy humor predominates in us. Such sadness is not actually vicious in itself, but our enemy makes great use of it so as to plot and prepare a thousand temptations in our souls. . . . Finally, there is sadness brought upon us by various misfortunes of human life.[56]

The devout were able to moderate that sadness, but in the world it often changed into despair. It then became the devil's instrument, because "the evil one is pleased with sadness and melancholy, because he is sad and melancholy himself, and will be so for all eternity; and therefore he wishes everyone to be like himself."[57]

For François de Sales, the only justification for suicide was "the glory of the truth." The suicides of classical antiquity had no value for him. In a chapter of the *Treatise on the Love of God* devoted to the question, he contests the virtue of the Stoics: How can anyone call people virtuous when they recommend killing oneself when life becomes unbearable? Seneca and others acted purely out of pride and vanity; Lucretius was wrong to kill himself, as St. Augustine showed. As for Cato, he was a desperate man, not a sage. Only the Christian martyrs who died willingly were admirable because they acted neither out of vanity nor out of egotism.

I freely admit, Theotimus, that Cato had a certain firm courage, and that in him such firmness was worthy of praise. But anyone wishing to follow his example must do so in a just and good cause, not by killing himself but by suffering death because true virtue demands this, not out of vainglory but for the glory of the truth. Such was the case with our martyrs who with invincible hearts performed so many miracles of constancy and valor that the Catos, the Horatii, the Senecas, the Lucretias, and the Arrias deserve no consideration in comparison with them.[58]

François de Sales was nonetheless touched to some extent by the morbid ambiguity of the spirituality of mystical detachment. He admitted that spirituality can lead to death, and he had difficulty explaining that such a death is not tantamount to suicide. Mystics, he wrote, do not die of grief, they die because of grief—a somewhat unconvincing distinction.

Among sacred lovers there are some who so completely devote themselves to exercises of divine love that its holy fire devours and consumes their life. Sometimes grief keeps the afflicted from drinking, eating, and sleeping so long that finally they become so weak and ill that they die. Hence people say they die of grief. This is not true, since they die of loss of strength and inanition. However, it remains true that since their weakness arises from grief, we must admit that if they do not actually die of grief, they die because of grief and for grief. Thus, my dear Theotimus, when the ardor of holy love is intense, it makes so many assaults upon the heart, wounds it so many times, causes such languors within it, melts it so constantly, and bears it off into so many raptures and ecstasies that by such means the soul is almost entirely taken up with God. It cannot furnish enough help to nature to ensure proper digestion and nourishment. Little by little the vital animal forces begin to fail, life is cut short, and death ensues. O God, Theotimus, how happy is such a death![59]

It is hard not to see this view as a counteragent to suicide or a substitute for it. Malebranche later shared the same discomfort when he noted the ambiguity of mystical behavior. He states, "We cannot be perfectly united to God without abandoning the interests of the body, without scorning it, sacrificing it, and losing it." How can one avoid the accusation that this was a voluntary death? Malebranche finds this impossible. We cannot unite with God without sacrificing our bodies, but we have no right to sacrifice them. Malebranche simply notes the problem, then smoothly moves on to a completely different issue:

This is not to say that it would be permissible for us to take our own life, nor even to ruin our health. For our body is not ours—it is God's, it is the state's, our family's, our friends'. We ought to conserve it in its strength and vigor, according to the use we are obliged to make of it. But we ought not to conserve it against the order of God and at the expense of other men. We must expose it to danger for the good of the state, and not fear to weaken it, ruin it, or destroy it in order to carry out the orders of God.[60]

The Ambiguity of Jansenism

Where voluntary death was concerned, Jansenism was perhaps the most ambiguous of the spiritual currents born of the crisis of the years 1580–1620. It formally condemned suicide, but replaced it with an ideal for life based on such a strong insistence on the absolute that death was the only way to achieve that ideal, a notion that is illustrated to perfection in the tragedies of Jean Racine. In this sense, the Jansenist ideal was a very unsatisfactory substitute for suicide; it rejected the homicidal act but kept the desire for death, thus generating a perpetual anxiety.

Jansenists categorically rejected the suicide of both pagans and Christians. Pagans were filled with pride and deserved no admiration, Antoine Arnauld said, in substance, and he was unable to imagine the least trace of grandeur in anyone who did not share the Christian faith. He wrote of the death of Diogenes, "All that this story shows is that a creature of glory was prideful unto death." As for Aristotle, it was undeniable that he committed suicide, because that was the fashion "in those miserable centuries of darkness and blindness."[61] Aristotle was damned beyond appeal. Pierre Nicole attacked Cato: "Let the Eulogies and Praises, wherewith the Philosophers, even to envy, heighten and raise the Death of *Cato*, be as great and pompous as they will, 'twas but a real effective weakness that carryed him to that Brutality, which they look on as the height of human generosity." Nicole attempted (somewhat childishly) to ridicule Cato: He was a coward who killed himself because he was afraid to look the emperor in the face. "We ought to say, that out of pittiful weakness he could not stand an Object which all the Women and Children of *Rome* could gaze at without trouble; and that his dread was so violent, that it forced him to leave this life by the greatest of all crimes."[62]

The Jansenists adopted a stand opposed to that of the Jesuit casuists, whom they accused, on this point as on others, of a relaxed morality; by carrying the refinement of distinctions to excess, the Jesuits ended up legitimizing certain suicides. One publication, the *Troisième écrit des curés de Paris,* insinuated that for the Jesuits, reason alone determined whether one could kill oneself. At that point, "could one not say, with even more color, that all the pagans who killed themselves, and especially those who did so only after having asked the magistrates' permission, as was the practice in certain cities, did not violate [the Mosaic] commandment? . . . We discover with horror what strange results can be born of that principle." In 1672 Joannes Sinnichius (John Sinnich) attacked "relaxed opinions" that excused suicide.

Subtlety was not the Jansenists' forte. In their pursuit of the absolute they refused all compromise with low earthly concerns. Pascal's horrified reaction to Montaigne's doubts is a familiar tale: "Montaigne's faults are grievous . . . [as are] his sentiments on suicide, on death. . . . One cannot excuse his wholly heathen sentiments concerning death; for we must say goodbye to piety if we have no desire for at least a Christian death. Now throughout his book he thinks only of a soft and easy death."[63] In the *Entretiens avec M. de Saci,* Pascal attacked Epictetus and the "diabolical pride" that led him to state "that we can kill ourselves when we are so persecuted as to think that God is calling us." The Stoic doctrine on suicide was based in pride.

Pascal was well aware that some people are led to commit suicide by a yearning for happiness: "This is the motivation for all men's acts, including [the acts of] those who are about to hang themselves," he wrote. But did the Jansenists comprehend that their uncompromising attitude and their demand that we limited, weak creatures attain the absolute could only be realized in death? Anyone who truly wanted to play the angel had little choice but to kill himself when he realized that he was playing the beast. And if anyone wanted to play the angel, it was the Jansenists: What could have been more frustrating for them than the implacable limits of human nature? By placing their demands too high, they were destined to perpetual failure. The Jansenists placed themselves at the center of an insoluble contradiction by rejecting voluntary death and by creating such high standards for living that they could only be satisfied by death.

Living in the world but playing no part in it and taking no joy from it was the Jansenist attitude. They set up a radical opposition between God and the world, asserting that it was impossible to transform the world in order to achieve authentic values here below, but that it was forbidden to transform the world in order to take refuge in the divine. The Jansenist's life showed a constant tension between these two irreconcilable extremes. An unbending demand for the absolute could not find contentment in human values, which are always imperfect and imply choice. By withdrawing from the world but remaining among the living, and by his refusal to engage in human enterprises, the Jansenist condemned himself to a profound solitude.

It is quite likely that after the 1620s Jansenism was to some extent a class phenomenon exclusive to the *noblesse de robe* and the high aristocracy, as Lucien Goldmann has so brilliantly argued.[64] This is secondary to our purpose, however. What is important to note here is that Jansenism, by its sweeping condemnation of the evil of this world, and its refusal of any hope of being able to change the world before the end of time, bore within it a fundamental temptation of death. Goldmann remarks, "To live in the world means living in ignorance of the nature of man; to understand this nature means realising that man cannot preserve the authentic values except by refusing life in this world, by choosing solitude and, in the last analysis, by choosing death."[65] Goldmann also quite rightly notes the profound similarity of Pascal's attitude and Faust's: The writer and the fictional character share a passion for universal knowledge and an awareness of its total vanity. They are torn, which leads Pascal to sink into a crucified acceptance of the mystery of an unreachable God, and Faust to contemplate suicide. The borderline between the two attitudes is thin; it takes very little to tip the balance to one side or the other.

In many ways, Faust's solution to the problem of suicide seems the more logical one and the only satisfactory one. This is what emerges, for example, in the tragedies of Racine, when the hero or heroine, understanding that an aspiration for the absolute cannot be reconciled with the world, chooses suicide. Andromaque, Junie, Bérénice, and Phèdre resolve their conflicts in death. Caught between an evil world incapable of reform, an always absent God, and a yearning for the absolute, these women have no way out but self-annihilation. Since they are pagans, they rush to embrace the void. That was Jansenism's natural penchant, held in check by St. Augustine's prohibition. As Goldmann states, "*Phèdre* represents . . . the tragedy of the hope that men can live in the world without concessions, hopes, or compromises, and the tragedy of the recognition that this hope is doomed to disillusion. . . . *Phèdre* raises the whole problem of why the attempt to live in this world is inevitably a failure, and is thus nearer than any other of Racine's plays to the vision of the *Pensées*."[66]

Authentic Jansenism was thus deeply ambiguous. By taking logical reflection on the human condition as far as it could, it reached an impasse: On one side there was a radically evil world that no acts could improve; on the other side there was an elusive God whose grace was restricted to a small number of elect; in the middle there was humankind, alone, thirsting for the absolute and aware that the absolute was unattainable.[67] Jansenism created an existential context in which nothingness was the only way out. But it also refused that way out in the name of a God who is absolute master of life, thus it closed humankind into a terrestrial trap. The only barrier to suicide was faith, a faith that Jansenism rendered fragile by making God into a being whose principle characteristic was absence—a being one continues to seek even when one has already found him, as Pascal put it. The frontier between that being and nonbeing is highly tenuous, and the minute the dividing line became unclear, the only obstacle to suicide disappeared. The Jansenist attitude directly prepared the atheistic philosophies of despair of the nineteenth century. It was a potential agent for suicide.

The question of the legitimacy of voluntary death, raised during the crisis of 1580–1620, remained a topic of debate within the educated elites throughout the seventeenth century. Although the number of actual suicides does not seem to have varied significantly, thought patterns slowly changed. The political and religious authorities retained their globally negative and repressive attitude toward suicide, but ever widening circles within society felt concern over the problem.

Unlike the Renaissance, the Grand Siècle had a pessimistic vision of humankind and of the world, and it shifted its hopes to the next world. In many respects, it was a century of prohibitions and frustrations. The move by the power structure to take back control of culture and politics was reflected in an increased insistence on moral rigidity and in a chilly formalism. Both marked the classical spirit in all domains. This world is evil and must be disciplined in expectation of the only true life in the next world. Life in this world is but a brief voyage that should be made with total detachment, one's eyes fixed on its ardently desired goal—death and eternal life. In the painful obstacle course that is daily life, it is forbidden to cheat and take a shortcut to the other world.

But spiritual life offered a palliative to the frustrations of the soul that aspired to eternal happiness, in the form of "annihilation" and withdrawal from the world. These substitutes for voluntary death were available only to an infinitely small minority, however; the prohibition on self-killing remained in full force for the mass of the people, and guilty verdicts for suicide were frequent. Individuals had a duty to the state and to society; they had to respect the law, both divine and natural, that commanded them to live at any cost. In spite of this, the trend in jurisprudence was toward greater indulgence in cases involving extreme misfortune and madness. Special consideration was shown to the ecclesiastical and noble elite for its honor and respectability, which means that there were hardly any sentences of culpable suicide among them, thus reinforcing a dual and hierarchical moral standard.

This was the situation when the question of suicide was raised again during the second crisis of conscience in Europe between 1680 and 1720. A critical spirit and rationalism, clashing head-on with the established churches, worked to weaken irreparably the most effective prohibitions on suicide—that is, the spiritual ones. At the same time, terrible crises of subsistence and economic catastrophes heightened the appeal of voluntary death. It was a crucial period and, incidentally, the one that saw the birth of the term *suicide*.

PART III

The Enlightenment

Suicide Updated and Guilt-Free

EIGHT

The Birth of the English Malady

1680–1720

From Thomas Creech to George Cheyne:
The English Malady

In 1700, exactly one century after the appearance of *Hamlet,* an Oxford scholar named Thomas Creech, who had translated the works of Lucretius, hanged himself. The event caused a considerable stir in the academic world, and it became a mythic tale that some found admirable but that others found horrifying. Some people interested in presenting Creech's death as a model of philosophical suicide circulated the rumor that shortly before his death he had read Donne's *Biathanatos,* holding the book in one hand and a rope in the other. Voltaire reported that Creech had written on the margins of his manuscript of his commentary on Lucretius, "N.B. Must hang myself when I have finished," which led Voltaire to remark, "He kept his word with himself so that he might have the pleasure of ending like his author. If he had undertaken a commentary upon Ovid he would have lived longer." One hostile observer noted that Creech had "died as he had lived, like a true atheist." The real story is much simpler: The translator of Lucretius killed himself for love because the parents of his beloved had rejected his suit. Nonetheless, colleagues and rivals claimed that errors he had made in his translation had plunged him into despair.[1]

It is not by chance that Creech's thoughts turned to suicide. The idea had been in the air for some time. Moreover, the link between Creech and Lucretius seemed a concrete example of a current of thought that those who upheld traditional morality found alarming. Beginning around 1680, the debate on suicide had taken on a new life in England: Tracts, pro and con, were published, and discussion was animated, encouraged, and punctuated by notorious cases.

On 13 July 1683 Arthur Capel, earl of Essex, who had been arrested and imprisoned in the Tower of London for plotting against the crown, cut his throat. In October 1684 a famous Baptist preacher, John Child, who had recently abjured his faith, calling upon his fellow Baptists to rejoin the Anglican Church, killed himself. In the same year one Thomas Law put an end to his days after losing his post as a chaplain. In 1685 one of the duke of Monmouth's lieutenants, Robert Long, committed suicide in Newgate Prison. In 1689 John Temple, the secretary of war, threw himself off London Bridge into the Thames. Temple was the son of Sir William Temple, a famous statesman, and had been humiliated by the failure of his negotiations to end the Irish rebellion. A note found in his pocket stated, "My folly in undertaking what I could not execute has done the king great prejudice, which cannot be stop'd no easier way for me than this: May his undertaking prosper, may he have a blessing."[2]

Creech's suicide in 1700 was followed soon after (in 1701) by that of a high aristocrat, the earl of Bath, whose son Charles Grenville, the new earl, imitated him two weeks later. In the following year (1702) Francis Godolphin, a cousin of the lord treasurer and a wealthy man who was happily married with a family, cut his throat for no apparent reason. On 4 January 1704 George Edwards, a well-off Essex man, killed himself by rigging up an elaborate mechanism for setting off three pistols at once. The affair caused a great stir when John Smith, an Anglican minister, published a pamphlet in which he presented Edwards's suicide as symbolic of the catastrophic results of "atheism."[3] In reality, the unfortunate Edwards was above all a victim of the intolerance of his milieu. An extremely pious man, he had drifted toward a rationalist religion after reading philosophical works. Doubting the truth of Scripture, he declared that the universality of religious beliefs did not prove the existence of God and that because some men were black and some white, all men could not have descended from Adam. When the congregation of his church turned against him, and even his wife rejected him, Edwards chose to kill himself. He was about forty years old. Smith saw his death as the result of the spread of neo-Epicurean ideas.

Word of all these suicides was circulated, with commentary, by the press. The accounts made a strong impression. In 1702 John Evelyn noted in his diary, " 'Tis . . . sad to Consider how many of this Nation have murdered themselves of late years 15 or 16 in my remembrance."[4] Evelyn's remark coincides with the beginning of a rise in the number of suicides reported in the bills of mortality, which by that date were being reprinted in the newspapers. Famous suicides seemed to reflect and illustrate a rising tide, as well as a deep and specifically English penchant.

Thus the myth of the "English malady" was born. It was made official by the publication of *The English Malady, or, A Treatise of Nervous Diseases of all Kinds* (1733) by George Cheyne, a physician. Cheyne explained that he had been urged to write his treatise by friends worried "by the late Frequency and daily Encrease of wanton and uncommon self-murders."[5] Since he had not read Fontenelle's *Dent d'or* (or had not retained its moral, that one should verify facts before seeking their cause), Dr. Cheyne analyzed why the English should kill themselves more than people of other nations. From then on the notion that England was the land of suicide was accepted as fact; the idea was well planted in the minds of the elites of Europe and no longer open to question. The quintessentially Enlightenment myth did not decline until the appearance of modern statistical techniques.

Cheyne explained that the suicidal tendencies of the English were tied, on the one hand, to the progress of atheism and the philosophic spirit among the English and, on the other hand, to the melancholy temperament of an island people living in unfavorable geographical and climatic conditions. Climatic determinism was in fashion at the time. Montesquieu later made broad use of it, and the idea was so well implanted that its influence was unconscious. Soon after he arrived in London in 1727, César de Saussure declared himself depressed by the weather, adding that if he had been an Englishman he would certainly have committed suicide.[6]

The Birth of the Word 'Suicide'

It was also in England that the end result of this malady was first called *suicide*. Up to now I have used the word anachronistically, for simplicity's sake: The term was actually coined in the seventeenth century, which in itself suggests evolving opinion and an increasing amount of debate on the topic. Like English, French too had only had paraphrases for killing oneself that display a redundancy emphasizing the exceptional and reprehensible nature of the act: *s'occir soi-même, se tuer soi-même, être homicide de soi-même, être meurtrier de soi-même,* or *se défaire.*

The appearance of the neologism reflects a desire to distinguish between homicide of oneself and killing another, and it is in its Latin form that the term was used in Sir Thomas Browne's *Religio medici,* a work written around 1636 but not published until 1642 (see chapter 6). In this work Browne took care to distinguish Christian "self-killing," an act that merits total condemnation, from the pagan *suicidium* of Cato. The term, founded on the Latin *sui* (of oneself) and *caedes* (murder), also appeared independently in the works of the casuists. Thus in 1652 a paragraph of Juan Caramuel's *Theologia moralis fundamentalis* was titled, "De suicidio." During the 1650s the neologism spread to English with the works of the lexicographer Thomas Blount and those of Walter Charleton, the editor of Epicurus. The term was sufficiently widespread in 1658 for Edward Phillips, John Milton's nephew, to place it in his *General Dictionary,* although with a fantastic etymology that expressed his own negative opinion: "*Suicide* . . . should be derived from *Sus,* a Sow, [rather] then from the pronoun *Sui* . . . as it were a Swinish part for a man to kill himself."[7]

The term *suicide* first appears in French in 1734, when it was used by Abbé Prévost, who was in England at the time and was writing for his review, *Le Pour et le Contre.*[8] Prévost contributed to spreading the myth of an "English malady" by repeating such stories as the one about a Chelsea clergyman who attempted to kill himself and was saved by a gentleman. When asked the reasons for his act, the would-be suicide stated, "I admit that it is a weakness; there would be more firmness of soul to supporting life with all its miseries than in voluntarily giving oneself death. But in order to support life, one must be able to maintain it. I haven't the necessary. I will die of hunger in three days. It isn't changing the order of heaven to move the moment up a bit." The gentleman then took the clergyman into his house but was unable to prevent him from subsequently drowning himself. The clergyman was a highly honorable man, Prévost noted, but was ruined by his own imprudence. Above all, he had been a great admirer of William Tyndale and Anthony Collins. The English, Prévost added, sang his praises.[9]

In his discussion of George Cheyne's book, *The English Malady,* which had recently been published, Abbé Prévost gave Cheyne's reasons for the high incidence of suicide in England: If the English commit suicide, it is because they heat their houses with peat coal, eat half-cooked roast beef, and are too licentious. Prévost did not seem persuaded.[10]

The term *suicide* was not commonly used in France until the mid-eighteenth century, however, and the verb, *se suicider,* was always either redundant or a pleonasm, which shows that the idea of a crime against oneself persisted. The most logical verb construction, *je suicide,* was never used in French. English has no verb at all: *suicide* is a noun, and it needs to be attached to an active verb, *to commit suicide.* Other languages use a double form or a paraphrase as well: German, for example, uses *sich den Tod geben,* or *sich töten.* It was also during the eighteenth century that the English term *suicide* passed into Spanish, Italian, and Portuguese.[11]

Statistics and the Press

How can we explain the success of the idea of suicide as an "English malady" during the years 1680–1720? The chief causes of its vogue seem to have been the combined effect of improved statistical techniques, sociocultural evolution among the aristocracy, a climate of intense religious rivalry, and the astonishing growth of the press, all of which operated in an overall atmosphere of a crisis in traditional values, the second one in the century.

English public opinion was struck by a spectacular rise in the number of reported suicides after 1680. Our principal source of statistical information, the London bills of mortality, shows a rise from an average suicide rate of 18 per year in the decade 1680–90 to 20 per year in 1690–1700, 25 in 1700–1710, 30 in 1710–20, 42 in 1720–30, and more than 50 in 1730–40, with a few peaks of more than 60 suicides per year.[12]

It is hardly surprising that some observers expressed concern. In 1698 William Congreve wrote, "Are there not more Self-murderers, and melancholick Lunaticks in *England,* heard of in one Year, than in a greater part of *Europe* besides?" In 1705 John Evelyn stated that "never was it known that so many made themselves away as of these late years among us, among both men of quality and others."[13]

The impression made by the raw figures was much strengthened by the rise of a popular press that reached an increasingly broad public in the late seventeenth century. The major newspapers are estimated to have published some 15,000 copies per issue, and by 1704 many of them appeared two or three times weekly.[14] Not only did newspapers publish the bills of mortality figures, they also printed articles on the most interesting, strangest, or most striking cases of suicide, inquiring into their circumstances and causes. Thus the public became familiar with a kind of human-interest story that until then had seemed exceptional. Beyond the raw numbers, newspaper readers retained the notion that suicide was a permanent part of urban life, and commentaries, both written and oral, maintained and amplified the impression that the situation was serious.

The press also contributed to secularizing the way suicide was viewed by presenting it in an exclusively human light. The articles published were usually neutral in tone, thus accustoming readers to seeing suicide as the result of social or psychological circumstances. Slowly but surely, public opinion came to see suicide as less culpable than before and to categorize it among ordinary social scourges afflicting people who were more victims than criminals.

Still, it would be a mistake to minimize the importance of the figures furnished by the bills of mortality. We obviously need to take into account the overall increase in the population of London, which at least doubled between 1650 and 1750 (but more complete census figures undoubtedly account for some of the apparent increase). Is population growth enough to explain a suicide rate in 1730 that was three and a half times higher than it had been in 1680? This seems even more improbable because it suggests that the suicide rate should have continued to swell after 1730, given that the London population continued to grow. The curve stabilizes after 1730, however, even tending to decline, until it returns to some 30 suicides a year in the 1780s.

This means that contemporary impressions were not totally erroneous: There was undeniably a rise in the suicide rate between 1680 and 1720–30. Where they were mistaken was in thinking that these trends were exclusively English.[15] On the Continent a number of observers noted the same phenomenon. The Princess Palatine was among them. In 1696 she limited her remarks to repeating what the exiled Queen Mary II had reported. The princess stated, "Suicides are very common among the English. Our queen of England told me that during the entire time she remained in that country, not a single day went by without someone, man or woman, hanging themselves, stabbing themselves, or blowing their brains out." By 1699, however, the princess realized that suicide was becoming more common in France.[16] Like many others, she blamed a growing spirit of atheism: "Religion is so dead in this country that all the young men desire to be considered atheists, but what is stranger is that the same people who are atheists at Paris play pious at Court. It is maintained also that all the cases of suicide, and lately we have had a great many, are the result of atheism. . . . Last Monday, moreover, a lawyer shot himself in his bed."[17]

These indications, vague as they are, come from the years 1680–90. In 1720 the princess recorded that suicides had increased in the early eighteenth century. "The fashion in Paris is now to slough off one's life: Most drown themselves, many throw themselves out of windows and break their necks, others stab themselves, and all because of accursed money."[18] The collapse of John Law's "system" had indeed brought on a temporary increase in the number of suicides, but even at the end of the seventeenth century, Father Bernard Lamy asserted that increased numbers of people had chosen to imitate Atticus and kill themselves: "It is an effect of Epicureanism."[19]

New and Old Causes for Suicide

Suicide thus seems to have been a widespread phenomenon, although one cannot call it epidemic or speak of a wave of suicides. Only the first financial crises, which struck an imprudent, risk-prone, and unprepared capitalist world, caused exceptional peaks in the suicide rate. In France, the years 1720–21 saw the crisis of Law's system and the collapse of the South Sea Company (known as the South Sea Bubble). Suicides in London increased dramatically from 27 in 1720 to 52 in 1721, of which 6 occurred during one week in January.[20] The newspapers echoed these dramas: On 22 April 1721 the *Weekly Journal* reported that a gentlewoman had thrown herself from a window because of losses she had sustained in the South Sea Company; on 20 May a tradesman grown melancholy at the prospect of poverty followed her example. In November a London merchant, James Milner, violently attacked the directors of the company in the House of Commons, then shot himself in the head. Since speculation was more developed in England than in France, crises and bankruptcies were also more numerous, and now and then someone committed suicide, as did one treasury official who hanged himself in Worcester in 1720 after losing considerable amounts of money. At times the mere idea of bankruptcy was enough to make someone kill himself: One wealthy merchant whose fortune was evaluated at £60,000 nonetheless hanged himself in January 1721.[21]

It is obvious that the development of capitalism made a sizable contribution to the rise in the suicide rate during this period. Instability and insecurity are an integral part of capitalism, which is founded on individualism, acceptance of risk, and competition. The solidarity systems of guilds and corporations had disappeared, leaving the individual to face financial ruin alone; bankruptcies were frequent, in part because control of economic mechanisms was still rudimentary and errors were often made. Bankruptcies were also merciless, and the fallen businessman could expect no pity from his contemporaries. England entered the era of laissez-faire economics, an age in which audacity paid and opportunities of all sorts opened up: Companies sprouted up everywhere, but failure rates ran as high as hopes. Aggressive capitalism then moved to the Continent. In France after 1715 banking and finance offered the best possibilities for speculation, and rude awakenings were often cruel. In the absence of guarantees and stable structures, the businessman of the early eighteenth century was necessarily vulnerable, and his position was fragile. It is little wonder that businessmen furnished a new contingent to traditional suicides.

Poverty, which had always been one of the prime causes of suicide, also increased in the years 1680–1720. Food shortages, terrible winters, dysentery, typhoid fever, and wars sorely tried the populations of Europe. Two wide-spread conflicts, the War of the Augsburg League and the War of Spanish Succession, dragged on for over twenty years. There was famine in 1693–94, a financial crisis in 1697–98, a *grand hyver* (terrible winter) in 1709–10; another financial crisis struck in 1713–14, and an epidemic of dysentery in 1719. These were the years of misery that Marcel Lachiver describes.[22] When poverty did not bring death by starvation, it could push the wretched to suicide. The newspapers in England reported many such cases: One London woman drowned herself and her two children in 1717 after the parish refused to raise her allowance.[23]

The press also reported cases of ordinary suicide due to unrequited love, conjugal problems, family quarrels, personal losses, rape, shame, and re-morse—the usual litany of human misery. It is quite possible that there were more such cases than before, thanks to an incipient relaxation of family ties, an early sign of the disintegration of the extended family in the modern age. Traditional solidarities slowly fell apart, accelerated by the growth of cities. The individual became increasingly isolated, even when surrounded by urban gregariousness and promiscuity.

An increased urbanism occurred earlier in England than elsewhere and was remarked on there sooner. Most of the examples of suicide reported in the newspapers were urban. On 26 April 1718 the *Weekly Journal* reported that a London woman had hanged herself after quarreling with her husband; on 5 October 1717 the same paper published news of the suicide by stabbing and hanging of a Southwark milkman guilty of raping his stepdaughter. Rural suicides were more likely to be the result of some sudden misadventure. On 1 March 1718, the *Weekly Journal* tells us, a Wiltshire farmer accidentally killed his son. On learning of the tragedy, his wife ran out of the house, leaving her eighteen-month-old child on the table. The child fell off and was killed, upon which the farmer killed himself. A more banal case occurred in Finchley in 1684, when a man driven to despair by a broken engagement killed himself after attempting to murder his ex-fiancée.[24]

Suicide and the English Aristocracy

The years 1680–1720 saw an unusual number of aristocratic suicides, to the point that suicide seemed a genuine fashion. They helped intensify the debate on voluntary death.

Some years after the restoration of Charles II in 1660, at a moment when the waves of violent religious struggles of the mid-century were beginning to abate, the nobility and the refined society of London began to show more indulgence toward suicide. In 1672 William Ramesey composed something like a treatise on good manners or a manual for gentlemen, *The Gentleman's Companion,* in which he preached compassion for suicides. We should not condemn them, he wrote, "for 'tis possible even for Gods elect, having their Judgments and Reasons depraved by madness, deep melancholly, or [some]how otherwise affected by Diseases of some sorts, to be their own executioners."[25] In 1690 the jurist Roger North, whose cousin Sir Henry North had committed suicide in 1671, declared that justice was too severe in the cases of voluntary homicide.

The news of famous deaths, amply diffused by the press, accredited the idea of a "fashionable" suicide obeying a code of honor similar to the one that governed duels. In both cases the instrument of choice was the pistol or the sword; suicide by hanging was profoundly scorned. Charles Moore, who gathered a good many anecdotes about suicide in his *Full Inquiry into the Subject of Suicide* (1790), reported the comment of one nobleman on a gentlemen who had hanged himself, " 'What a low-minded wretch, to apply the halter! Had he shot himself, like a gentleman, I could have forgiven him.' "[26]

Records show that between 1660 and 1714, peers, knights, and gentlemen accounted for 10 percent of the suicides in England, but 70 percent of suicides with pistols. Only 20 percent of nobles hanged themselves, whereas 65 percent of suicides in other social categories did so.[27] Death by dagger or sword increased after the beginning of the eighteenth century with the growing popularity of Cato. In 1709 Jonathan Swift wrote an article for the *Tatler* praising Cato above all other pagans, and in 1713 Joseph Addison's highly successful tragedy, *Cato,* presented the protagonist's death as a glorious apotheosis. The *Gentleman's Magazine* reported in 1737 that the poet Eustace Budgell had left behind an incomplete couplet before flinging himself into the Thames: "What Cato did and Addison approved, / Cannot be wrong."[28]

In 1711 William Withers treated the "art of suicide" with irony and macabre humor, providing a satiric guide to voluntary death for persons of the better social classes. Withers subscribed to the notion of an "English malady": "In a Nation Renown'd as ours is, for such Great and frequent Examples of *Heroic Death* as none of our Neighbours can boast of, no Body should yet have taken into Consideration the Miscarriages that often happen in so *Serious* an Affair, merely for want of a *Conduct,* answerable to our Native *Intrepidity.* "[29]

Withers's basic rules were these: Choose a clean, efficient method, and leave a suicide note that your widow can read and reread later.

It seems as if the English aristocracy's lenient attitude toward suicide lay in the higher social classes' desire to distance themselves from the religious excesses of the preceding period. Twenty years after the death of Cromwell, when the exaggerations of Puritanism were a thing of the past, a skeptical generation made much of its suspicion of all forms of supernatural intervention in this world. This was the generation of John Locke, one that had suffered from religious conflicts, from extremism, and from the fanaticism of both sides. In reaction it adopted a moderate, if not tepid, religious attitude, withdrawn and hostile to all excess. It was at the same period that High Church Anglicanism first flourished, as is reflected in the new churches of London reconstructed by Christopher Wren after the great fire of 1666. Anglicanism was a religion for the prosperous; it was a muted, comfortable religion where good taste reigned and worship took place in sanctuaries with high windows, thick cushions, and velvet and gilt everywhere. The churches smelled more of wax than of incense and, halfway between churches and salons, they purveyed a religion for people of good company that banished God and the supernatural from ordinary conversation. Among the better society of London in the years 1680–1720, inflammatory invective against suicide as an act inspired by the devil was scorned as a shocking relic of more fanatical times. The devil was no longer seen as having a hand in human behavior, and voluntary death might be an honorable choice under certain circumstances, if one followed the proper etiquette. Charles Moore attributed the evolution of noble attitudes toward suicide to a reaction against the "affectation of piety and bigotry of puritanism in Cromwell's day."[30]

The question of voluntary death was, in fact, at the center of polemics between Anglicans and Puritans. In 1684, after the suicide of John Child, the Baptist (mentioned earlier) who had converted to Anglicanism, pamphlets circulated declaring that his conversion had resulted from persecution and his death was the work of the devil. Benjamin Dennis and Thomas Plant said as much in a fifty-page work published in 1688 and reissued in 1715, 1718, 1734, and 1770.[31] The aim of the pamphlet was to strengthen Puritan communities, which were under pressure from the established church (the Church of England), by showing that Child's apostasy was the result of a diabolical suggestion that had, quite logically, ended in suicide.

Other happenings added fuel to the polemics, and they too were exploited for political purposes. One example is the suicide in 1683 of the earl of Essex, a man prominent in the Whig party. Discussion of such voluntary deaths helped spread England's reputation as the land of suicide. Treatises favorable to indulgence toward suicide flourished as well. In 1680 Charles Blount, a deist, praised Donne's *Biathanatos* (Blount committed suicide four years later). Blount's treatise, *The Two First Books of Philostratus,* was reprinted in 1700, a further sign that literature of the sort had readers. New translations of Montaigne in 1685 and of Charron in 1697 furnished skeptics with fresh arguments. In 1695 the freethinker Charles Gildon took up the defense of his late friend Blount and enlarged the debate to a theoretical plane. Blount, Gildon wrote, died like a philosopher, in conformity with the precepts of nature and reason. He suffered from an impossible love and preferred to die rather than prolong his suffering. Nature and reason have never demanded that we enjoy evil, Gildon continued, citing Epicurus. To say that we are like soldiers who must not quit our posts is absurd because soldiers have chosen their profession, but we have not asked to be born. Finally, Gildon stated, the argument of suicide as a crime against society is equally vain: A person who emigrates also weakens his country, and someone who kills himself does no more harm to his country than the émigré.[32]

This way of reasoning infuriated the champions of traditional morality. They too wrote one treatise after another, which—paradoxically—contributed to reinforcing the myth of the "English malady" when word of them reached foreign shores. In 1674 Thomas Philipot published a work sharply attacking the influence of Donne's *Biathanatos,* and in 1699 Charles Leslie attacked Blount and Gildon, accusing the deists of having set up self-murder "as a Principle."[33]

Treatises against Suicide

In 1700, the year Thomas Creech died, John Adams published a treatise, *An Essay concerning Self-Murther,* that proved a landmark in the history of the controversy on suicide.[34] What was original about Adams's book was that it attacked suicide on a completely philosophical plane, abandoning the purely religious and theological arguments that had been reiterated ever since St. Augustine. The work inaugurated a strategy for the Anglican clergy of fighting their adversaries on their own terrain, but this was in fact a victory for the defenders of tolerance of suicide, henceforth considered a purely human affair.

The clergy's position was particularly fragile, since once they had given up the prohibition of suicide by divine decree, it was difficult for them to prove, in strictly human terms, that taking one's own life was prohibited. This was, however, what Adams set out to do. His first objective was to show that suicide is a violation of humankind's obligation toward God, something even the deists admitted. Adams followed the reasoning of John Locke, a providential but compromising ally: God created humankind, so we are his property; thus we have only a right of use over our lives, not a right of absolute ownership. Adams's second point was that suicide violates natural law. Here Adams had to make a pact with the devil and use Thomas Hobbes, a writer suspected of atheism, as his authority. His third point was that suicide violates the rights of society because it does not contribute to the public good, an argument he borrowed from a Latin treatise published by Richard Cumberland in 1672.[35] Finally, Adams added a practical argument: that permitting suicide would be equivalent to destroying all human laws because the death penalty, which is the gravest sanction available against those who break the law, would no longer have any force. For that same reason, an anonymous treatise published in 1728 argued, posthumous punishments for both dueling and suicide should be maintained.[36]

The major spiritualist philosophers became concerned over the apparent progress of the "English malady," and they hastened to reinforce traditional morality. In 1706 Samuel Clarke published *A Discourse Concerning the Unchangeable Obligations of Natural Religion,* in which he attacked Gildon, calling his reasoning "weak and childish," citing all the usual authorities, and repeating the analogy of the soldier who must not leave his post.[37] The great George Berkeley spoke with scorn and anger of the more or less atheist "minute philosophers" who spread the notion of tolerance of suicide but lacked the courage to act on their principles and kill themselves. A much more modest clerical figure than Bishop Berkeley, John Prince, wrote a refutation of Donne's and Gildon's works in 1709.[38]

Such works met with little success in enlightened circles. Thomas Hearne reported that in 1705 an Oxford professor failed to find a publisher for his refutation of Donne's *Biathanatos,* whereupon his colleagues mocked him, declaring that no one wanted to read such a book.[39] New ideas were in fashion. Cato, Epicurus, and Lucretius had become heroes once again, and it was chic to be broad-minded about suicide and oppose the clergy. Saint-Évremond, who remained at the center of a brilliant libertine circle in London until his death in 1703, shared and spread an Epicurean indulgence.

The opponents of suicide nonetheless scored a few isolated successes. One was Charles Gildon's retraction in 1705. Gildon had been shaken by Charles Leslie's attack in 1699, in which Leslie accused him of having written an apology for self-murder. This was an unfair accusation, but one that the adversaries of suicide frequently used to silence their opponents. Defending a right to suicide did not mean advocating suicide. When the champions of traditional morality refused to make that distinction, they implicitly accused the partisans of tolerance of encouraging suicide. By charging them, in the eyes of public opinion, with an undeserved responsibility for advocating suicide, they hoped to press hard on their conscience, bring them around to remorse, and force them into silence. Thanks in part to such tactics, discourse on voluntary death was timid, rare, and discreet. For the same reason, the authors of treatises calling for tolerance toward suicide often took fright at the responsibility their opponents thrust upon them and either destroyed their writings (as Justus Lipsius did) or gave up all thought of publishing them (as did John Donne and David Hume, whose books on the subject were published posthumously). Gildon made an official retraction, and in 1705 he wrote that he was now "perfectly convinc'd, that *Suicide* is not Lawful."[40]

Growing Tolerance in England and France

No change occurred in the legal sphere in the years 1680–1720. The law remained as severe as always, and belief in the intervention of the devil had not completely disappeared from either the popular mind or religious attitudes. Nonconformist circles tenaciously clung to such beliefs. In 1677 Richard Gilpin reaffirmed in his *Daemonologia sacra, or, A Treatise on Satan's Temptations* that it was the devil who manipulated people's thoughts and sentiments in order to push them to suicide.[41] In 1709 John Prince wrote that Satan "is very often the Author (or chief Agent) of this abominable Sin of Self-murder."[42] When an apprentice, Thomas Burridge, attempted suicide in 1712, his fellow dissenters attributed his gesture to Satan's possession of his spirit and organized a prayer vigil to deliver him.[43] That same year Jane Wenham was convicted of witchcraft, and one of the proofs of her guilt was that she had used supernatural means to urge two girls to drown themselves. In 1726 Isaac Watts declared that the devil is behind all suicides.[44] Some authors, such as Charles Wheatly (writing in 1715), even thought that madness was no excuse, and that the body of a madman who had committed suicide should receive the same punishment as other suicides.[45]

The stricter attitude, which by this time was the minority opinion, stood in contrast to a strong trend among judges to hand down *non compos mentis* decisions—verdicts that recognized that the suicide was insane at the moment of committing the fatal act. This more lenient attitude made spectacular progress, particularly in the years 1680–1720: The proportion of suicide cases tried before the King's Bench and judged not guilty for reasons of insanity rose from 10.5 percent in 1675–79 to 44.1 percent in 1705–9. In certain cities (Norwich for one) such verdicts accounted for over 90 percent of decisions.[46]

There were several reasons for this change. For one thing, as we have seen, English coroners' juries, responsible for examining cases of suicide, were always loath to ruin the families of the deceased by handing up *felo de se* verdicts. In 1693 a statute confirmed their opposition and made it easier to arrive at more clement verdicts. The new law stated that forfeitures would henceforth be made, not in favor of the crown, but rather in favor of persons who held royal patents giving them the right to the goods of suicides. This change had two results. First, local communities, which were much more opposed to a patent-holding noble in their own locality than they were to the crown, showed even less enthusiasm for enriching the gentlefolk to the detriment of the peasantry. Second, the crown, which now had no interest in the outcome of coroners' inquests, no longer sought to ascertain the equity of the verdicts or intervene in the proceedings. This left coroners and coroners' juries much freer of control, and they took advantage of their freedom to exonerate a majority of suicides.

One flagrant case occurred in 1698 in Cumberland, on the lands of the duke of Somerset. John Atkinson slit his throat after declaring he had been forsaken by God. He died three days later. The somewhat hasty coroner's inquest came to a verdict of natural death. The duke, who held a right to the forfeited property of felons, was furious and ordered a second inquest. The body was dug up and a second jury called. Its members were sternly reminded of the duke's rights and of the meaning of a *felo de se* verdict, perhaps with the implication that Atkinson's death fell into that category. No mention was made of the possibility of a *non compos mentis* verdict, but in spite of the talking-to they had been given, that was the verdict the jury brought in.[47]

Even when they handed up a *felo de se* verdict, coroners' juries usually took care to undervalue the suicide's wealth so as to avoid plunging the family into poverty. Whereas in 1670–74 more than 30 percent of the estates forfeited had a value of more than one pound sterling, this category represented no more than 6.7 percent of estates between 1710 and 1714, thus suggesting that the immense majority of suicides who were judged guilty were poverty-stricken. In 1704 Daniel Defoe noted that public opinion was increasingly hostile to the forfeiture of suicides' goods: "The Children," he wrote, "should [not] be starv'd because the Father has destroy'd himself."[48]

Among the aristocracy in England, suicides were regularly attributed to madness or accident. Thus the suicide of Charles Grenville, earl of Bath, was put down to being "unfortunately killed by the casual going off of a Pistol."[49] The overall tendency was toward leniency, and the coroners' juries, whose members became better educated, more enlightened, and increasingly open to the new ideas, were less and less inclined to judge suicides guilty.

We can see the same tendency on the Continent, where it operated on several different levels. Jurists in France continued to argue for leniency: In 1715 Antoine Bruneau declared that the insane should be exonerated when they kill themselves, as should the unfortunate, which left only those who kill themselves out of simple weariness with life.[50] In 1719 Philippe Bornier returned to Pierre Ayrault's arguments to protest inflicting penalties on the bodies of suicides.[51] The explanation of suicide as a direct result of insanity made spectacular advances. According to Michel Foucault, it was at this time that people became aware that madness had reached the level of a social phenomenon and that the same awareness led to the movement for enclosure of the insane and the founding of asylums. Foucault says, "We need to take into account the entire period of the installation of internment, which extended roughly from 1680 to 1720, and during which growth was extremely rapid, much more rapid than that of the population in general."[52] At the Salpêtrière hospital in Paris the number of inmates rose from 3,059 in 1690 to 6,704 in 1790, and at the Bicêtre it rose from 2,000 to 3,874 over those years.

During the same period, a connection was made between melancholia and madness, in particular by the physician Thomas Willis, whose complete works were published in Lyons in 1681. Melancholia, Willis wrote, is "a madness without fever or frenzy, accompanied by fear and sadness."[53] Animal spirits become "obscure, opaque, shadowy" when they are agitated, and the images they carry to the brain are veiled with "shadows and with shades." The individual grows sad and prone to morbid, even suicidal reactions.

Under the cover of fiction, literature continued to present ancient suicide as praiseworthy. The protagonists of *Andronic* (1685) and *Tridate* (1691), tragedies by Jean Galbert de Campistron, for example, kill themselves because of an incestuous love. As part of his great project to establish a moral code independent of religion, Pierre Bayle stated in his *Dictionnaire historique et critique,* "Lucretia's act should excite only sentiments of compassion and admiration." He went on to declare that St. Augustine was unjust when he condemned her in the name of a Christianity that she could not have known. Bayle rejected the idea that Lucretia killed herself (as Jacques Du Rondel had suggested in 1685) for pagan religious reasons, sacrificing to the Eumenides. Reason alone could justify heroic sacrifice.

For Saint-Évremond, the suicide of Petronius was a worthy, simple, serene, and deliberate death:

As for his death, after examining it well, either I am mistaken or it is the finest of antiquity. In the death of Cato I find emotional hurt and even anger. Despair over the affairs of the republic, loss of liberty, [and] hatred of Caesar helped his resolution much, and I do not know whether his wild nature had not perhaps reached the point of madness when he ripped out his entrails. Socrates died as a true sage and with a good measure of indifference; still, he sought to satisfy himself concerning his condition in the other life and did not succeed in doing so; he reasoned about it in prison with his friends ceaselessly and fairly weakly, and to tell the truth, death was for him a considerable object. Petronius alone brought softness and nonchalance into his death. . . . He not only continued his usual occupations, setting some of his slaves free, punishing others; he indulged in the things that amused him, and his soul at the point of such an arduous separation was more touched by the sweetness and smoothness of verse than by all the sentiments of the philosophers. Petronius at his death leaves us only an image of life: No action, no word, no circumstance shows the travail of a dying man. For him dying was truly ceasing to live.[54]

The Return of Noble and Ecclesiastical Suicide in France

In France as in England, aristocratic suicides increased. Authors of memoirs reported them with not the least hint of blame or reprobation, as if voluntary death had become a common occurrence in noble milieus. Not only were such events reported in the same neutral tone as natural deaths, but at no moment is there mention of the confiscation of goods, even less of ignominious punishments visited on the cadaver. Burial took place in utterly normal fashion, in consecrated ground, and with the saying of a solemn mass. There is no hint of laws or religious prohibitions of suicide. Freedom to kill oneself seems to have continued to be a privilege of the nobility.

The duc de Saint-Simon is typical in this respect, despite his severity and his Jansenist cast of mind. He speaks of twelve suicides in his *Memoirs*.[55] One of their principal causes is debt: To commit suicide for gambling debts one could not repay was an honorable way out. This was why, as Saint-Simon declares, "everyone pitied him and I regretted it much" when Louis de Belcastel, seigneur de Permillac, a gentleman of the chamber to the duc de Lorraine, shot himself in the head in May 1699. Saint-Simon gives a good account of Belcastel, adding that the poor man had killed himself "for having lost all he did not have, nor could have had, since he had been a high-stakes, assiduous gambler all his life." Saint-Simon expresses similar regrets about another inveterate gambler, Péchot de Saint-Adon, who killed himself at Brussels in 1706, according to Dangeau, of an overdose of opium. Saint-Simon remarks, "Everyone pitied him; he was brave, a good conversationalist, and although low-born, made for good company."[56] It speaks volumes about the gap between ecclesiastical discourse and aristocratic attitudes that the court should pity the people who had ruined themselves gambling, a practice that the Church condemned, and who had killed themselves, an act deserving of eternal damnation.

Saint-Simon is less indulgent about the comte de Monastérol, who killed himself in 1718. What he condemns, though, is not Monastérol's suicide but the fact that he betrayed his sovereign, the elector of Bavaria, by misappropriating funds to gamble with. Ordered to account for the missing sums, "at the end of his rope, and backed into a corner, he got himself out of it one morning by a pistol shot to the head in his room. He left innumerable debts, nothing to pay them with, and accounts in disorder that showed plainly how greatly he had abused the confidence and the kindness of the elector. That prince, who had always liked him, wanted to hush up the catastrophe, and he had it rumored that Monastérol had died suddenly" (6:641).

Fierce ambitions clashed at court, and some courtiers committed suicide when their career hopes were dashed. One such was the marquis de Silly, a man "of an unbridled ambition, with absolutely no trace of anything to constrain him, which made him an extremely dangerous man, but one who was exceptionally clever at hiding that fact" (2:485). In 1727, when Silly's hopes had proven vain, he killed himself by throwing himself out of a window of his chateau. There was no mention of confiscation; his sister inherited his entire fortune. Similarly, in 1706 the marquis de Maulévrier was crushed when he was rejected because of his bad reputation. Saint-Simon tells us:

Beside himself with fury on realizing that this opinion had definitively ruined all the plans of his ambition, his dominant passion, he gave himself over to despair. Although his wife watched over him with extreme care, as did several very good friends and his domestics, on Good Friday of that year he managed to give them the slip for a moment around eight in the morning, went into a passageway behind his apartment, opened the window, and threw himself into the courtyard, crushing his head on the paving stones. Such was the catastrophe of an ambitious man, whose utterly foolish and dangerous passions reached their height, turned his head, and took away his life. A tragic victim of himself. (2:710)

Saint-Simon attributes some of the other suicides he reports to insanity. In 1693, for instance, he writes: "On Sunday 29 November, the king, on leaving his evening devotions, learned from the baron de Beauvais that La Vauguyon had killed himself in his bed that morning with two pistol shots to the throat, having got rid of his domestics with the pretext of sending them to mass" (1:109). Saint-Simon then relates the count's odd behavior: He seems not to have been quite right in the head, since it was his habit to play constantly with his pistols, and he regularly threatened his valets with them. That did not prevent him from being a diplomat, in fact ambassador to Spain. In 1716 Saint-Simon speaks of Abbé de Brancas, a somewhat "crack-brained" man with "a highly deranged head" who had thrown himself into the Seine (6:42). Although he was fished out by some boatmen, he died a few hours later. In 1736 the marquis de Pellevé also drowned himself in the Seine at the Moulin de Javel (2:702).

In 1692 Saint-Simon mentions the suicide of Séron, the personal physician of Louvois, insinuating that he might have poisoned his master (5:499). In 1714 he speaks of the vice-bailiff of Alençon, who had killed himself dramatically after losing a lawsuit, stabbing himself in the presence of the *chancelier* as the latter was getting into his carriage. Saint-Simon comments:

He [the vice-bailiff] asked him to review his case and appoint a *rapporteur* [counsel for the defense]. The *chancelier* explained, gently and goodheartedly, that [the man] had every right to appeal, should there be good cause, but that review was unheard of, after which he started to get into his carriage. As he did so, this unfortunate man exclaimed that he knew a shorter way out of his troubles, at the same time stabbing himself twice with a dagger. At the cries of the lackeys, the *chancelier* got down from the carriage, had [the man] carried to a room, and sent for a surgeon he knew and a confessor. The man confessed tranquilly enough and died an hour later. (4:731)

Edmond Barbier mentions in his journal, in an entry dated 11 May 1721, the suicide of Monsieur de La Goupillière, a *conseiller* at the Parlement de Paris, a man thirty-four years old who had shot himself in the mouth during a quarrel with the *procureur* of the Parlement. Barbier comments:

His mind was a little off, which it was said came from his family. His mother had been declared legally incapacitated by reason of dementia, and he had a brother who merited the same. . . . Some attributed his derangement to the affairs of the age; others to a mistress, the daughter of a cabinetmaker, with whom he had had children and to whom he had promised marriage, but whom he no longer frequented and who had threatened to have him killed.[57]

Whatever his sanity, La Goupillière was buried in the normal fashion on 13 May. Similarly, when a gentleman had killed himself in 1685 because the king had not granted his petition, Louvois had *lettres de grâce* sent to the Châtelet to avoid having the corpse hanged.[58]

Tallemant des Réaux, who died in 1690, mentions several suicides of nobles and even *grands bourgeois* that entailed no legal pursuits. They include a *président* of the *chambre des comptes* of Montpellier who killed himself when his mistress died, the daughter of a gentleman in La Beauce who drowned herself because her father opposed her marriage, a *président des Enquêtes* who threatened to throw himself out of a window on his wife's death, and a gentleman from Argouges who drowned himself for his mistress's beautiful eyes. A rejected suitor might also use suicide as a form of blackmail.[59] The blackmail attempt was not always successful: Mathieu Marais relates that one d'Autray, who was in love with Madame d'Avergne, the ex-mistress of the regent, wrote the lady that he would kill himself if she did not share his passion. "In response, she sent him a Capuchin friar so he would not die without confession."[60]

Suicide came to be regarded as more banal in ecclesiastical circles as well. Some clerics even admitted to an admiration for it. Abbé de Bellegard wrote that Lucretia "is a model that the ladies should always have before their eyes," and Abbé de Saint-Réal stated that among the famous suicides "there are some who have given real demonstrations of grandeur and intrepidity."[61] Other clerics even substituted deeds for talk, especially love-stricken abbés, a type not infrequent at the time. Tallemant mentions Abbé du Tot, who would have bled to death if his mistress, Mademoiselle du Languetot, had not intervened, and Abbé Calvières, who starved himself to death at the demise of Mademoiselle de Gouffoulens.[62]

Marais relates in a journal entry for 1 February 1723 the suicide of Abbé François Raguenet, who had slit his throat with a razor. A wealthy and learned cleric and the author of a life of Cromwell, Raguenet was perfectly sane, and he seems to have killed himself out of lassitude for life, making his death one of the first philosophical suicides of the century. No penalties were incurred:

He was fully in his right mind [and] very well off, enjoying an income of ten to twelve thousand livres. . . . [He had] much money and many books, [and was] only a bit philosophical and fond of retiring into his study. He sent away his two lackeys after dinner, left the key in the door, put on his dressing gown and his nightcap, then delivered himself of his life, of which he was apparently weary. This was a nasty end for a proper man. . . . He was buried as fast as possible, and his estate was delivered to his heirs.[63]

When a seminarist killed himself in 1707, he was passed off as insane.[64] In 1719 Abbé Fleury, a priest from Orléans, committed suicide after an unfortunate series of circumstances that showed that even spirits steeped in piety are not immune to despair. A respected pastor much esteemed by his parishioners, Fleury was arrested during the night of 24–25 April 1718 and imprisoned in the Bastille because he had expressed his opposition to the papal bull *Unigenitus*. He was accused of forging a letter to the regent in the name of his bishop. He was declared innocent, but the order for his release was somehow lost. Desperate, he starved himself to death, dying on 16 April 1719. Far from eliciting criticism, his death made him all the more popular locally, and quatrains circulated to the effect that "he blossomed by dying, and he vanquished by his death." His body was not taken back to Orléans for fear of setting off a riot.[65]

Voluntary Death Neutralized

Abbé Fleury's story is yet another illustration of changing attitudes toward suicide. Although in principle suicide was still prohibited and was vigorously condemned, in real life everything depended on the circumstances, on the suicide's social class, and on his or her motives. A certain relativism began to be the rule, and we have indications that the social and intellectual elites no longer found the idea of voluntary self-homicide shocking.

Suicide almost became something to joke about. Louis Racine relates that one day Boileau, Molière, and Chapelle set off merrily to drown themselves in the Seine.[66] Elsewhere, Racine presents as a simple case of excessive temperament the suicide of a young woman who had poisoned herself because she had been falsely accused of being pregnant. Her act seemed to him unreasonable, and he concludes, "That is the humor of the people of this country, and they carry passion to the nth degree."[67] Guy Patin, who mentions five suicides in his letters, takes a light view of the question: "When she takes antimony prepared the court's way, she will be immediately expedited," he writes of one young woman.[68] In 1699 the Princess Palatine seems almost admiring of the young duc de Berry, a spoiled brat given to temper tantrums who tried to crack his skull with a stone when one of his governors disciplined him for nearly shooting his brother while they were hunting.[69] The princess speaks harshly of suicide elsewhere, however.

We find the same inconsistency in Madame de Sévigné. She has not one word of reproach for Vatel, and she says jokingly of Lauzun's attempted escape from prison: "Do you think he'll break his head against the wall?" As old age approached, Madame de Sévigné was less sure that suicide deserved condemnation. In 1689, when she was seventy-three, she wrote to her daughter, Madame de Grignan:

I cannot, however, refrain from calculating and reflecting, and I find the conditions of life are very hard. It seems to me that I have been dragged against my will to the fatal period, when *old age* must be endured; I see it, I have attained it; and I would, at least, contrive not to go beyond it, not to advance in the road of infirmities, pain, loss of memory, *disfigurements* which are ready to lay hold of me; and I hear a voice which says, "You must go on, in spite of yourself; or, if you will not, you must die, an alternative at which nature recoils." Such, however, is the fate of those who have reached a certain period. But a return to the will of God, and to that universal law which is imposed upon us, restores reason to its place, and makes us call in patience to our aid.[70]

Seven years later, in 1696, the aging and weary marquise reached the point of desiring death: "As for me, I am no longer good for anything; I have played my role and, for my taste, I would never wish for such a long life. It is rare that the end and the dregs are not humiliating. But we are happy that it is God's will that regulates it, as with all things of this world: Everything is better in his hands than in our own."[71]

Resignation did not come easily to the marquise. She accepted "the end and the dregs" and the humiliations of old age, and she drank that draft to the last drop, but refusal was not far off. Some of her contemporaries recalled Seneca's pronouncement that you have to be a real drunkard to drink the dregs after the wine.[72] This was what happened to Lioterais, whose end Tallemant relates. When "he was old and life began to be a burden to him, he spent six months openly deliberating how he should die. One fine morning, while reading Seneca, he took out his razor and slit his throat."[73] This is clear proof of a change in attitudes and a wide gap between moral theory and practice: Lioterais had been openly contemplating suicide for six months without prompting any sort of reaction.

Tallemant spoke of other voluntary deaths as well. There were those of an artisan who was in love with the maréchale de Thémines, a man who had learned that his mistress was going to take the veil, and a young woman abandoned by her fiancé who starved to death next to a pond. There was also a certain Thomas, who had been his sister's lover and had murdered her, and who was interred by the parish priest in the section of the cemetery reserved for stillborn children. In 1672 the *Mercure galant* pitied the fate of a woman who first killed her unfaithful husband, then herself. Mathieu Marais told of several suicides under the regency, in particular in 1722. He wrote on 14 April of that year, "The misfortunes of the times are turning everybody's heads. . . . La Mazé, once a girl at the Opéra and a very pretty woman who had 3,000 livres of income in city [real estate] but who had been ruined by the system [of John Law], drowned herself in the middle of the day at La Grenouillère. She was wearing rouge, with beauty patches and flesh-colored silk stockings, and was all dressed up as if for a wedding." On 7 May Marais wrote, "Comte de Guiscard, a gambler by profession, drowned himself; another man hanged himself and made a very short testament in which he said, 'I have three stock shares, which I give to the regent, and my soul to the devil.' A cabaret owner of the rue Montmartre stabbed himself three times in the stomach because his mistress had been unfaithful. When they put a device on him [to stop the flow of blood], he tore it off and said, 'I didn't kill myself in order not to die.' "[74]

Suicide in Prison: A Government Concern

People's consciences were troubled and their minds were upset. This was particularly true in prisons, asylums of despair where the detainees, faced with perpetual imprisonment, at times with dreadful torture, often chose to kill themselves. Abbé Fleury was not the only one; Saint-Simon mentions a forger who cracked his skull against the walls of his cell in the Bastille in 1714. In 1717 a soldier who had assassinated Abbé de Bonneuil stabbed himself when he was arrested.[75]

After the 1690s the number of prisoners' suicides apparently alarmed the government of Louis XIV, given that suicides fed rumors and caused unpleasant reports to spread about conditions of detention.[76] The *lettres de cachet* and the penitentiary system were already highly unpopular, and the government had every interest in not adding to their bad reputation. In 1702 Father François d'Aix de La Chaize, the king's confessor, assigned a Jesuit to investigate the rumored brutal treatment of prisoners in the Bastille. Although he was not permitted access to the prison itself, the Jesuit worked for seven months to gather what information he could, after which he wrote a memoir that was transmitted to the king and to the chancellor, Louis Phélypeaux de Pontchartrain. Pontchartrain demanded an explanation from Saint-Mars, the governor of the Bastille, who did his best to reassure the minister, stating that everything was just fine in his establishment and that so far no prisoner had complained. Pontchartrain was nonetheless disturbed, not about the fate of the prisoners, but because confidential information had been passed through the prison walls. Had prison guards been indiscreet? The chancellor decided to find out who had talked. He wrote to Father de La Chaize:

Since that religious of your Company was refused entry into the Bastille, how does it happen that in seven months he was able to be so perfectly instructed in all its deepest secrets, as it appears from his memoir? His Majesty has commanded me to ask you this question, and he would be very happy to know who are the persons who may have said all these things. This is not an indifferent matter, since such persons may address themselves to others less discreet than the religious and make bad use of [what they learn].[77]

Every effort was made to stifle any alarming news. When a prisoner in the Bastille attempted to stab himself in 1691, the administration intervened "to try to put him back into the right path."[78] In 1696, when a Marseilles burgher who refused to pay the head tax was arrested, he killed himself, to the great embarrassment of the administration. The authorities decided to declare him insane—wasn't refusal to pay taxes a sign of madness? In the interest of avoiding scandal, the *intendant* wrote to the *contrôleur général:* "I have written to the king's prosecutor and to the judge ordinary that if it be absolutely necessary to conduct procedures concerning this fatal accident, they must consult with the magistrates to agree on the time and the manner so as to avoid a commotion they seem to fear." The *contrôleur général* gave orders "not to pursue the madman for killing himself." He was buried in secret.[79] In 1702 a wigmaker's apprentice who had strangled himself was refused absolution, and his body was dragged on a hurdle. Chancellor Pontchartrain was not happy. He wrote the prosecutor: "You were right to say to the commissioner not to make any mention in the dispositions of the witnesses of the refusal of absolution to this unhappy man. I beg of you to tell me who are the persons whom you consulted before making your decision to have the body dragged on a hurdle."[80]

In 1704 a prisoner in the Bastille named Vinache cut his throat. The marquis d'Argenson, who commanded the Paris police, intervened immediately to avoid an inquest and to keep the event secret, as was customary "every time such unfortunate things happen in the Bastille," as he wrote to the *procureur général.* The public was not to be alarmed. Argenson stated: "I always believe that deaths such as his are best hushed up, and every time such unfortunate things happen in the Bastille I have proposed to keep knowledge of them away from a public that is all too ready to exaggerate accidents of the sort and to attribute them to a governmental barbarity that it does not know but presupposes."[81] We read between the lines that prisoner suicides were frequent.

If the government sought to camouflage "accidents" that occurred in its jails, it also wanted to see that the penalties against ordinary suicide were applied. A royal declaration of 1712 stated that "crimes that cause deaths very often remain unpunished, either because the officers of justice fail to receive the instructions that should be given to them or because those same officers are negligent or dissimulate. The persons who have an interest in keeping the causes and circumstances of these deaths from being known [operate] by secret and precipitous interments, telling the clergy facts counter to the truth."[82] The law required that in every case of suspected suicide, the judge was to draw up a report, place a seal on the forehead of the cadaver, call in surgeons for a medical report, and hear witnesses.

Even more than the Ordonnance criminelle of 1670, the 1712 royal decree reflected the growing concern of the political authorities about what it is only somewhat exaggerated to call a suicide psychosis. In France no figures exist to confirm the rumors and the memorialists' impressions. Still, the frequency of allusions to suicide in the years 1680–1720, added to what we have seen in England, is troubling. If it was in the state's interest to conceal word of prison suicides, and if voluntary deaths among the clergy and the nobility went unremarked and unpunished, it was also in the state's interest to reduce the number of suicides among the people, given that suicides weakened the strength and the morale of the nation. The state could think of only one way to reduce the number of popular suicides—dissuasion through severe punishment. It saw the courts' growing indulgence toward the crime of suicide and their facilitation of dissimulation as simply encouraging voluntary deaths. If the respectability and honor of the clergy and the nobility put them above common morality, ordinary people must be made to understand that for them, suicide signified confiscation of possessions, posthumous punishment for the body, and hell for the soul.

Despite exceptions, commoners' suicides continued to be punished severely, particularly in the provinces and especially among the lower classes, who provided good examples at little social and political cost. In April 1684 the body of a cobbler from Angers was dragged on a hurdle, then hanged by the feet after he had killed himself "in despair, in his house." In Château-Gontier in 1718 Marie Jaguelin, a poor girl six months pregnant, poisoned herself out of shame. The unfortunate girl did not realize that only the nobility could kill themselves with impunity. Her cadaver was disinterred, brought to trial, sentenced, then dragged on a hurdle face down. When the group reached the town square, the executioner slit her womb and extracted what remained of the foetus, which was buried in the section of the cemetery reserved to the unbaptized. Marie's lacerated body was hanged by the feet and left, ignominiously exposed to the public gaze, until it rotted. It was eventually burned, and the ashes were thrown to the winds.[83]

The Casuists: A Harsher Stance

During this same time the Church maintained its strict condemnation of suicide, and the casuists continued to explore all possible circumstances for suicide, block all loopholes, and close all avenues of escape. On occasion, their efforts to be exhaustive led them to consider eventualities so exceptional as to approach the ridiculous. Behind their harder attitude and their universal reprobation we sense their need for reinforcements in the face of an increasing threat.

In his *Theologia moralis practica* (1680), Innocent Le Masson went so far as to assert that a man who is driven by his suffering to accuse himself of a crime he has not committed is guilty of suicide. In his *De jure et justitia* (1687) François de Coco forbade even actions that many casuists of the early age had authorized, such as throwing oneself off a tower in flames, blowing up one's ship when there was no hope of salvation, or throwing oneself in the water, to certain death, in order to baptize a drowning infant. In his *Theologia speculatrix et practica* (1662–63) Jean-Baptiste Du Hamel condemned all voluntary death. In 1694 Natalis Alexander (Noël Alexandre) wrote in his *Theologia dogmatica et moralis,* "All those who turn violent hands against themselves meet with eternal damnation." Returning to the case of the doomed ship, Alexander reiterated that it is forbidden to blow up the ship or to throw oneself in the water with no hope of survival. The prisoner condemned to death by starvation who refuses food brought to him in secret and the debauchee who shortens his life by his excesses are also guilty. In 1695 the bishop of Grenoble published a *Théologie morale* that absolutely condemned all types of suicide, which he called "the most criminal" of all murders because it is a crime against humanity and against human nature, which is "offended in the person of every man." What is more, the bishop added, "homicide of oneself is much more contrary to charity than the other homicides because well-organized charity must always begin at home, with oneself." Paul Laymann's *Theologia moralis* (first published in 1625 and republished in 1703) reiterated an unconditional condemnation of suicide, as did François Genet's work with the same title, published in 1706. Also in 1706, Franciscus Henno's *Tractatus moralis* returned to the case of plunging into the water to baptize an unbaptized infant who is drowning; he forbade the would-be rescuer from doing so if there were no chance of his getting out alive. In another case, Henno stated that someone on board a ship who has a fatal and contagious disease has no right to throw himself overboard to save his fellow-passengers.

Jean Pontas was one of the most famous casuists of the age. Born in

Normandy in 1638, he was a doctor of both civil and canon law, the author of many works, and *sous-pénitencier* of the Cathedral of Notre-Dame in Paris. In 1715 he published his *Dictionnaire des cas de conscience,* an authoritative work that was republished in 1724, 1726, 1730; it was translated into Latin in Geneva in 1731 and 1732, in Augsburg in 1733, and in Venice in 1738, and it was republished in the nineteenth century by Jacques-Paul Migne with commentary by Pierre Collet.[84] Pontas found no guiltless way to kill oneself, and he rejected all pretexts. He also cited a vast number of utterly exceptional cases: For example, a magistrate who has sovereign authority and who commits a crime punishable by death does not have the right to kill himself; a mortally wounded soldier who is begging to be put out of his misery cannot be killed as an act of mercy.

Canon law, diocesan statutes, and synodal ordinances confirmed this extreme severity. Claude Fleury writes, for example, that refusing Christian burial to suicides is necessary in order to inspire "terror in the living." Terrorizing the living to keep them from killing themselves was the best way society's leaders could devise for persuading people to remain alive! The more stringent attitudes reveal their profound failure. If a growing number of men and women found existence on this earth an unbearable calamity, it was in part because those who were responsible for the organization of this life had shown themselves incompetent. Rather than seeking to ameliorate living conditions in this world, the theorists attempted to persuade the faithful that their fate would be still worse if they tried to quit it. Everyone must patiently wait deliverance.

Nor did the theorists look kindly on settling in to enjoy this life. Death was still desirable. The old ambivalence remained: The Christian should be persuaded that this world is bad (hence it does not need to be too comfortable) and death is desirable, but that same believer must absolutely refuse to bring about his or her own death. This centuries-old balancing act was becoming increasingly difficult. Two crises of conscience marked the coming of the modern spirit and profoundly weakened traditional attitudes. First, in the years 1580–1620, the question had been whether it was better to be or not to be. Second, in 1680–1720, after a century of reflection, many people began to answer that question by opting for action, some of them choosing to be transported immediately to the next world, others choosing to work to improve conditions in this world. Both tendencies worried the Church, whose interest lay in maintaining the tension between remaining in this world and aspiring to the next.

Spiritual Substitutes and Practical Tolerance

Certain spiritual currents of thought found a compromise that I have called a substitute for suicide. The spirituality of annihilation continued to permit its adepts to get as close as possible to death without taking the final step, thus stifling the desire for death or deceiving it by seeming to satisfy it. This is what we find in Claude-François Milley's devotion to "nothingness." Milley (1688–1720) was a Jesuit, and his dates coincide nearly perfectly with those of the European crisis of conscience. He died caring for plague victims in Marseilles. He wrote in 1709: "Ours is no longer a time for living; the death of all things natural must be our lot" and "We must be suspended between heaven and earth; we must no longer look at ourselves." Hence we are nothing, a quasi-void. What was needed, as Jean Deprun puts it, was to turn the void *in* oneself into a void *for* oneself.[85] Let us persuade ourselves that we are nothing; let us annihilate ourselves, Father Milley declared. "What more could a little nothing do than to annihilate itself before Being? Is that not the proper and natural order? Nothing must be nothing and not think itself something."[86]

We can better appreciate the troubling and terribly ambiguous nature of those words if we compare them to the last sentence in the testament of Abbé Jean Meslier, an atheist priest who probably starved himself to death in 1729. Meslier declared: "The dead among whom I am about to go are no longer burdened with anything and no longer care about anything. Thus I will end with nothing, but also I am now scarcely more than nothing, and soon I shall be nothing."[87] To be nothing was what the pious Abbé Milley sought by remaining in this life and the materialist Meslier found by slipping into death. Their discourse is nearly identical. More than ever, the spirituality of annihilation seems a substitute for suicide.

Quietism, which reached its height in those same years between 1680 and 1720, was equally fraught with ambiguity. A need for annihilation, for a complete stripping away of the self, is at the origin of pure love. Such an attitude also brought its share of anguish and despair: Maine de Biran wrote, "The most painful way to die for oneself is to die for all that is the most intimate . . . to feel oneself die by what contains intellectual and moral life."[88] Fénelon too felt a strong attraction to annihilation, which, in his sensitive soul, came from disgust with oneself. Paul Hazard tells us, "This tortured soul, this heart so prone to weariness and sadness, brooded with sorrow on something he could not explain, deep down in his moral nature. The sight turned him sick, for what he saw was a swarm of reptiles."[89] That is why Madame Guyon's suggestion of complete abandonment, a total stripping away, and indifference to all things appealed so to Fénelon.

Quietism had a more alarming aspect, however, as the vigilant Bossuet pointed out in his *Écrits sur les maximes des saints.* Fénelon's way to total abandonment and sloughing off everything might pass through deepest despair. Fénelon asserted, citing the case of François de Sales, who went through a profound crisis before finding his spiritual equilibrium, that it might be salutary to let the penitent think that he was damned and that God had no intention of saving him. This, Bossuet declared, was both a pernicious doctrine, because it suggested belief in the heretical idea of denying that God intends to save everyone, and a dangerous doctrine, because it ran the enormous risk of "making a soul succumb to the temptation of despair. The temptation to despair consists in inducing the soul to believe invincibly that there is no salvation for it . . . which is the height of despair because [the soul] believes it invincibly."[90] Whereas for Fénelon, acceptance of the certitude of eternal damnation represented the utmost and absolute self-sacrifice and opened the door to quietude, Bossuet considered it "an act of true despair and the height of impiety." What concerned Bossuet was the ambiguity of the spiritual currents that flirted with despair, annihilation, and a desire for death.

Bossuet sought to maintain a balance that must necessarily underlie Christian life. We are in a vale of tears, where we should give thanks for our trials while aspiring to the eternal happiness of the next world. Admittedly, life is merely a preparation for death: "A Christian is never alive on this earth because he is always mortified here, and mortification is a trial, an apprenticeship, a beginning of death," Bossuet declared in the *Oraison funèbre de Marie-Thérèse d'Autriche.* We must desire that death without ever seizing it, but if that salutary tension is to exist, we must continue to hope for salvation.

Bossuet and Fénelon agreed in an approval of certain biblical suicides—Samson's, for one. They even went a step further, since Bossuet came close to approving of voluntary deaths for honor: "I do not doubt that a right-thinking man [un homme de bien] can prefer [honor] to his life, and that he even ought to do so in certain circumstances."[91] Fénelon praised Christian voluntary martyrs, and in his *Dialogues des morts* he had Cato pronounce an eloquent discourse justifying his suicide.

By the end of the seventeenth century an entire network of seminaries labored to form a clergy that would conform to the Christian ideals of the Catholic Reform; what was wanted was a clergy that would operate in the world without being of the world. The priest should mortify his flesh, humiliate his spirit, die to himself by killing his self-love, and desire death. Louis Tronson, the director of the seminary of Saint-Sulpice in Paris, recommended this examination of conscience to his seminary students:

Let us examine if we hate ourselves and our flesh as true penitents must. Have we regarded ourselves as having within us a horrifying fund of terrifying malignity that encourages us always to offend God? And have we treated ourselves with all the rigor that a slave, ever ready for revolt and rebellion, would deserve? Have we been happy to be poorly fed, ill dressed, occupied with low employments, subject to many infirmities, lacking in any talent, only good for being scorned and rejected by everyone— and to have been so in the conviction that we legitimately merit all these states, and that they were not harsh enough for sinners who desire being held in execration by all creatures? Have we had great aversion for our flesh as being our greatest enemy, mistrusting it, watching over its every movement, taking great care to persecute it ceaselessly without desiring peace with it or even a truce? Have we embraced the zeal of the apostle, making [our flesh] bear the punishments it merits and ardently desiring to be separated from it?[92]

When they left the seminary, the fledgling priests would have to confront cases of suicide in their parishes. They needed to be prepared for that eventuality. Matthieu Beuvelet's *Instructions sur le Manuel . . . pour servir à ceux qui dans les séminaires se préparent à l'administration des sacremens* long remained the manual most used on the parish level.[93] Although it might seem surprising, unlike the casuists and the authors of treatises on moral theology, Beuvelet recommends a degree of tolerance in practical situations. Christian burial must be refused to "those who out of despair or rage (but not madness) have procured their own deaths, unless before dying they gave some sign of repentance." He adds that one witness suffices to establish that sign, and his or her word is not to be questioned. The passage deliberately suggests that the priest should always adopt the most charitable attitude and grant Christian burial after even the smallest indication of repentance. With one stroke of the pen, Beuvelet nullified hundreds of volumes of abstract moral preachments and casuistry; whatever the circumstances, one could always suppose madness or repentance. That option explains why families easily obtained decent burial for their suicides and why so few suicides were judged guilty. Guilty verdicts did exist, as we have seen, but they were for extreme and particularly desperate cases. All texts are only worth what application makes of them. Theoretical rigor, which is often necessary for dissuasion, proved much more supple when it was applied to a practical situation.

The Dilemma Clarified

The second European crisis of conscience (1680–1720) marked a turning point where voluntary death was concerned. The question, "To be or not to be?" had arisen between the years 1580 and 1620; despite the authorities' attempts to stifle it, the seventeenth century reflected on the question. The first answers began to appear in the years 1680–1720—answers that began to worry society's leaders and that grew more insistent during the eighteenth century.

The great majority of intellectuals chose "to be." On the condition that such "being"—that is, life—be worth living, which was far from true for the multitude. After Bayle and Fontenelle, voices began to be raised to demand a reorganization of this world to make it more livable for a greater number of human beings. Those who thought it could be made a better place began to challenge privilege, injustice, and institutions. The seductive idea of terrestrial happiness appeared. Religion needs to be made more smiling, the earl of Shaftesbury wrote, in a mood that reflects the inspiration of devout humanism. We need to be joyful, to indulge in humor: A melancholy attitude toward religion was what made it so tragic and created so many lugubrious catastrophes. Religion should instead be treated with good manners and cheerfulness.

Institutions soon came under attack, sometimes with good humor. Montesquieu's *Lettres persanes* (*Persian Letters*) were published in 1721, but they were simply a prelude to the more substantial fare that Voltaire, Diderot, Holbach, and others provided. The message of the philosophes was that we are indeed eager "to be," but on the condition that this world be refashioned, making it a sojourn of delight, not a vale of tears.

A small minority of intellectuals preferred the other choice, "not to be." They preferred to leave this life immediately, or the minute it became unbearable, and they fully intended to be able to do so in full liberty. Some began to demand the right to choose and to give their own answers to the fundamental question, "To be or not to be." That liberty of choice took center stage in the eighteenth century.

The authorities—the religious authorities in particular—thought that a liberty of the sort was impossible. Their position became extremely delicate, however, because they rejected both what the partisans of being and what the partisans of nonbeing had to offer. To make our stay on this earth too agreeable was to put an end to aspirations to eternal salvation in the next world, which was the motive force of morality; to authorize humans to dispose of their own lives was to frustrate the divine plan and to do away with the indispensable trials that permit us to earn our way to heaven. For those of that frame of mind there was no choice, only the obligation to be unhappy in the hope of eventual happiness. The best that one could do in this world was to administer our ephemeral unhappiness. This solution was less and less acceptable in a century whose aspirations were reflected in its own version of Hamlet's question: "To be happy or not to be."

NINE

The Debate on Suicide
in the Enlightenment

From Morality to Medicine

"To be or not to be?" The question that had been posed as the Renaissance declined and that was discussed endlessly in the salons and the intellectual circles of the seventeenth century became a topic of public debate in the eighteenth century. The question emerged from Latin treatises and muted controversy to blossom in the light of day, despite governmental efforts to stifle it. Never before had people talked so much about voluntary death, never before had so much been written about it: Many thinkers hastened to take a stand on it, and entire treatises were written, pro or con. The question had become a social reality, and it finally had a name of its own, *suicide*. For some Frenchmen it was even an elegant fashion, like everything else that supposedly originated in England. In London in the 1780s public debates were organized on the subject: The *Times* of 27 February 1786 announced a debate on the topic, "Is suicide an act of courage?" It cost sixpence to attend. In 1789 the same newspaper declared that suicide was "at present a general subject of conversation among all ranks of people." Another debate was organized following the suicide of a Frenchman in Greenwich Park: So many people attended and such a great stir was caused that it ran far overtime.[1]

A topic situated at the point where religion, justice, and mores meet, and one that had become a burning question, was bound to attract the interest of the philosophers. They all wrote on suicide at one point or another, and their writings made the debate even more heated, to the point that their critics held them responsible for a supposed rise in the number of voluntary deaths. The partisans of traditional morality, alarmed and bewildered by what seemed to them an increase in suicides, attacked deism, freethinking, and the philosophical spirit.

Treatises on Suicide: Expressions of Growing Concern

The number of treatises against suicide published after the mid-eighteenth century gives a good indication of the traditionalists' concern.[2] The first of these was *Les Lettres persanes convaincues d'impiété* (1751) by Abbé Jean-Baptiste Gaultier. The work repeated all the old arguments: To kill oneself is a crime against God, society, and the laws. The same year, an anonymous treatise *Les hommes* declared that merely "to have some traits in common" with those who defended voluntary death was shameful. In 1755 "le Chevalier de C." published a work entitled *L'honneur considéré en lui-même* in which he reduced suicides to three categories: the falsely courageous (who were despicable), the desperate, and the hypochondriacs (who inspired horror). Again, as good soldiers, we must occupy our posts to the end; God has put a love of life in us like a "secret order" that works toward our preservation. In 1756 Gabriel Gauchat declared in *Lettres critiques, ou, Analyse et réfutation de divers écrits modernes contre la religion* that tolerating suicide was equivalent to permitting all murder. Suicide destroys both families and countries; it is not even courageous, as killing oneself is "very easy." The severity of the laws regarding suicide must be maintained, Gauchat insisted, in particular, the punishment inflicted on cadavers. Claude Dupin agreed with this in *Observations sur . . . l'Esprit des lois* (1757), where he called for "severe laws."

Also in 1757, a collective work with the evocative title *La religion vengée* argued at great length to refute defenses of suicide. The book is divided into two sections, each of which covers ten points. First come ten arguments against voluntary death:

It dishonors human nature.

Since we have no right to kill someone who is making us suffer, we have no right to kill ourselves because we are suffering.

Suicide goes against our desire for happiness because it leads us to damnation.

We are not proprietors of our own lives.

We cannot desert the post God and nature have assigned to us.

If suicide were permitted to those who suffer too much, all suicides would be tolerated, because the idea of unbearable suffering is relative and varies from one individual to another.

The sovereign has rights over our life.

Society is harmed by suicide.

Suicide is forbidden in all the most enlightened nations.

Nature requires of us that we love life.

After this come ten objections that partisans of suicide might make, each one followed by a response:

The law does not forbid suicide, as there are always exceptions. (*Response:* The exceptions are offered precisely to defend life.)

The search for happiness is more important than love of life. (*Response:* Suicide brings on eternal unhappiness.)

Our body is contemptible. (*Response:* By preserving it we have an opportunity to suffer, hence to advance in virtue.)

The soul is in no way harmed by killing oneself, as it is immortal. (*Response:* By killing oneself, one deprives the soul of the pleasure of virtue.)

Life is a boon, but one can renounce a boon if the price to be paid for it is too high. (*Response:* The price for eternal happiness is never too high.)

Suicide permits avoidance of crimes. (*Response:* That is as good as saying that one can poison oneself to avoid illness.)

All peoples practice suicide. (*Response:* All enlightened peoples condemn it.)

Nature urges us to flee evil. (*Response:* If God wanted to call us to him he would simply have us die.)

Killing oneself is an act of courage. (*Response:* It is an act of weakness or madness.)

When God, the proprietor of the house that is our body, ruins that house by destroying our health, it is a sign that it is time for the tenant to leave the premises. (*Response:* We are not the tenants of our bodies but the guardians.)

This heterogeneous enumeration concludes by reiterating that suicide is always a crime, even when committed by illustrious pagans. The author approves of penal sanctions and declares them effective: "The intention of the legislators was to frighten, and up to a certain point their desires have met with success."

In 1761 Louis Antoine de Caraccioli stated in *La grandeur d'âme* that one must be "truly imbecilic" to find the least grandeur in suicide. It sends us to hell, and even if we are not absolutely sure it does, it is stupid to run such a risk.

In 1763 Jean-Georges Lefranc de Pompignan criticized the philosophers' admiration for the suicides of classical antiquity. In 1765 Samuel Formey, who was a Protestant, condemned all suicides in the name of natural law in his *Principes de morale*. According to him, the Catholic arguments of the soldier sticking to his post and those of obligatory obedience to the Mosaic commandment were not very effective because in certain cases the same arguments could be turned around to argue in favor of suicide. Only those who kill themselves "because their patience is exhausted or who are driven to despair by illness" can perhaps be excused. In his *Traité de morale, ou, Devoirs de l'homme envers Dieu, envers la société et envers lui-même* (1767), Lacroix taxed Cato and Brutus with "stupid pride" and attributed their suicides to weakness.

In 1771 Flexier de Reval attacked "children of pleasure" who seek to excuse all suicides, and in *Les Contradictions du livre intitulé De la philosophie de la nature,* Simon de La Boissière opposed drawing any distinction between good and bad suicides, because doing so could only contribute to "diminishing the horror that such an attack on oneself should arouse." Suicide was always proof of "vileness of soul." Augustin Barruel and *La petite encyclopédie* denounced their contemporaries' tolerance of voluntary death. Still in 1771, Joseph-Nicolas Camuset's *Principes contre l'incrédulité, à l'occasion du "Système de la nature"* and Giovanni da Castiglione's *Observations sur le livre intitulé "Système de la nature"* attacked Holbach and reasserted that suicide is an offense to God and society.

In 1772 Father d'Audierne condemned all forms of suicide, direct or indirect, in his *Instructions militaires:* Blowing up a ship or a fortress (and oneself with it) so as to keep them from falling into enemy hands is a sin against God, one's country, nature, and civil and canon laws. We have no right to sacrifice our lives to save someone else, and even less to avoid poverty, escape temptation, or save our honor.

In Amsterdam in 1773 Jean Dumas, a Protestant, published an indictment against all forms of voluntary death, *Traité du suicide, ou, Du meurtre volontaire de soi-même.* In it he attempted to refute all the philosophic arguments in favor of suicide, singling out Cesare Beccaria, who had argued in favor of eliminating penal sanctions for suicide. For Dumas as for Formey (also a Protestant), suicide should be punished because it was a crime, and the punishments inflicted ought to be sufficient to impress people and discourage imitations. In 1774 Charles Louis Richard attacked the suicides of classical antiquity, Pythagoras in particular, in his *Défense de la religion.* In another work, *Exposition de la doctrine des philosophes modernes* (1785), Richard connected suicide, parricide, and regicide.

Dictionaries and encyclopedias printed vigorously hostile opinions in their entries under *suicide*. The *Dictionnaire de Trévoux* states concisely, "Suicide is the system of cowards, who have neither the patience to endure themselves nor the courage to bear the burden of a misfortune, and by stabbing himself Cato proved he was more the first among extravagants than the first among Romans." A Christian who killed himself out of fear of eternal punishment was raving mad, and anyone who did so for philosophic reasons was a fool. The dictionary goes on to flail at bad examples given in literature, in the theater, and by prominent figures.

The *Encyclopédie méthodique,* the 1782–1832 edition in some two hundred volumes developed from the enterprise founded by Diderot and d'Alembert, was no more favorable. More precisely, it expressed two different opinions— yet another proof of the heterogeneous nature of an enterprise that is too often thought of as a monolithic block of philosophe propaganda. The *Encyclopédie méthodique* treats suicide in two different articles, written by different authors. The entry under *suicide* in the volumes entitled *Jurisprudence* simply recalls the punishments inflicted on suicides and notes past excesses and absurdities.[3] Beneath its apparent neutrality, however, the article is clearly critical: "Today the cadavers of those who have killed themselves are sentenced to be dragged face down on a hurdle, then hanged by the feet; they are deprived of burial." When possible, the article continues, suicides are tried immediately "to make the example of their punishment more striking." When this proves impossible, "because of the dreadful odor emitted by the cadaver," the guilty person is put on trial in memoriam. Such procedures apply, however, only to "those who kill themselves in cold blood, with complete use of reason, and out of fear of torture." Those who kill themselves "in dementia [en démence]" or even "those whose minds are subject to wandering [sujets à des égarements d'esprit]" do not receive such penalties, and in case of doubt insanity is presumed. The article recalls that in ancient Rome, committing suicide out of distaste for life was considered "a trait of philosophy and heroism," and goods were confiscated only when the suicide was a condemned criminal. This was clearly a criticism of current practice.

Religious Opposition

The article on suicide that appears in the volumes of the *Encyclopédie méthodique* subheaded *Théologie* is totally different in tone from the one published under *Jurisprudence*.[4] The entry was written by Abbé Nicolas-Sylvestre Bergier, canon of Notre-Dame and confessor to Monsieur, the king's brother.

Bergier had already written several works in which he attacked the philosophes. In one of these, *Examen du matérialisme, ou Réfutation du Système de la nature* (1771), he praised the dissuasive force of the severest possible penalties for suicide. His encyclopedia article is a veritable indictment of voluntary death.

Bergier sets the tone from the start, defining suicide as "the act of killing oneself to deliver oneself of an ill one hasn't the courage to bear." The article notes the increasing frequency of suicide: "Our public papers have related the multitude of suicides that have occurred in our century; hardly a one can be found that does not derive, directly or indirectly, from libertinage." At least the Romans killed themselves for valid reasons; now "it is when we have lost our money, or in the excess of a mad passion for an object that is not worth the trouble." The philosophical spirit is furthering the scourge of suicide: "In our days, the abuse of philosophy has gone so far as to try to apologize for this crime." There are "some unbelievers" who claim that suicide is not prohibited by either natural law or divine law, and who base that statement on the attitude, approved by the Church fathers, of certain martyrs.

Abbé Bergier took it upon himself to refute such ideas. God gives us life, he insists, which is a boon, "whatever the peevish reasoners say," and only God can dispose of it. We receive life in order to serve society, and every individual is useful to that end: "When [a person] serves simply to give an example of forbearance, that in itself would be much, and nothing can excuse him from it." Those who kill themselves lack virtue, for they are incapable of bearing suffering. Moreover, people with suicidal tendencies are quite capable of killing others: They are potential criminals. The evils we endure are always deserved, and we have no right to elude them.

Bergier then responds to objections. First he insists that when suicide deprives society of one of its members, it is a more serious matter than clerical celibacy, which deprives it only of hypothetical members. Next he treats the old question of whether Jesus committed suicide, a question raised in the age of the Church fathers and revived in the age of the philosophes as a way to embarrass the Church. Holbach, for instance, wrote in his *Système de la nature:* "Christianity, and the civil laws of Christians, are very inconsistent in censuring *suicide.* . . . The *Messiah,* or the son of the Christians' God, if it be true that he died of his own accord, was evidently a *suicide.* The same may be said of those penitents who have made it a merit of gradually destroying themselves."[5] Jean Barbeyrac, Jean Le Rond d'Alembert, Delisle de Sales, Guillaume Dubois de Rochefort, and Johann Bernhard Merian all raised the problem, and Bergier answers it as best he can. Jesus, he states, gave his life to save the lives of all humanity; his death was not a suicide but a sacrifice. Moreover, He knew He would rise again. In his *Examen du matérialisme,* Bergier adds an unfortunate argument: Jesus did not commit suicide, he states, "unless one wishes to accuse Socrates of the same crime"—a parallel that many champions of traditional morality were drawing.

As for the Christian martyrs, Bergier continues, one cannot speak of suicide in their case, as their intention was not to destroy themselves but to demonstrate to their persecutors that persecutions were in vain: "Heroic charity" did much to put an end to persecution. Virgins (St. Pelagia, for example) who killed themselves to avoid being raped acted well, for if they let themselves be ravished they faced the "danger of consenting to sin and succumbing to the weakness of nature": Death was preferable to risking the least suspicion of carnal pleasure.

Bergier draws distinctions among biblical suicides. Abimelech, Saul, Ahithophel, and Zimri were reprobates; Razis died for the same reasons as the Christian martyrs; Samson and Eleazar sacrificed their lives for their nations, thus were not true suicides. Aside from these quite special cases, the Mosaic commandment stood as an absolute: "Thou shalt not kill"—unless, of course, society demands it, as in wartime or by judicial decree.

The casuists remained just as systematically opposed to suicide as they had been in former years. Nonetheless, St. Alfonso de' Liguori suggests a certain number of exceptions, though for truly extraordinary circumstances. In his *Instruction pratique pour les confesseurs* he recalls, "It is not permitted to anyone to kill himself directly and deliberately without authority or divine inspiration, by which fact several martyrs have caused their own deaths without sin. Thus tightrope walkers (that is, those who walk balancing on ropes attached to high places), those who swallow poisons, or those who permit themselves to be bitten by vipers in peril of their lives commit a great sin."[6]

Returning to the casuists of the sixteenth and seventeenth centuries, Alfonso adds:

It is at times permitted to expose one's life to peril for a just cause, following the doctrine common to many doctors [of the Church]. Thus the soldier must not leave his post even though he sees that death will strike him (that opinion is general). It is permitted to give one's food to a friend who is in distress, as with the floating log, where one cedes to another the possibility of being saved. . . . It is in fact more probable, for there is a great difference between giving oneself death and ceasing to defend one's life, which is permissible when there is a just cause. . . . It is permissible in case of fire to jump out of a window, provided that this give hope of escaping imminent death.

Similarly, Alfonso declares:

It is legitimate to set fire to one's ship, even at peril of one's own life, when the general good demands that it not fall into enemy hands. . . . Although a young girl cannot give herself death, she can nonetheless expose herself to danger rather than be raped, and that does not seem improbable, if it is out of love of chastity as well as because of the danger of sin that emerges from such occasions. It is permissible for a guilty detainee not to flee when he can, and even to present himself before the judge to be sentenced, even when the penalty would be death.

Alfonso writes concerning mortification of the flesh: "It is permitted to mortify oneself by fasting and penitence out of love of virtue, even if one must necessarily shorten one's life by several years (provided, however, that such penitence not be indiscreet), because there is a difference between positively shortening one's life and permitting it to be shortened out of affection for virtue." Here he left himself open to criticism from the philosophes, Holbach in particular, who hastened to note the relationship between mortification of the flesh and suicide. Finally, Alfonso admits, "We are in no way held to preserve our lives (unless it is necessary to the general good) by extraordinary or extremely painful means such as the amputation of a leg, the extraction of a stone, or other similar remedies."

Theologians and moralists usually linked the question of mutilation to suicide. They disagreed profoundly about castration, a mutilation commonly practiced on the request of bishops who had an interest in providing high voices for their cathedral choirs. The greatest number of castrati were in the pontifical chapel, where the custom continued to the late nineteenth century. Alfonso de' Liguori expresses some reservations, but he permits the practice "provided, however, the child consent to it and that he not risk his life, because the preservation of the voice for those who are extremely poor can be of great importance to them and change their fate; because the eunuchs can seem useful to the general good by contributing, by their singing, to retaining the faithful within the churches; and because, in a word, that operation has degenerated into a habit and is authorized by a number of prelates."

Writings about Suicide in England

Whether it was rigid (Abbé Bergier) or flexible (Alfonso de' Liguori), Roman Catholic opinion worried that ideas favorable to suicide were making headway. The Protestant world reacted in much the same way. In England the Nonconformists who came after the Puritans accused the deists of demoralizing society. Richard Steele and Thomas Beach bitterly criticized high society's cult of Cato.[7] In 1730 John Henley wrote a *Cato Condemned, or The Case and History of Self-Murder,* published in London.[8] George Berkeley attributed the rise in suicides to "the minute philosophy": "As the minute philosophy prevails, we daily see more examples of suicide," he declared in *Alciphron*.[9] George Cheyne, the author of *The English Malady,* also held the propagandists for ancient suicide responsible for a rising suicide rate. John Wesley, the founder of Methodism, suggested that penalties against suicide should be strengthened and that suicides' bodies should be left to rot on the gallows. Other writers suggested that the cadavers be used for clinical dissections. Some clergy refused to bury the bodies of suicides, even when the deceased had been declared insane.[10] For many of the clergy, Satan was still at work, tempting a growing number of men and women to kill themselves. Isaac Watts repeated this stance in 1726 in *A Defense Against the Temptation to Self-Murder.*[11] In 1754 an anonymous *Discourse upon Self-Murder* recommended fasting and prayer to combat the temptation of suicide, and in 1755 Francis Ayscough gave a sermon entitled "A Discourse against Self-Murder," in which he held the devil responsible for the crime of suicide.[12]

Sinister events reinforced such beliefs. The *London Evening Post* of 11 September 1760 revealed that a notorious murderer, Francis David Stirn, had committed suicide in prison after writing on his cell wall, "O Lucifer, Son of the Morning! How art thou brought down to Hell, to the side of this pit." In 1765 a coachman left a suicide note in the form of a warning, "Never let the Devil get the upper hand of you." In 1783 a woman drowned herself after writing that she had struggled with the devil for several days. In 1792, before poisoning himself, John Abbot got up in the middle of the night and was heard to say, "Oh, here is the Devil [who] has got hold of me; pray for me, pray for me."[13] On other occasions the ghosts of suicides were heard to complain of their eternal torture.

The Methodists were particularly persuaded that Satan had a role in suicides. Wesley related several cases in his journal, the *Arminian Magazine*. In 1763, for instance, Richard Rodda declared, "The devil likewise tempted me to destroy myself. One day, when I had a razor in my hand, he told me that [it] was a fit instrument for the purpose. He likewise added, if I did, I should be happy for ever. But something within answered, No murderer hath eternal life abiding in him. . . . At length I threw the razor on the ground, and fell on my knees. God soon heard me, and rebuked the destroyer."[14]

The *Arminian Magazine* abounded in tales of this sort. Methodist preachers also spoke of their encounters with the devil in their autobiographies. John

Valton, a former Roman Catholic and the son of French immigrants, on several occasions was tempted by Satan to hang himself, as was the poet William Cowper, an evangelical given to lofty flights of fancy.[15]

The Anglicans accused the Methodists of promoting suicide by spreading terror of hell. In August 1743 the *Norwich Gazette* held a Methodist preacher named Balls responsible for the death of a woman of unsteady mind, and John Jones, an Anglican, accused John Berridge of driving his listeners mad with despair by his preaching, and of having caused the suicide of eight persons.[16]

The *Times* repeated these accusations: On 3 May 1788 it stated that "the numerous suicides committed in and about London" were to be attributed to Methodist preaching. On 4 April of the same year, the *Times* published a letter written by a preacher in Daverhill who complained of being held responsible for the suicide of a woman in his congregation because he had preached that they would all be damned if they failed to act on his words.[17] Several physicians who specialized in mental illness confirmed this view: Alexander Crichton and William Pargeter declared that the Methodists favored suicidal melancholy by their obsession with hell and eternal happiness.[18]

The complexity of the religious scene in England made debate on suicide both more confused and more lively than elsewhere. The myth of an "English malady" was solidly entrenched, and it opened the way to an increasing number of accusatory writings that sought to assign responsibility for the phenomenon. These in turn encouraged the myth: Discussion about suicide in England was taken as proof that England was more affected than other lands. It is true that England produced a larger number of treatises exclusively devoted to voluntary death than continental countries, where the question was usually treated within much broader works on morality or social criticism. Precisely because voluntary death was seen as one point in a vast whole, the terms *suicide* and *self-murder* rarely appeared in the titles of books printed on the Continent. In England, it was a topic in itself.

Accusations in England were unfocused and contradictory, however: On the one hand, the rise in the number of suicides was blamed on the demoralizing influence of freethinking, the philosophical spirit, and the atheism of some members of the aristocracy; on the other hand, its cause was seen as an eschatological despair stimulated by excessive religious zeal, exaltation, and fanaticism among Nonconformist and sectarian groups. Between these two extremes the Anglican clergy offered a model of equilibrium. Anglicanism favored a reasonable and national religion that was hostile to all excess and encouraged psychological and social harmony, the best guarantee against suicide.

The Philosophes: A Favorable View of Suicide?

On the Continent, and in France in particular, the situation was in appearance simpler and more Manichaean. Two armed camps stood opposed: that of traditional morality, which was defended jointly by the Roman Catholic Church and the absolutist state, and that of a supple, critical, rational morality based on human rather than religious values, which was defended by the champions of the "philosophic spirit." The first accused the second of fomenting demoralization, of corrupting mores by undermining the divine foundation of morality, and of favoring free suicide, which brought on the dissolution of society.

This view is a caricature that does not stand up to closer scrutiny. The men who were called philosophes during the Enlightenment were in reality far from being apologists for suicide. Their position on the problem fluctuated widely, and it defies all systemization. What is more, the philosophes themselves refused to be considered supporters of voluntary death. If people kill themselves, they insisted, it is not because of philosophical arguments but because they are suffering, physically or mentally. Holbach, who was among the writers most tolerant of suicide, insists on this point.

Many persons will not fail to consider as dangerous these maxims, which, in spite of the received prejudices, authorize the unhappy to cut the thread of life; but *maxims* will never induce a man to adopt such a violent resolution: it is a temperament soured by chagrin, a bilious constitution, a melancholy habit, a defect in the organization, a derangement in the whole machine, it is in fact necessity, and not reasonable speculations, that breed in man the design of destroying himself. Nothing invites him to this step so long as reason remains with him, or whilst he yet possesses hope—that sovereign balm for every evil.[19]

A glance at the biographies of the *maîtres à penser* of eighteenth-century France proves that they had little interest in providing examples of suicidal conduct. How many philosophes killed themselves? None of the better known ones, until 1794, when Chamfort committed suicide for reasons that had little to do with philosophy. The other philosophe suicides—and there are very few of them—involve obscure figures (Pidansat de Mairobert, for instance). The suicide of Johannes Robeck, a Swede, caused quite a stir, but it was an isolated case. Robeck was little known, moreover. A Lutheran who converted to Catholicism (at one time he even attempted to join the Society of Jesus), he seems to have been of somewhat fragile mind. In 1735 he wrote a treatise in Latin justifying suicide, *De morte voluntaria philosophorum et bonorum vivorum*. After he had completed the mansucript, he donned his best clothes, rented a small boat in Bremen, rowed out to sea, and disappeared. His body was found on shore several days later; his treatise was published the following year.[20]

This was a spectacular case, but is it a viable model for the philosophic attitude? The philosophers of the Enlightenment loved life too much to imitate such a desperate act. Even Rousseau, who so often looked on the worst side of things, was not tempted by the adventure. When the philosophes were faced with Hamlet's dilemma, they chose "to be." They were by no means ready to die for ideas. Martyrdom and sacrifice of one's life were rather marks of the fanaticism that they fought against: "I would much prefer to be the confessor of the truth, not of martyrdom," Montesquieu wrote. Voltaire concurred: "I would not like to augment the number of the martyrs." Voltaire had only sarcasm for exalted minds of all camps who let themselves be killed to defend their ideas: Polyeucte was just as much of a fool as the fanatical opponents of religion, who were "people with no sense who should be confined to asylums." Nor did Voltaire admire the famous suicides of classical antiquity: In *Candide,* Cunégonde takes pains not to imitate Lucretia. For other writers—Jean-François Regnard, for one—Lucretia was even the object of bawdy pleasantries.

Even Socrates came in for criticism. In 1763 the audience watching one tragedy applauded Crito when he advised Socrates to flee.[21] Socrates had few imitators in the eighteenth century. When Frederick II of Prussia threatened the philosopher Christian Wolf with hanging if he did not resign from the University of Halle, where he was accused of teaching irreligion, Wolf left forthwith. Alberto Radicati, a Piedmontese who had emigrated to England, wrote:

It is a maxim generally accepted in this enlightened century that a wise man should never expose himself to any danger in the aim of instructing the common people or refuting a predominant opinion, no matter how pernicious for society. The patriotic ideas that were the pride of the heroes of antiquity are now regarded as ridiculous and chimerical. Those famous Greeks and Romans . . . would now pass for madmen, unworthy of living because of the bad example they would give people.[22]

In short, the philosophes preached the same practical attitude—let us keep on living—as the Church, although for different reasons. Like the clergy, they also condemned dueling, a substitute for suicide and an aristocratic vice. Holbach compared dueling to human sacrifice, and d'Argens likened it to cannibalism; Diderot bitterly criticized "the sanguinary laws of a point of honor" as something that must be fought, even at the price of making use of religious prejudices. Voltaire, Rousseau, Bernardin de Saint-Pierre, and Sedaine all violently opposed dueling, and they accused the clergy of being altogether too accommodating on that score. They expressed satisfaction at the decline in frequency (cowardice aiding) of such ritual murders, and they called for severer measures against dueling. A Paris judge, François Gorguereau, put such demands into systematic form in a treatise published in 1791.[23]

Another point of convergence between the philosophes and the Church—though again, their reasons differed—was that although death was not to be sought, neither was it to be feared. The philosophes accused the clergy of inculcating fear of death (and the judgment that followed immediately) within a broader pastoral policy of encouraging fear of hell. In reaction, the philosophes did their best to combat the macabre and its system of images. "Death is nothing," Glenat wrote in 1757 in his *Contre les craintes de la mort.* Holbach attempted to strip death of its mythic aspects in his *Réflexions sur les craintes de la mort* and his *Système de la nature.* Voltaire did the same in 1766 in *Sophronime et Adelos.* Holbach proposed replacing the image of death—a terrifying and inaccurate vision—with the idea of death—an intellectual notion. It was Christian death that was terrible and inhumane. Sylvain Maréchal wrote: "On his deathbed, like a criminal, [a dying man] trembles at the approach of the supreme judge. The idea of a rewarding or vengeful God prevents him from indulging in the last effusions of nature. He coldly turns away his family and his friends in order to dispose himself to appear before the supreme tribunal."[24]

The clergy and the philosophes agreed, however, that death does us a great service by ridding us of the miseries of this life. Holbach attempted to persuade the readers of his *Réflexions sur les craintes de la mort* that "it is good to establish some principles that will diminish our attachment to life and, consequently, make us regard death with more indifference." Death, he continued, cuts short old age and its misery; the sum of all the woes of this life outweighs the good things; even people who are wealthy and honored are unhappy, because they are exposed to envy and agitated by passions; "one in ten thousand" is happy. Thus death "cannot but grant them an often advantageous revolution."

The philosophes were divided when it came to the next world, but they all were reassuring. Those who believed in God declared themselves convinced of his goodness. Montesquieu wrote, "I seek immortality, and it is within me. My soul, extend yourself! Precipitate yourself into immensity! Return into the great Being." The deists' God did not promise eternal hell; He was not a vengeful God. Thus, as Rousseau assured his readers, we can pass to the great beyond in all confidence. The materialists were equally confident. La Mettrie wrote, "Death is the end of everything; after it—I repeat—an abyss, an eternal void. All is said, all is done; the sum totals of good and evil things are equal; no more cares, no more roles to play: The farce is over."[25] Death was the gate to the void, and nothingness was by its essence unimaginable. Its most reassuring comparison was sleep, however, a dreamless sleep with no risk of the bad dreams that gave Hamlet such pause.

If that were true, why hesitate? In the final analysis the philosophes' position was ambivalent. They had little enthusiasm for suicide, but they also made death less fearsome, which meant that the only way they could justify a desire to live was by presenting existence as basically positive—something not all of them felt they could do, as we have seen with Holbach. In reality, all the philosophes found it difficult to reach a coherent position. Hamlet's dilemma still lurked behind a self-assured façade, behind their somewhat forced optimism, and behind their sarcasms and their nonchalance.

Literary Suicide: An Epicurean Refinement or an Exorcism?

In a century in appearance so lightweight, the intellectuals' fascination with death was a very troubling characteristic (a point that Robert Favre makes in *La mort au siècle des Lumières*). The macabre is present throughout eighteenth-century literature, and stories of suicides, often in horrible circumstances, are frequent. Still, authors who claimed to be liberated from superstition and who spoke incessantly of voluntary death hardly ever put an end to their own days. Are we to see this dialectic of attraction and repulsion as a way that some writers used to exorcise suicidal tendencies and others used to frighten themselves and make the pleasures of life even more enjoyable—a supreme Epicurean refinement? Favre suggests as much, and it is not impossible.

Characters in eighteenth-century literature kill themselves by the hundreds with not a word of authorial repoach. It would be nearly impossible to recapitulate all the voluntary deaths scattered through the novels of Bastide, Bernardin de Saint-Pierre, Charpentier, Madame de Charrière, Diderot, Dubois-Fontanelle, Florian, La Dixmerie, La Haye, Léonard, Lesage, Loaisel de Tréogate, Louvet, Mademoiselle de Lussan, Marivaux, Marmontel, Mouhy, Prévost, Regnard, Rétif de La Bretonne, Madame de Riccoboni, Madame de Tencin, Madame de Villedieu, and Voltaire. In his brief overview of literary suicides in the eighteenth century, Albert Bayet classifies them as altruistic suicides, suicides to preserve honor, suicides out of remorse and to expiate crimes and faults, and suicides for love. In a similar review of dramatic works, Bayet concludes: "Thus tragedy taught the same moral stance at its decline as it had at its birth. Abbé Desfontaines was right to reproach it for minimizing 'the horror of suicide.' Not only do the plays we have just seen fail to show [suicide] as an object of horror, they present it as the normal, elegant, or obligatory solution in certain well-defined cases."[26]

Eighteenth-century tragedy, like seventeenth-century drama, provides sonorous phrases about the beauty of suicide:

> Quand on a tout perdu, quand on n'a plus d'espoir,
> La vie est un opprobre, et la mort un devoir

(When all is lost, and not even hope remains, to live is shameful, and to die, our duty.)[27]

> Des héros désarmés c'est le dernier parti

(It is the last option of unarmed heroes.)[28]

> . . . La mort n'est qu'un instant
> Que le grand cœur défie, et que le lâche attend

(Death is but an instant that the great-hearted defy and the coward awaits.)[29]

> Lorsqu'un péril pressant nous laisse sans appui,
> C'est mériter la mort que l'attendre d'autrui

(When a pressing danger leaves us defenseless, we deserve death if we await it from others.)[30]

> Ne laissons point le peuple arbitre de mon sort,
> Et plutôt en chrétienne offrons-nous à la mort

(Let us not allow the people to decree my fate, but as a Christian woman offer ourself to death.)[31]

> Les criminels tremblants sont traînés au supplice.
> Les mortels généreux disposent de leur sort.
> Pourquoi des mains d'un maître attendre ici la mort?
> L'homme était-il donc né pour tant de dépendance?

(Criminals are dragged to punishment; but generous minds are masters of their own fate: Why meet it from the hands of Genghis? Were we born thus on others' wills?)[32]

Voltaire allows Alzire to give the best summary of the sentiments of eighteenth-century tragedy:

Quoi, ce Dieu que je sers me laisse sans secours!
Il défend à mes mains d'attenter sur mes jours!

. . .

Eh! quel crime est-ce donc devant ce Dieu jaloux
De hâter un moment qu'il nous prépare à tous?
Quoi, du calice amer d'un malheur si durable
Il faut boire à longs traits la lie insupportable?
Ce corps vil et mortel est-il donc si sacré
Que l'esprit qui le meut ne le quitte à son gré?
(Alas! Alzire, the new God thou servest
Withholds thy hand, and says thou must not finish
Thy hated life. . . . Is it a crime to hasten on, perhaps
A few short years, the universal doom
Appointed for us all? and must we drink
The bitter cup of sorrow to the dregs?
In this vile body is there aught so sacred
That the free spirit should not leave at will
Its homely mansion?)[33]

Even authors with a reputation for having a light touch at times permitted themselves dark thoughts, as did Marivaux in *Le Spectateur français*.[34] Amusing works such as Montesquieu's *Les lettres persanes* are full of massacres and morbid passages, to the point that Favre speaks of "frenzies of torture and blood."[35] Moreover, rumors circulated about the supposedly atrocious deaths of actual people: Rousseau's purported suicide, Prévost's death in an autopsy, Gilbert's madness, Voltaire's deathbed agony.

Literature also gave full rein to the theme of illusory death. It is as if authors were seeking to terrify their readers. As Favre puts it, "We see everywhere false suicides, deceptive dangers, failed assassinations, premature burials miraculously remedied, providential lethargies, interrupted executions, pardons granted against all verisimilitude, false ghosts."[36] False suicide was not only a literary device: Some artists and authors themselves sought death-defying thrills. Hubert Robert was fond of terrifying himself by climbing about the ruins of the Coliseum in Rome or by deliberately losing his way in the Roman catacombs. Others simulated hangings, seeking the aphrodisiac effects the physicians Bichat and Cabanis had claimed in their writings.[37] The marquis de Sade used the same device in his novels, *La nouvelle Justine* among others. Favre states, "Tasting death in order to arrive at a heightened sense of existence and to increase the enjoyment of being alive was an experience that literature made available to everyone. . . . Was this not in reality the very ancient desire to travel to the land of the dead and return?[38]

All imaginable means were used to evoke death: The fashion for ruins, tombs, and the sort of funerary monuments that adorned parks *à l'anglaise* favored hedonistic meditations on the flight of time and the emptiness of life; revery in some wild place (Senancour recommended the Alps) or an autumnal landscape permitted communion with "the terrible necessity that forms only to dissolve." According to Feucher d'Artaize, reflection on the many woes that cast their shadow over the human condition was a way to "make death less hideous." A desire for death was among the sentiments most often expressed in intellectual circles in the eighteenth century, from Jean-Jacques Barthélemy, who wrote in 1763, "I confess to you that I am weary of living and that I would have no difficulty in ending it," to Rousseau, who declared in 1770, "If I were offered the choice here below of what I wanted to be I would answer, 'dead.'"

A complementary theme was deploring ever having been born and having come into this unhappy world. When Gilbert stated, "Woe to those who bore me," he was only one of many authors who echoed Job's "Perish the day on which I was born." The least one could do was to refuse to have children: "Why give life to someone who will resemble oneself?" Madame de Staël asks rhetorically.[39] Dorval, a character in one of Diderot's novels, is grieved at the thought of becoming a father and thrusting a child "into a chaos of prejudices, extravagances, vices, and miseries." Although he was opposed to suicide, Diderot, in a letter to Sophie Volland, gave a definition of life that many of his contemporaries seem to have shared:

To be born in imbecility amid pain and cries; to be the plaything of ignorance, error, want, illnesses, malice, and the passions; to pursue a return to imbecility from the moment one first stammers to the moment one drivels; to live among worthless people and charlatans of all sorts; to fade away surrounded by one man who takes your pulse and another who bothers your head; not to know from whence one comes, why one has come, where one goes—that is what people call the greatest gift our parents and nature have given us: life.[40]

This is a surprising attitude that upsets the traditional image of the Enlightenment. As we learn from Robert Favre, however, the eighteenth century was pessimist. The century that prepared the way for romanticism flirted with the idea of death, and suicide was naturally a favorite topic in a highly popular sort of reflection, which at times seems a turbid literary game, among the elegant people who took pride in grasping the novelties that crossed the

English Channel. Even authors who officially declared their opposition to voluntary death did not escape that contagion.

The case of Abbé Prévost provides a good example. He was an odd sort of "abbé," when you come to think of it, having led a life that was far from religious, as did certain other eighteenth-century men of the cloth, from Jean Meslier to Abbé Sieyès. As a young man, Prévost, who had attended a Jesuit school, first joined the army, then joined the Society of Jesus, which he left to pursue an adventure involving a woman. He then rejoined the army. After a phase of fairly joyous living, he joined the Benedictine Order. For a time he preached and taught theology, but under threat of a *lettre de cachet* he left the monastery and went to England. There he found a post as a tutor, but lost it over yet another question involving a woman, and left for Holland. He then returned to England, where he lived with a beautiful adventuress. Eventually he returned to France under the protection of the prince de Conti, whose almoner he became. He soon ran up enormous debts, and when imprisonment in the Bastille seemed likely, he fled, first to Brussels, then to Frankfurt. By the time he returned to Paris he had earned a formidable literary reputation. He also returned (more or less) to the ecclesiastical life. He died of apoplexy in 1763 in the Forest of Chantilly.

Prévost's contemporaries were struck by the macabre and bloody character of the novels and short stories of this ambiguous and baffling author, who seemed both horrified and fascinated by death. In Prévost's works people kill one another and themselves with both horror and delight; suicides are innumerable and as if inevitable, dictated by fate. In his moralistic works, however, Prévost strictly condemned suicide. His review, *Le Pour et le Contre,* printed stories that were often tragic and that carried highly traditional moral lessons that might seem surprising from the pen of the author of *Manon Lescaut.*

In 1734 the suicide of an English clergyman prompted Prévost to write "Reflection on Suicide." In this piece he shows that voluntary death is in all cases a grave fault. If a would-be suicide is Christian he should fear damnation; besides, killing oneself is senseless. "The Christian who kills himself is a madman." A philosopher is a fool to put an end to his days. What can he expect by killing himself? "This desire, taken simply in itself, is an absurdity and in accordance with no reasonable lights." Will suicide increase one's pleasures? Anyone who expects pleasures from chance has little hope of satisfaction, and he abandons what is certain for what is highly uncertain. If we await pleasures from God, we have no hope whatsoever of succeeding, because we force the Creator's hand. Should we get rid of our woes? That is totally illusory; to make that happen, death would have to be followed by nothingness, "which is perhaps the most unlikely of all chimeras." Anyone tempted to kill himself would do better to expect punishment by aggravated troubles. "The author of these reflections concludes from them that praising those who voluntarily kill themselves grants esteem to fools or madmen."[41]

Prévost is a strange figure who seems to float in incoherence. One might well wonder what he expected of a world beyond death that he refused to see as nothingness. Between the many suicides he depicts in his novels and the abstract suicide that he condemns in *Le Pour et le Contre,* which one exorcises the other? We may have to accept Prévost's ambiguity. Like his epoch, he hesitated between life and death, refinement and vulgarity, and faith and atheism.

Montesquieu's Explanations

All the philosophes had an interest in suicide, but although some of them clearly condemned it and others scandalized their contemporaries by demanding full liberty to dispose of one's life, most of them—including all the best-known ones—raised questions, hesitated, contradicted one another, and split hairs.

Montesquieu's attitude illustrates this fondness for nuances. He considered the problem of suicide on three occasions and from different angles. In 1721 he treated the question in the seventy-sixth of the *Lettres persanes,* where he vigorously criticizes judiciary repression of suicide:

European laws are ferocious against those who kill themselves. They are, so to speak, made to die twice, for they are hauled ignominiously through the streets, proclaimed infamous, and their property is confiscated. It seems to me, Ibben, that these laws are most unjust. If I am laden with sorrow, misery, and contempt, why should anyone want to prevent me from putting an end to my cares and cruelly deprive me of a remedy which lies in my hands?[42]

Montesquieu attempts to show that suicide neither harms society nor hinders Providence. Society, he says, is founded on mutual advantage, and if I no longer gain any advantage from that contract, I am free to withdraw. Life has been given me as a good; if I no longer feel that it is good, I can give it back. To the objection that separating a soul and a body that God has joined together thwarts Providence and upsets the order of nature, he responds, through Usbek:

When my soul shall be separated from my body, will there be any less order and arrangement in the universe? Do you believe that any new combination will be less perfect or less dependent upon the general laws, or that the universe will have lost something, or that the works of God will be less great or, rather, less immense? Do you think that my body, having become a blade of wheat, a worm, or a piece of lawn, would be changed into a work less worthy of nature, and would my soul, freed of everything terrestrial, become less sublime?[43]

In reality, Montesquieu insists, it is our pride that persuades us that we are so very important that our death would change the order of nature.

This letter says nothing about motivations for suicide; it simply shows that suicide is not a crime. In the 1754 edition of the *Lettres persanes,* however, Montesquieu prudently added a seventy-seventh letter. In Ibben's short, timid, and formal response to Usbek he states that our woes serve to expiate our offenses, and that we should submit ourselves to the Creator who joined our souls to our bodies.

In 1734 Montesquieu returned to the subject of suicide in his *Consider-ations sur les causes de la grandeur des Romains et de leur décadence.* In this work he examines Roman suicides but seems not to share the enthusiasm of classical antiquity's most fervent admirers. He weighs various cases: "Brutus and Cassius killed themselves with inexcusable precipitation, and we cannot read this chapter in their lives without pitying the republic which was thus abandoned. Cato had killed himself at the end of the tragedy; these began it, in a sense, by their death."[44]

Why, Montesquieu wonders, did so many Romans kill themselves? His answer: They did so because of the influence of Stoicism; because the custom of granting a triumph to a victorious general and the existence of slavery made generals unable to bear defeat; because Romans wanted to avoid criminal prosecution and the confiscation of their property; because of "a kind of point of honor" and the "great opportunity for heroism" that suicide offered. Montesquieu adds that some Romans, carried away by their emotions, committed suicide without really thinking of death. He makes no value judgments, but rather ends this passage with a psychological analysis of suicidal tendencies. Suicide, he explains, is by no means an attempt to seek death; it is a supreme act of self-love. "Self-love, the love of our own preservation, is transformed in so many ways, and acts by such contrary principles, that it leads us to sacrifice our being for the love of our being. And such is the value we set on ourselves that we consent to cease living because of a natural and obscure instinct that makes us love ourselves more than our very life."[45]

Fourteen years later, Montesquieu attempted a medical diagnosis of suicide. When he examines the *maladie anglaise* in *De l'esprit des lois,* he does not question the reality of the disease, but simply attributes it to the influence of the English climate on physiology:

We do not find in history that the Romans ever killed themselves without a cause; but the English are apt to commit suicide most unaccountably; they destroy themselves even in the bosom of happiness. This action among the Romans was the effect of education, being connected with their principles and customs; among the English it is the consequence of a distemper, being connected with the physical state of the machine, and independent of every other cause. In all probability it is a defect of the filtration of the nervous juice: The machine, whose motive faculties are often unexerted, is weary of itself; the soul feels no pain, but a certain uneasiness in existing. Pain is a local sensation, which leads us to the desire of seeing an end of it; the burden of life, which prompts us to the desire of ceasing to exist, is an evil confined to no particular part.[46]

This analysis permits Montesquieu to offer a criticism of society, and he remarks that "it is evident that the civil laws of some countries may have reasons for branding suicide with infamy; but in England it cannot be punished without punishing the effects of madness."[47] As we have seen, this is not totally accurate. Far from writing a defense of voluntary death, Montesquieu thus limits himself to analyzing the reasons that lead individuals to suicide in certain civilizations and to demanding that criminal pursuits for suicide be abolished.

Voltaire: "Amiable People Ought Not to Kill Themselves"

Voltaire, who amused himself at Lucretia's expense, was no more enthusiastic about suicide than Montesquieu. His sarcasm was directed at the religious and civil punishment of the cadaver and at the penalties inflicted on the suicides' families. Suicide in itself intrigued Voltaire; it awakened his curiosity much more than his sympathy. He spoke of it often, informed himself about it, and sought the reasons that lead certain people to leave a life to which he himself was so attached. By temperament Voltaire was little inclined toward voluntary death, except in moments when he found the spectacle of human folly particularly depressing. "I wish for death," he wrote in 1753. After telling, over and over again, the horrors that filled both the history of the past and contemporary events, he arrived at the conclusion that this life is nauseating and absurd, "full of sound and fury, signifying nothing." At times he himself took on Shakespearean tones to denounce existence as a voyage that, although unbearable, is still hard to quit. Humanity is but a "horrible assemblage of unlucky criminals" living on a ridiculous little globe that "contains only cadavers." Earth is an anthill where survival of the whole is all that counts: "We are ants, ceaselessly being crushed, who renew ourselves; in order for these ants to rebuild their dwellings, and in order for them to invent something resembling a polity and a morale, how many centuries of barbarity!"[48]

To have a vision of humanity as lucid as Voltaire's and not cede to the temptation of nihilism shows proof of an exceptional temperament. At times Voltaire himself seemed surprised. He wrote in 1764, quoting La Fontaine's "Le Bûcheron et la mort," "Mieux vaut souffrir que mourir, / C'est la devise des hommes" (Better to suffer than die; that's man's motto).

The motto might seem the height of absurdity: Why insist on remaining a spectator (worse, an actor) in an odious drama? If anyone had a thousand reasons for committing philosophical suicide, it was Voltaire, yet he never thought of taking that way out (any more than the twentieth-century existentialists did). Those who proclaim the absurdity of the world most loudly are not the ones who leave it voluntarily; rather, suicides are those who are the most attached to the world's values. Probably lucidity helps those who proclaim life's absurdity to avoid disillusionment, which is the source of despair. If we can believe Frederick II, Voltaire did once attempt to kill himself, but the affair was soon forgotten. He attributed his gesture to "either constancy, cowardice, or philosophy," and he lived on to age eighty-four. His principal stimulants were irony, sarcasm, and a determination to denounce the history of the world as an odious farce. He wanted to "make men return to themselves, and make them feel that they are in effect only victims of death, who should at least console one another."[49] Deriding one's fellows was the best way to avoid sharing their absurdity: "I always take to my bed in the hope of making fun of humankind when I awake. When I no longer have that faculty it will be a certain sign that I should leave."[50] This was a powerful remedy for despair, as Diderot recognized when he thanked Voltaire, who had just completed the *Essai sur les mœurs,* for having taught him "indignation."

Voltaire's longest discussion of voluntary death is found in the *Dictionnaire philosophique,* the entry "De Caton, du suicide." In this article he sketches out an analysis, based on actual cases, of why people kill themselves. Were suicidal tendencies in part hereditary? He tells us that on 17 October 1769, "I was almost an eye-witness of a suicide." The victim was a "man of a serious profession, of mature years, of regular conduct, without passions, and above indigence." He had left a "written apology for his voluntary death," Voltaire tells us, which was not made public for fear of setting off a wave of other suicides. As it happened, his father and a brother had killed themselves at the same age. Voltaire wonders "that nature should so dispose the organs of a whole race that at a certain age each individual of that family will have a passion for self-destruction—this is a problem which all the sagacity of the most attentive anatomists cannot resolve. The effect is certainly all physical, but it belongs to occult physics. Indeed, what principle is not occult?"[51] What Voltaire calls "occult" here may have been a presentiment of genetic coding.

Voltaire gives other examples as well. Philip Mordaunt, a cousin of the earl of Peterborough and a young man twenty-seven years of age—"handsome, well made, rich, of noble blood, with the highest pretensions"—shot himself in the head because "his soul was tired of his body."[52] Richard and Bridget Smith, simple folk, hanged themselves and left a note expressing their confidence in God's mercy. Lord Scarborough killed himself because he was caught in an impossible situation between a mistress whom he loved but could not marry and a fiancée he esteemed, to whom he had promised marriage. The most common causes for suicide seem to have been weariness of existence, poverty, and unrequited love. These examples all came from England, but Voltaire, more clairvoyant than Montesquieu, accords no credit to climate or to the myth of the English malady as explanations of English suicide. This was an illusion, he writes, due to the fact that English gazettes could report suicides freely, whereas French newspapers were censored and could not write on the subject. If all French cases were known, he adds, "we should, in this particular, have the misfortune to rival the English."[53] There was no reason to take fright, however, and no epidemic of suicides was imminent. "Against this, nature has too well provided. Hope and fear are the powerful agents which she often employs to stay the hand of the unhappy individual about to strike at his own breast." Humankind is made in such a way that we prefer to endure all manner of suffering rather than do away with ourselves. "The apostles of suicide tell us that it is quite allowable to quit one's house when one is tired of it. Agreed, but most men would prefer sleeping in a mean house to lying in the open air."[54] The Old Woman in *Candide* is of a like opinion: "I have been a hundred times upon the point of killing myself, but still I was fond of life. This ridiculous weakness is, perhaps, one of the dangerous principles implanted in our nature. For what can be more absurd than to persist in carrying a burden of which we wish to be eased?"[55]

The instinct of self-preservation is so strong that extraordinary force of character is needed to kill oneself. This is why Voltaire rejects the accusation of cowardice, an accusation frequently made against suicides: "None but a strong mind can thus surmount the most powerful instinct of nature. This strength is sometimes that of frenzy, but a frantic man is not weak."[56] Voltaire was capable of recognizing the grandeur of soul of the famous suicides of ancient Rome, a grandeur so inconceivable that he permits himself to doubt the historical truth of such acts: "We do not, indeed, see how Codrus or Curtius could be condemned." Cato was admittedly the eternal honor of Rome, but the story of Lucretia was pure fable. As for Lucretius, Voltaire has Memmius say, "He would have suffered and he suffers no longer. He made use of the right to leave his house when it was about to collapse. Live as long as you have a just hope; die when you lose it. That was his rule; it is also mine." Arria was "sublime," and Voltaire compares the suicide of two lovers in Lyons to that of Paetus and Arria. To give the other side of the story, Voltaire reports that Cardinal Dubois was heard to mutter to himself, "Kill thyself! Coward, thou darest not."[57]

Still, Voltaire was capable of seeing suicide in another perspective, in particular when it was young women who "hang and drown themselves for love." They would do better to "listen to the voice of hope, for changes are as frequent in love as in other affairs."[58] In a letter to Madame du Deffand written in 1754, Voltaire speaks about "an eighteen-year old girl whose head had been turned by the Jesuits and who departed for the next world to rid herself of them." He remarks, "This will not be my course of action, at least not soon, because I have arranged life annuities for myself with two sovereigns, and I would be inconsolable if my death were to enrich two crowned heads."[59]

Voltaire uses the same light tone to speak of the letter on suicide in Rousseau's *La nouvelle Héloïse:* "His instructions are admirable. First he proposes to us that we kill ourselves, and he claims that St. Augustine was the first person who ever imagined it was not nice to kill oneself. The minute we are bored, according to him, we should die. But Master Jean-Jacques, it's even worse when we bore others! What should we do then? Answer me. To believe you, all the common people of Paris should run to bid adieu to this world."[60]

According to Voltaire, many suicides were due to madness, still others displayed a "sickness" that induced people to kill themselves for trivial reasons. One thing that favored the development of suicidal tendencies was idleness, thus "an almost infallible means of saving yourself from the desire of self-destruction is always to have something to do." This was why more people killed themselves in the city: "The laborer has no time to be melancholy; none kill themselves but the idle. . . . The remedy is a little exercise, music, hunting, the play, or an agreeable woman." In any event, Voltaire adds, if you have decided to kill yourself, wait a week before putting your resolution into effect. It would be surprising if the instinct of self-preservation did not win out in that time.[61]

When friends were tempted to put an end to their days, Voltaire scolded them. "Amiable people ought not to kill themselves; that is only for unsociable spirits like Cato [and] Brutus. . . . Companionable people ought to live," he wrote concerning an Englishman named Crawford.[62] On several occasions, Voltaire comforted Madame du Deffand, who had melancholy tendencies. When he learned of the suicide of an acquaintance, he deplored it, and he was much affected by news of the death of his friend Jean-Robert Tronchin. He tried to be understanding: "In general, I blame no one," he wrote.[63] On one occasion he visibly refrained from criticizing one of his former Jesuit teachers, but he put a pinch of malice in his insistence: "I have no intention of closely inspecting the motives of my former prefect, Father Benassès, a Jesuit, who bade us good-night in the evening and, the next morning after saying his mass and sealing a few letters, threw himself from the third story. Everyone has his own reasons for his behavior."

In this domain as in others, liberty was, in the final analysis, the height of wisdom for Voltaire. "I once received a circular letter from an Englishman, in which he offered a prize to any one who should most satisfactorily prove that there are occasions on which a man might kill himself. I made no answer: I had nothing to prove to him. He had only to examine whether he liked better to die than to live."[64]

Suicide was for Voltaire a question of individual liberty. It harmed neither God nor society. When the Huron asks Gordon, "Do you then think that any one upon earth hath the right and power to prevent my putting an end to my life?" Voltaire tells us:

Gordon took care to avoid making a parade of those common-place declamations and arguments which are relied on to prove that we are not allowed to exercise our liberty in ceasing to be when we are in a wretched situation; that we should not leave the house when we can no longer remain in it; that a man is like a soldier at his post; as if it signified to the Being of beings whether the conjunction of the particles of matter were in one spot or another. Impotent reasons, to which a firm and concentrated despair disdains to listen, and to which Cato replied only with the use of a poniard![65]

Suicide does not harm society: "If suicide wrongs society, I wonder whether the voluntary homicides, legitimated by all the laws, that are committed in wartime do not wrong the human race even more."[66] Voltaire states that after all "the Republic will do without me as it did before I was born."

Returning to the contrast between Montaigne and Pascal on the subject of suicide, Voltaire drives home his argument:

Speaking philosophically, what harm does a man do to society who departs from it when he can no longer serve it? An old man has the stone and suffers intolerable pain. He is told, "If you don't have yourself cut, you are going to die; if you are cut, you will be able to continue in your dotage, to dribble, and shuffle along for a year, a burden to yourself and to others." I suppose the old fellow would choose to be no longer a burden to anybody. This is pretty much the kind of circumstance Montaigne is talking about.[67]

Neither the authentic Christian texts nor Roman laws prohibited suicide. Voltaire returns to this point in his *Commentaire sur le livre Des délits et des peines,* a work that refers to Cesare Beccaria's *Dei delitti e delle pene* (*On Crimes and Punishments,* 1764). Voltaire makes use (though for his own purposes) of Duvergier de Hauranne's *Question royalle,* which showed that the prohibition on killing is subject to all sorts of exceptions the minute those who enjoy positions of authority in society feel that leniency is required. Moreover, sacrificing one's life to save the state, the homeland, or the sovereign was generally approved: Why, then, should suicide for personal reasons be prohibited? "I seek not to apologize for an act which the laws condemn, but neither the Old Testament, nor the New has ever forbidden man to depart this life when it has become insupportable to him. No Roman law condemned self-murder."[68]

Hence punishments visited on the cadaver and on the victim's family were odious:

We still drag on a sledge and drive a stake through the body of a man who has died a voluntary death; we do all we can to make his memory infamous; we dishonor his family as far as we are able; we punish the son for having lost his father, and the widow for being deprived of her husband. We even confiscate the property of the deceased, which is robbing the living of the patrimony which of right belongs to them. This custom is derived from our canon law, which deprives of Christian burial such as die a voluntary death. Hence it is concluded that we cannot inherit from a man who is judged to have no inheritance in heaven. The canon law, under the head "*De Poenitentia,*" assures us that Judas committed a greater crime in strangling himself than in selling our Lord Jesus Christ.[69]

Voltaire is in his element here as he denounces the absurdity of the criminal laws of the ancien régime and points out their iniquity. He returns to the topic in *Prix de la justice et de l'humanité,* where he declares that suicides "care little, when they are good and dead, whether the law in England orders they be dragged in the streets [and buried] with a stave driven through their bodies, or whether, in other states, the fine criminal judges have them hanged by their feet and confiscate their wealth. Their heirs take it much to heart, however. Does it not seem to you cruel and unjust to despoil a child of his father's estate just because he is an orphan?"[70]

There are other passages in a similar vein in Voltaire's writings.[71] Still, the fact remains that Voltaire was no apologist for suicide. He advised his friends against it, but he sympathized with those who took that route.

Hesitation among the Philosophes

Diderot was firmly against suicide. Admittedly, he recalled in the *Encyclopédie* that the Bible contains positive examples of voluntary death, that martyrs like St. Pelagia and St. Apollonia were "true suicides," that Christ's death was voluntary, that mortification of the flesh shortens life, and that John Donne found ways to speak favorably of suicide. Diderot also recognized the grandeur of the suicides of ancient Rome, and he wrote, echoing Seneca, that "to take away Cato's dagger is to envy him his immortality."

Diderot is the presumed author of an article in the *Encyclopédie* that repeats the traditional arguments: God has given us life and has put in us an instinct for self-preservation; destroying oneself is destroying God's work; no one is useless in society, and it is not sure that life is a greater misfortune than death. Like the casuists, the article condemns all suicides, including those committed out of ignorance, for they come from failing to master one's passions.

Although the authorship of the article is in doubt, the viewpoint it expresses reappears in two works clearly by Diderot. In *La Marquise de Claye et Saint-Alban,* Diderot categorically rejects all temptation to philosophical suicide. "Distaste for life is false and exists only in a deranged or poorly organized head. What is more, it is only momentary." He adds that everyone has obligations to family and friends, an argument he repeats in the *Essai sur les règnes de Claude et de Néron:* "It is rare that one harms only oneself." Diderot is sensitive to the charge that the philosophes favored suicide, and he asks them to adopt a responsible attitude. For him, Cato and Seneca rendered no service to the cause of philosophy. He does his best to dissuade anyone who declares his intention to kill himself. Diderot was highly ambivalent about one would-be suicide in literature, young Desbrosses. The suicides in Diderot's novels are victims of overwhelming despair, or they are so abominable that they inspire an aversion to suicide.

One way to reduce the number of suicides was to encourage optimism, confidence, enthusiasm for life, and hope by improving social, political, and cultural conditions; the way to put a stop to an exaltation of death and a yearning for the next world was to combat injustice, tyranny, ignorance, and superstition in this world. Diderot declares:

These are the principal causes of suicide. If the government's operations thrust a large number of subjects into sudden poverty, we must expect suicides. Many others will rid themselves of life whenever an abuse of pleasures leads to boredom, whenever luxury and the nation's bad habits make work more frightening than death, whenever lugubrious superstitions and a gloomy climate combine to produce and maintain melancholy, [and] whenever part-philosophical, part-theological opinions inspire a scorn of death.[72]

We find the same mix of condemnation and comprehension in d'Alembert. Reasoning in the name of a "purely human" morality, d'Alembert stresses the antisocial aspect of suicide, but adds, "One wonders if this reason for preserving one's days will have sufficient power over a wretch overwhelmed by misfortune for whom pain and misery have made life a burden. We respond that in such a case, that reason must be strengthened by other, more powerful ones, which revelation will add to it."[73] In any event, d'Alembert continues, it is vain and iniquitous "to inflict penalties on an action from which nature alone is sufficient to guard us" and on a guilty party who cannot be punished. Suicide is blameworthy, but it is not punishable; it must be considered "at times as an action of pure insanity, a sickness that it would be unjust to punish because it supposes that the soul of the guilty person is in a state where he can no longer be useful to society, and at [other] times as a courageous action that, speaking in human terms, requires a firm and far from ordinary soul."[74] To say that suicide is an act of cowardice is just as ridiculous as accusing a man of cowardice when he dies braving the enemy rather than face the shame of fleeing. D'Alembert's message is thus ambivalent: He excuses voluntary death but advises against it.

La Mettrie is even more bewildering. In his *Anti-Sénèque* he seems to agree with the Stoics, declaring that "it is a violation of nature to maintain [life] for one's own torment. . . . When [life] is utterly without good and, to the contrary, is besieged by terrible ills, must one await an ignominious death?"[75] In his *Système d'Épicure*, on the other hand, La Mettrie attacks the "monster" who breaks all ties and kills himself:

No, I will not be the corrupter of the innate pleasure one takes in life. . . . I will make humble people see the great good that religion promises to anyone who has the patience to bear what one great man has called *le mal de vivre*. . . . The others, those for whom religion is only what it is—a fable—and whom one cannot retain by broken ties, I will try to seduce with generous sentiments. I will show them a wife, a mistress in tears, [and] desolate children. . . . What sort of monster is someone who, afflicted with a momentary pain, tears himself away from his family, his friends, and his homeland, and has no other aim but to deliver himself from his most sacred duties?[76]

The marquis d'Argens was more coherent. He stated that "the crime of such People as murder themselves is inexcusable, look upon it in whatever light you will." Suicide endangers society; we should recoil with horror before "a crime that opens the door to all sorts of evils" and that "covers the memory of those who commit suicide with shame and infamy."[77]

Johann Bernhard Merian was just as categorical. In a study published by the Berlin Academy he states that all suicides result from mental illness. For him, there is no such thing as philosophical suicide, because when people kill themselves, even in voluntary martyrdom, they suffer despair, which is a form of "delirium." Merian's view totally excludes religious remedies for suicide. Everyone has seen "atrabilious imbeciles" who do not dare commit suicide because they fear hell, but who commit crimes in order to get themselves put to death. The best solution, Merian continues, is still the penalties currently in effect, which are an "excellent deterrent" to suicide. Such penalties do indeed affect families—that is, innocent people—but "one individual or one family is nothing when society is at stake."[78] These are somewhat startling words for a philosophe.

In a position totally opposed to Merian's, Delisle de Sales thought it odious to punish suicides and their families. In a *Mémoire addressé aux législateurs par la veuve d'un citoyen puni pour crime de suicide* he lashed out at absurd laws that do nothing to prevent people from killing themselves and that take innocent people whom society has ostracized and throw them onto the street. He exclaimed, "If only we could make policies that would prevent suicides rather than punish them! If at least the tortures inflicted for the crime did not always fall on innocent people!" Turning to the act of suicide, Delisle de Sales declared that we cannot place "all the actions of this sort either in the class of crimes or in that of virtues." In general, the suicides of classical antiquity had valid reasons for killing themselves, and "the ashes of those famous patriots will always be respected even by the philosopher who disavows them." Still, phrases such as "the fanaticism of love of homeland" hint that he had serious reservations.

What was the criterion for a "good" suicide? Delisle de Sales stated, "In general, the public interest should lead to suicide or at least justify it." Far from clarifying the situation, that principle led him to indecisive casuistic hairsplitting. Although Demosthenes and Cato were "magnificent citizens," they were wrong. Similarly, a widow who killed herself so that people would speak about her was wrong, but if she did so out of love or because of grief, that was somewhat different: "I do not justify such a suicide, but my sensitive heart grows indignant about putting a love heroine next to Robeck and the anglomanes."[79]

Helvétius and d'Argenson felt a similar embarrassment. Everything depended on the suicide's motives. Helvétius wrote, "Two persons throw themselves into the sea. Both Sappho and Curtius did so, but one did it to put an end to the torments of love, and the other to save Rome; Sappho was therefore a fool and Curtius a hero. In vain have some philosophers given the name of folly to both of these actions; the public sees clearer than they, and never gives the name of fool to those from whom it receives an advantage."[80] Those who kill themselves out of weariness with life deserve to be considered wise and courageous. For d'Argenson, the suicides of classical antiquity, who followed Stoic principles, were admirable, but his own contemporaries "almost always" killed themselves for bad reasons.[81]

Vauvenargues scorned death, but he thought that "despair is the greatest of our errors" and that it was "more deceitful than hope." Maupertuis was generally opposed to suicide, which all Christians ought to consider a crime. Outside of Christendom, however, it was a different question. The Stoics used suicide as a remedy to ill fortune, Maupertuis stated, and that same remedy was still available to victims of their fellow humans: "A ship returning from the Guinea Coast is full of Catos who would rather die than outlive their freedom." Suicide, he continued, is perhaps the most reasonable solution, for there is "neither glory nor reason in remaining prey to misfortunes that one can escape with merely momentary pain." We are so attached to life that the act of killing ourselves cannot ever be a mark of cowardice. As for Christians, if they are truly persuaded that suicide leads to eternal damnation, their only choice is to remain in this life; the contrary would be proof of insanity.[82]

In March 1757 the newspaper *Le Conservateur* published a long article on old age ("De la vieillesse") that distinguished between the attitudes of the Christian and those of someone guided "by human reason alone." Beneath an apparent deference to Christianity, the author used a light, bantering tone to demonstrate that religious discourse was unreasonable. This was a common technique among the philosophes, and it never failed to send the champions of traditional morality into a frenzy. Indeed, the article caused a furor. The author wondered aloud whether anything could be more reasonable than killing oneself, rather than enduring the irreversible sufferings of old age.

Should not the state itself force us to do so, if it were truly interested in assuring our happiness?

If at the age of eighty one had the same firmness of purpose as at thirty, few men would not make that decision. I am not speaking of the divine law that makes it the duty of each one of us to remain at his post until it may please the sovereign Being to remove us; that reason is highly specific, and in discourses like mine one must, as much as possible, make use of general reasons only. . . . Should not politics, which strive to assure us peace and happiness, force us to take recourse [in suicide] when it is the only way to end our misery?

In any event, the article continued, God had other plans: May his will be done. "His mercy has placed us in this world and intends us to remain here as long as it may please him. Let us await old age as one of life's greatest tribulations, [and] as a happy opportunity to expiate our crimes and to avoid letting a fleeting urge lead us into eternal torment."[83]

Dubois-Fontanelle had a more general view of suicide, and he sought ways to reduce the number of its victims. Calling current legislation "savage," he claimed that it is useless to publicize suicides—indeed, he said, publicity encourages suicide and has a bad influence on public morality. "It would perhaps be better to stifle these events, which afflict humanity, and not give them publicity by procedures that remedy neither the past nor the future and that fall upon the living." Dubois-Fontanelle's stance (stifle news of suicides, dissimulate them, close one's eyes to them, establish a wall of silence around them) was in fact just what the royal government was already doing. It was to be the prevailing attitude throughout the nineteenth and twentieth centuries. Suicide must be left in oblivion, which was where it had been for centuries since the Renaissance. It must be a taboo--one of the few remaining in modern society. The method may not have been courageous, or even effective, but it was practical. What else was one to do? Moral precepts and reasoned arguments had little hold on minds that "offer traces of insanity of a more or less strange sort." The only true remedy was to "make men happy." Was this an admission that there was no solution to the problem of suicide? Dubois-Fontanelle made a pro forma suggestion: "The great remedy needed for suicide is in the hands of the government. It consists in supervising mores, stopping excessive luxury, [and] putting an end to public disasters that augment and aggravate individual disasters."[84]

Many other philosophes and moralists joined the battle about suicide on one side or the other, and more often than not, on both sides at once. Marmontel praised Cato in one text, but elsewhere he denounced the "captious sophisms" of Montesquieu, calling them "frivolous palliatives for the blindest fury."[85] Le Noble drew a distinction between a "worldly morality" that sees Cato's act as cowardly and a "human morality" that sees a virtuous side to suicide.[86] Robinet admitted that an individual might legitimately sacrifice his life for others, but he also declared suicide an offense to God, nature, and society.[87] Denesle wrote that those who justify suicide "are indistinguishable from assassins," that lovers "who play with ropes or give themselves potions" are mad, and that Cato, Brutus, Otho, and Porcia were guilty of a crime, but he also stated that Otho was a hero, since he sacrificed himself to stave off civil war in Rome.[88] Feucher d'Artaize declared that "suicide is simply the cowardly side of courage," but he also recognized that "it is a dreadful benefit of our high development; a refinement of liberty," and he praised Arria and Cato (whom he nevertheless criticized for displaying a bit too much caution before killing himself).[89] Toussaint allowed suicide when motivated by a virtuous act. Barbeyrac saw it as an act of courage in itself but a moral weakness. Camuset called Cato a "Pygmy" in wisdom. Lévèque gave suicide a physiological explanation (it was due to a shortage of active spirits in the nerve fluid). Chevignard saw it as an act of madness: "To kill oneself is the height of folly. What can be its motivations? Despair or cowardice."

Suicide and Madness

Many of the philosophes were nonetheless moving toward the idea that suicide was a result of madness or physiological malfunction, hence it belonged under the category of medicine more than under those of justice or religion. Eighteenth-century scientific works helped to relieve suicide of guilt.

Explanations of suicide on the basis of climate moved in this direction, and Montesquieu was not the only writer to advance them. For George Cheyne, a fresh, humid, and unstable ocean climate helps small drops of water penetrate the fibers of the human body, making them lose firmness and predisposing the mind to suicidal madness. Another explanation was based on the supposed influence of the moon. The idea of "lunatism" (or lunacy), which was common in the sixteenth and seventeenth centuries but less frequent in the eighteenth century,[90] resurfaced in the 1780s, but in a form that linked it to meteorology. In the treatises of Giuseppe Toaldo (1770; French translation, 1784) and Joseph Daquin (1792), the influence of the moon on the atmosphere was presented as one cause for derangement of the brain in people who were so predisposed.[91]

All exaggerated emotions or excessive physical and mental activity were considered as physiological sources of perturbation for the brain and encouragements for melancholia and suicidal mania. Even the *Encyclopédie* (in the entry "Manie") notes such origins for suicide as "passions of the soul, contentions of the mind, forced studies, profound meditations, anger, sadness, fear, long and painful sorrows, love scorned."[92]

To read Jean-François Dufour's *Essai sur les opérations de l'entendement humain,* a work published in 1770, one might wonder how there could still be balanced people when nearly every physiological function led to hypochondria, melancholia, mania, hysteria, and madness:

The evident causes of melancholia are everything that concentrates, exhausts, and troubles these spirits: great and sudden frights or violent afflictions of the soul caused by transports of joy or by lively affections; long and profound meditations on a single object; a violent love, sleepless nights; all vehement exercise of an occupied mind, particularly at night; solitude, fear, hysterical fits, [and] everything that prevents the formation, repair, [and] circulation of various secretions and excretions of the blood, in particular in the spleen, pancreas, epiploon, stomach, mesentery, intestines, breasts, liver, uterus, [and] hemorrhoidal vessels; consequently, the hypochondriac illness, uncured serious illnesses, principally *frénésie* and *causus;* all medications or overabundant or suppressed excretions, hence sweat, milk, menses, lochia [postpartum discharges], ptyalism [excessive saliva] and repressed scabies. A low sperm count commonly produces the so-called erotic delirium or erotomania. [Other causes are] cold, earthy, tenacious, hard, dry, austere, or astringent foods; similar beverages; raw fruit; unfermented farinaceous substances; long-lasting and violent heat, which burns the blood; [and] gloomy, swampy, stagnant air.[93]

Excessive study, excessive piety, and excessive meditation, which affected the liquids in the human body, were among the most frequently mentioned causes of depressive melancholia. Robert James's *Medicinal Dictionary* (translated into French as *Dictionnaire universel de médecine* in 1746–48) gives a good description of this theory. The brain, the seat of all imaginative and intellectual functions, is thrown off balance if blood and humors circulate too irregularly, too rapidly, too slowly, or too violently. The same theory appears in Anne-Charles Lorry's *De melancholia et morbis melancholicis* (1765). Such a situation might lead to passive suicide by simple inertia and glum stupor, as in one case reported by the *Gazette salutaire* on 17 March 1763: "A soldier became melancholic because of his parents' rejection of a girl he desperately loved. He was distracted, complained of a severe headache, and of a continual heaviness in that part. He grew visibly thinner; his face turned pale and he became so weak that he voided his excrement without noticing it. . . . There was no delirium, although the patient gave no positive answers and seemed to be entirely absorbed. He never asked for either food or drink."[94]

In another explanation, the melancholiac was totally out of phase with the external world because his "fibers" were either slack or immobilized by too much tension. Buffon had yet another theory, still making the suicide a victim of his physiology. In the "Homo Duplex" section of his "Discours sur la nature des animaux," Buffon shows that our humor is commanded by the roles played by two contradictory principles: "The first is a bright luminary, attended with calmness and serenity, the salutary source of science, or reason, and of wisdom. The other is a false light, which shines only in tempest and obscurity, an impetuous torrent, which involves in its train nothing but passion and error."[95] When the second of these principles predominates, it produces "that condition or disease called *vapours.*" When the two principles exist in equal strength in an individual, the temptation to suicide arises: "This is the ultimate point of disgust, which makes a man abhor himself, and leaves no other desire but that of ceasing to exist, no other power but that of arming with fury against himself." When that happens, the will is powerless, stricken with "inconstancy, irresolution, and languor" and assailed by "doubts, inquietude, and remorse." When the individual falls into this "most miserable of all states" he is irresistibly led to suicide.[96] In similar fashion, Charles-Louis François d'Andry distinguished three melancholic states in his *Recherche sur la mélancolie* (Paris, 1785), two of which, manic delirium and hypochondria, led to voluntary death.

Hypochondria was a diagnosis that the eighteenth century took very seriously as an explanation of suicidal tendencies, particularly after the publication of Richard Blackmore's *Treatise of the Spleen and Vapours, or, Hypochondriacal and Hysterical Affections* (London, 1725). Blackmore defined hypochondria and hysteria as due to a "morbific constitution of the spirits." In the mid-century Robert Whytt included "depression, despair, melancholia, or even madness" among the symptoms of hypochondria.[97] In 1755 at Halle, Michael Alberti published his *De morbis imaginariis hypochondriacorum,* a work in which he established a link between hypochondria and a desire for death.

If suicidal tendencies were due to psychological and physiological difficulties, they could be treated, as Voltaire had suggested. Whytt advised using quinine as a good remedy for "weakness, discouragement, and depression." Tartar was a good detersive for a blocked circulatory system. "Insofar as I have observed it," Whytt stated, "soluble tartar is more useful in maniac or melancholic affections produced by harmful humors amassed in the primary canals, than for those produced by a flaw in the brain."[98] Friedrich Hermann Ludwig Muzell also prescribed tartar for "madness and melancholia," and Joseph Raulin claimed that chimney soot, wood lice, powdered lobster claw, and bezoard also cleared clogged arteries. François Doublet praised the virtues of showers.[99] Others suggested treating suicidal tendencies with travel, which might help to dissipate an idée fixe, with sojourns in the country, and with music. Physicians disagreed about the value of theatrical spectacles and novels, but most thought them harmful. The theater unleashed the imagination and was particularly harmful for women, who tend to become overly excited by imaginary emotions.

As we have seen, literature glorified suicide and frequently presented it as a noble and heroic act. Christian moralists had long denounced the pernicious influence of such fictions, and in the late eighteenth century some physicians and psychologists began to think they were right. Was not the world a sufficiently horrifying spectacle without inventing more of them under the pretext of depicting the passions? Beauchesne developed the idea that theater and novels perverted mores in *De l'influence des affections de l'âme dans les maladies nerveuses des femmes* (1783).

Excessive intellectual effort, which hardens the brain, was also thought to have harmful moral effects. In his *Avis aux gens de lettres sur leur santé* (1778) Samuel-André Tissot warned fellow-writers of the risks they were running. The physicians tended increasingly to blame religion, although the point was still disputed by some authors (Johan Karl Wilhelm Möhsen among them) who emphasized the therapeutic value of traditional religion. Religion, they said, reassured the faithful that their sins would be pardoned through confession and penitence, and would accompany them at all the key moments in their lives.[100] These considerations bore little weight for enlightened thinkers, who denounced a pastoral policy of fear for its devastating effect on fragile minds. In the entry under "Mélancholie" the *Encyclopédie* stated:

The intemperate impressions made by certain extravagant preachers, the excessive fears they inspire of the pains with which our religion threatens those who break its laws, produce astonishing revolutions in weak minds. At the hospital of Montélimar, several women were reported suffering from mania and melancholia as a result of a mission held in that city; these creatures were ceaselessly struck by the horrible images that had thoughtlessly been presented to them; they spoke of nothing but despair, revenge, punishment, etc., and one of them absolutely refused to undergo any cure, convinced that she was in Hell and that nothing could extinguish the fire she believed was devouring her.[101]

For the physician Philippe Pinel, religion was capable of pushing people to despair, folly, and suicide. The proof was that "examining the registers of the insane asylum at Bicêtre, we find inscribed there many priests and monks, as well as country people maddened by a frightening picture of the future."[102] The philosophes' accusations were probably to some degree undeserved, given that fear of hell declined among the faithful during the second half of the eighteenth century.[103] The theme of hellfire was to return in full force under the Restoration.

Whatever the reasons, however, people of the eighteenth century had the decided impression that the insane had increased in number, as Michel Foucault has amply demonstrated. In France several institutions specializing in the internment of the insane opened their doors toward the mid-century, and the number of internees grew steadily until the 1770s, when the curve flattened out. In the empire similar establishments opened (or reopened) in Frankfurt in 1728, near Bremen in 1764, in Brieg in Schleswig in 1784, and in Bayreuth in 1791; an asylum opened in Austria in Wurzburg in 1743. Michael MacDonald and Terence R. Murphy tell us that in England "after 1780 or so, as asylums and mad-doctors began to proliferate, evidence that a dead person had been confined to a madhouse or had been treated by a specialist in mental disease began to be heard at inquests as proof of suicide. Such testimony effectively immunized the deceased from a *felo de se* verdict, but it also virtually assured that he would be judged a suicide, no matter how frail the other evidence was."[104] England had quite a few madhouses. Liverpool, Manchester, and York all had asylums founded in 1777, and in London, St. Luke's Hospital, rebuilt after 1782, could hold 220 mental patients. By the end of the century, however, these institutions were inadequate to meeting the need. When they examined and cared for mental patients, it helped to reinforce the connection between madness and suicide, both among the medical profession and in public opinion. William Black estimated that 15 percent of the inmates of Bedlam had attempted suicide at least once.[105] A majority of intellectuals (Horace Walpole among them) thought that madness was a component in most suicides.

The connection between suicide and insanity furthered the notion that suicide should not be subject to criminal sanctions. Adam Smith, who was in general fiercely opposed to any arguments in favor of voluntary death, admitted, "There is, indeed, a species of melancholy . . . which seems to be accompanied with, what one may call, an irresistible appetite for self-destruction. . . . The unfortunate persons who perish in this miserable manner, are the proper objects, not of censure, but of commiseration. To attempt to punish them, when they are beyond the reach of human punishment, is not more absurd than it is unjust."[106] In 1788 William Rowley wrote, "Everyone who commits suicide is indubitably *non compos mentis,* and therefore suicide should ever be considered an act of insanity."[107]

Rowley's appeal fell on deaf ears, but what is important is that it had been made. It gave witness to a decisive change that had taken place in the late eighteenth century, partly in response to pressure from coroners' juries, and partly in response to discussion that the philosophes had launched and the sa-lons, the press, and books had circulated. The debate on suicide had touched all the thinking elite of the century of the Enlightenment, but opinions still varied. No philosophe came out as an apologist for suicide; almost all of them expressed reservations and embarrassment. Although they were pessimistic about the world and society, their pessimism made them more apt to urge people to change society than to invite them to flee it. As Robert Favre writes, "The philosophes simply expressed pessimistic reflections on life, but they did not carry ruminations on the difficulty of living to the point of disgust and despair."[108]

Still, the philosophes helped to decriminalize voluntary death and to make it seem a more ordinary event. They did so by stating that voluntary death had an essential connection with madness and by demanding the abolition of criminal punishment for it. All the philosophes agreed that it was odious and barbarous (or at the least absurd) to punish a corpse and inflict the real punishment on innocent survivors. Their campaign worked to dissociate suicide from crime. Moreover, a rising tide of deism indirectly contributed to reducing the fear of hell, which remained a powerful deterrent to suicide for many Christians. Weakening the fear of hell worked both ways, however, because feeling certain that one was on the way to hell could lead to suicide in some cases. Finally, most of the philosophes distinguished between ancient and Christian suicides, praising classical suicides as sacrifices for homeland and liberty. This means that in a dechristianized context (which is what they were working to create), suicide might be a noble act. Here the philosophes directly prepared the wave of political suicides that occurred during the French Revolution.

The philosophes themselves had no vocation for martyrdom, but that was because up to that time, such self-sacrifice had been connected with fanati-cism and religious superstition. When it came to defending great human-itarian principles, they proved themselves more open to sacrifice. Diderot expressed a courageous prudence in a letter to Sophie Volland: "When one hasn't the courage to acknowledge one's discourse, the only thing to do is remain silent. I don't want people to go in search of death, but I don't want them to flee it."

When the preromantic atmosphere that first arose in the 1770s combined the theme of virtue with a strong return to classical antiquity—David's *Oath of the Horatii* was painted in 1785—an entire generation took Cato, Lucretia, Brutus, and Arria for its models. Political upheavals added homeland and liberty to this combination, and the times were ripe for the Rolands, Charlotte Corday, Lucile Desmoulins, Nicolas-Joseph Beaurepaire, Adam Lux, Charles Romme, François-Noël Babeuf, and other suicidal patriots.

TEN

The Elite

From Philosophical Suicide to Romantic Suicide

During the eighteenth century new reasons for committing suicide spread within the cultivated elite, who had been won over to the philosophic movement and its tendency to defend voluntary death, usually by referring to a doctrine such as Epicureanism. Self-induced death was presented as the result of the coherent act of refusing life, should it bring more troubles than satisfactions. Such an attitude was above all aristocratic and English. With the aid of *anglomanie* (the French elite's admiration for all things English), suicide on philosophical grounds was thought a highly refined act. Beginning in the 1770s, however, young people began to be seduced by romantic enthusiasms: Thomas Chatterton's death in 1770 and Werther's fictional death in 1774 produced a fashion for the suicide of despairing lovers, a taste for solitude, *le vague à l'âme* (vague spiritual malaise), and complaints that time was fleeting.

In spite of a few notorious cases, however, suicide was committed more in words than in acts. People talked endlessly about voluntary death but killed themselves only rarely, and when they did, their motives were often less intellectual than salon conversations would lead one to think. True suicide continued to occur where it always had, in huts and shops, and always for the same simple reason, suffering.

The Smiths' Suicide

Philosophical statements on suicide were far from anodyne, but those who made them had sufficient means, culture, and equilibrium to adapt them to their own lives. The same was not necessarily true of those who listened to or read those statements. In 1732 Alberto Radicati, a Piedmontese nobleman living in exile in London, published a treatise of Epicurean inspiration, *A Philosophical Dissertation upon Death*. The world, Radicati stated, is governed only by the laws of matter and movement, and death is simply the transformation from one form of being into another. Nature has disposed the world to assure our happiness, and the moment happiness is out of our reach, she has "given to Men an intire Liberty to quit Life when it is become troublesome to them."[1]

In April 1732, several weeks after the publication of Radicati's book, a London bookbinder, Richard Smith, and his wife Bridget shot their two-year-old daughter and hanged themselves in their rooms. They left three letters, one of which, addressed to Richard's cousin Brindley, explained their act:

It was an inveterate Hatred we conceiv'd against Poverty and Rags; Evils that through a Train of unlucky Accidents were become inevitable; we appeal to all that ever knew us whether we were either idle or extravagant, [and we state that we have taken as much trouble to earn our living as any of our neighbors; but our cares have not had the same success. . . . We have concluded that the world cannot be without a first motor—that is, without the existence of an all-powerful being—but while recognizing the power of God we cannot but be persuaded that he is not implacable, that he does not resemble the perverse race of men, and that he does not take pleasure in the unhappiness of his creatures. In confidence of that, we remit our souls into his hands without being seized by terrible apprehensions, and we submit ourselves wholeheartedly to all that he shall be pleased, in his goodness, to ordain for us at the moment of our death. . . . Finally, we are not unaware of certain human laws made to inspire terror, but indifferent to what our bodies may become after our lives, we leave disposition of them to the wisdom of the judges.] . . . It is the Opinion of Naturalists, that our Bodies are at certain Stages of Life composed of new Matter; [so that a great number of people change body more often than they do clothing.] Now Divines are not able to inform us which of those several Bodies shall rise at the Resurrection, it is very probable that the deceased Body may be for ever silent as well as any other.[2]

Is the similarity between Richard Smith's statement and Radicati's book coincidental, or does it show direct influence? The Smiths' Epicurean naturalism has a troubling kinship with the *Philosophical Dissertation upon Death.* Their suicide received wide press coverage and was much discussed throughout Europe. Voltaire speaks of it in the entry on Cato and suicide in the *Philosophical Dictionary,* as does Diderot in his entry in the *Encyclopédie.* Conservative circles took alarm: A simple bookbinder could not have conceived such ideas independently; the popular classes were becoming infected with philosophical, deist, and Epicurean ideas, only the most negative aspects of which they retained. As the century progressed, many other works joined Radicati's and praised the suicides of classical antiquity. In 1733 appeared an anonymous work entitled *The Fair Suicide;* there were also the elegies of Alexander Pope; even Edward Gibbon praises voluntary death among the

Romans in *The Decline and Fall of the Roman Empire.* In 1726 Jonathan Swift expressed his disgust for the human condition in *Gulliver's Travels,* where a humanity that is already absurd and odious becomes immortal, but in the form of the horrible, stinking Struldbruggs whom Gulliver encounters in his travels.

David Hume's Treatise

One contribution to the philosophical literature that viewed suicide with a tolerant eye and that aroused intense interest was a treatise by David Hume. The work, first published in France in 1770, was scheduled for publication in England in 1777, along with another brief work, under the title *Essays on Suicide and the Immortality of the Soul.*[3] The troubled history of this text illustrates the passions that its subject matter aroused.

Hume's treatise, which is only twenty-two pages long, shows no great originality except in its discussion of the social aspects of suicide. The work is divided into three parts, in which Hume demonstrates that suicide does not contradict our duties to God, to our fellow humans, or to ourselves.

In the first part, Hume shows that suicide is not an offense to God because men

may employ every faculty with which they are endowed, in order to provide for their ease, happiness, or preservation. What is the meaning then of that principle, that a man who tired of life, and hunted by pain and misery, bravely overcomes all the natural terrors of death, and makes his escape from this cruel scene: that such a man I say, has incurred the indignation of his Creator by encroaching on the office of divine providence, and disturbing the order of the universe? (8–9)

Hume finds such an idea absurd. All created beings have received the power and the authorization to change the natural course of things in order to guarantee their well-being. Each one of our actions changes the course of nature, and killing oneself does not change it any more than any other voluntary act. "If I turn aside a stone which is falling upon my head, I disturb the course of nature." This means that "were the disposal of human life so much reserved as the peculiar province of the Almighty, that it were an encroachment on his right, for men to dispose of their own lives; it would be equally criminal to act for the preservation of life as for its destruction" (11).

We must submit to Providence. So be it. But "when I fall upon my own sword, therefore, I receive my death equally from the hands of the Deity as if it had proceeded from a lion, a precipice, or a fever. The submission which you require to providence, in every calamity that befalls me, excludes not human skill and industry, if possible by their means I can avoid or escape the calamity: And why may I not employ one remedy as well as another?" (13).

Superstition in France had led people to declare vaccination impious, because they claimed that producing a disease infringed on the role of Providence. Hume states, " 'Tis impious says the modern *European* superstition, to put a period to our own life, and thereby rebel against our Creator; and why not impious, say I, to build houses, cultivate the ground, or sail upon the ocean? In all these actions we employ our powers of mind and body, to produce some innovation in the course of nature" (15). As for the argument of the soldier who cannot quit his post, it is simply ridiculous. The various elements that compose our bodies will be incorporated into other wholes and continue to play a role: " 'Tis a kind of blasphemy to imagine that any created being can disturb the order of the world, or invade the business of Providence!" (17).

Hume then turns to the question of whether suicide harms society:

A man who retires from life does no harm to society: He only ceases to do good; which, if it is an injury, is of the lowest kind.—All our obligations to do good to society seem to imply something reciprocal. I receive the benefits of society, and therefore ought to promote its interests. . . . I am not obliged to do a small good to society at the expense of a great harm to myself; why then should I prolong a miserable existence, because of some frivolous advantage which the public may perhaps receive from me? (18–19).

Hume raises a question, however: "Suppose that it is no longer in my power to promote the interest of society, suppose that I am a burden to it, suppose that my life hinders some person from being much more useful to society. In such cases, my resignation of life must not only be innocent, but laudable" (19).

Is suicide an offense against oneself? Hume declares, "I believe that no man ever threw away life, while it was worth keeping." Suicide is our supreme remedy: " 'Tis the only way that we can then be useful to society, by setting an example, which if imitated, would preserve to every one his chance for happiness in life, and would effectually free him from all danger of misery" (21–22).

Hume adds in a final note that no text in Scripture prohibits suicide and that resignation to Providence implies only submission to unavoidable ills. "Thou shalt not kill" refers to killing other people, over whose lives we have no authority. In any event, Hume adds, the law of Moses has been abolished.

So much for the argument in the brief treatise on suicide that David Hume wrote around 1755 and intended to publish with a treatise on the immortality of the soul. When the proofs were ready and the book was about to be published, Hume decided to withdraw the two essays, and he took back the proof copies and destroyed them, just as Justus Lipsius and John Donne had done with their works a century and a half earlier. This last-minute change of heart has intrigued critics.[4] It is unlikely that Hume had been subjected to pressure. More probably, he measured the weakness and the banality of most of his arguments. Perhaps he felt a certain responsibility. Also, steady and universal reprobation may have seemed nearly a law of nature, too strong to combat. In the collective conscience, suicide was as much of a taboo as incest. Attacking that prohibition meant risking pursuit by the authorities and ostracism by a good portion of society. Were all these risks worth running for a work that would do little to enhance his reputation? Hume had little of the Don Quixote in him, and he chose not to tilt at the windmills of ineradicable prejudice that cluttered the landscape of the collective conscience.

A few proof copies of Hume's treatise escaped destruction. There is even a story that Hume lent one to a friend, who congratulated Hume before shooting himself in the head. The story is pure slander, but it shows the intensity of the emotions that the question prompted. One copy of the work reached France, where Holbach translated the essays into French. They were published anonymously in 1770. A year after Hume's death in 1776, the two essays were published in England, still anonymously. Hume's name appeared only on the 1783 edition, which also included Rousseau's two letters on suicide extracted from La nouvelle Héloïse.

The literary press greeted Hume's work with violent hostility. In 1783 the Critical Review called the essay "a little manual of infidelity" that contained principles corrosive to society and religion and that attempted to "frustrate our sublimest views and expectations." The Monthly Review also attacked Hume's publisher, who had prudently added a refutation of Hume's arguments. In 1784 the Gentleman's Magazine declared that the refutation was a weak antidote to the poison the work administered, and in the same year Bishop George Horne condemned Hume's essay in his Letters on Infidelity.[5]

The remarks of Hume's publisher are interesting, though unconvincing. Revealed truth, he declares, is the only real consolation for the human heart. If everyone were to apply Hume's ideas, humanity would soon cease to exist (an anticipation of Kant's argument). Moreover, "it is not only impossible for a man to decide, in any given period, of the progress of his existence, or what utility or consequence he may be to society; but without the faculty of prescience, it is even more impracticable for him to divine what purposes he may be intended to serve in the many mysterious revolations of futurity."[6]

Finally—and the argument was an important one—if everyone is master of his own life, he can delegate powers over his own existence to someone else, which was a notion whose consequences would be incalculable.

It was one thing to write a theoretical treatise defending or condemning suicide; it was quite another thing to be directly confronted by a possible suicide. When the comtesse de Boufflers complained that she was unhappy and threatened to kill herself, Hume wrote her (on 14 July 1764), not to congratulate her on her courageous resolution but to express his "terror": "If there are any obstacles to your happiness, I should wish they were of a nature that could be removed; and that they admitted of some other remedy that the one you sometimes mention, on which I cannot think without terror."[7]

Some years earlier, in 1746, Hume had been witness to the suicide of Major Alexander Forbes, who had slit his arteries. Hume had found Forbes, as he wrote to his brother on 4 October of that year, "wallowing in his own Blood" but still alive. Hume called a physician, who bandaged Forbes's wounds, and until Forbes died twenty-four hours later, the two men talked. Hume reports, "Never a man exprest a more steady Contempt of Life nor more determined philosophical Principles, suitable to his Exit. He beg'd of me to unloosen his Bandage & hasten his Death, as the last Act of Friendship I coud show him: But alas! we live not in Greek and Roman times."[8]

Thus when Hume was confronted with the application of his principles, he admitted they were no longer valid in modern times. He may have been troubled by a repressed fear of damnation, which might explain his refusal to publish his essay. Suicide is indeed a strictly personal and existential question.

I might remark that except for Johannes Robeck, authors of treatises on suicide did not commit suicide. Their works were not apologies for voluntary death; what they wanted to demonstrate was that when life becomes physically or mentally too burdensome, suicide is a legitimate option.

From Holbach to Chamfort: "Death Is the Only Remedy for Despair"

Holbach, a contemporary of Hume's, vigorously proclaimed the legitimacy of the option of suicide. In his *Système de la nature* he states from the outset that he is a materialist unencumbered by religious objections. In the chapter on suicide he says, "That the suicide should be punished in another world, and should repent of his precipitancy, he should outlive himself, and should carry with him into his future residence his organs, his senses, his memory, his ideas, his actual mode of existing, his determinate manner of thinking."[9]

Holbach's work appeared in 1770, the year in which Hume's treatise was published in France, quite possibly in Holbach's translation. The influence of English philosophy in *Système de la nature* is clear. Suicide, Holbach writes, in no way harms society, because we are linked to society by a pact that "supposes mutual advantages between the contracting parties. The citizen cannot be bound to his country, to his associates, but by the bonds of happiness. Are these bonds cut asunder? He is restored to liberty" (137). In any event, "what assistance or what advantage can society promise to itself from a miserable wretch reduced to despair, from a misanthrope overwhelmed with grief, from a wretch tormented with remorse, who has no longer any motive to render himself useful to others, who has abandoned himself, and who finds no more interest in preserving his life?" (138).

Holbach finds no more validity in the objection that suicide is an act against nature. People say that nature inscribes in us a love of life, but what if nature, for one reason or another, inspires in us a distaste for that same life? "If the same power that obliges all intelligent beings to cherish their existence, renders that of man so painful and so cruel that he finds it insupportable, he quits his species; order is destroyed for him, and he accomplishes a decree of nature that wills he shall no longer exist. This nature has laboured during thousands of years to form in the bowels of the earth the iron that must number his days" (136).

Nor is suicide a cowardly act. A person who resolves to commit suicide does so only "when nothing in this world has the faculty of rejoicing him—when no means are left of diverting his affliction. His misfortune, whatever it may be, for him is real" (138). It is in that unhappiness that one finds the strength to surmount the fear of death. Moreover, suicide should be evaluated in terms of a sickness prompted by woes or by excesses, which was why reasoning could neither lead to suicide nor prevent it: "Many persons will not fail to consider as dangerous these maxims, which, in spite of the received prejudices, authorize the unhappy to cut the thread of life; but *maxims* will never induce a man to adopt such a violent resolution; it is a temperament soured by chagrin, a bilious constitution, a melancholy habit, a defect in the organization, a derangement in the whole machine, it is in fact necessity, and not reasonable speculations, that breed in man the design of destroying himself" (138).

Philosophical suicide, Holbach argues, does not exist. Those who cite grand principles to justify their act are only masking their moral or physical suffering, consciously or unconsciously. In saying this, Holbach parried in advance any accusation that he was encouraging people to kill themselves.

Volumes of apologetics for suicide would not lead to one more death if people had no good reasons for killing themselves. On the other hand, it would be far preferable to have humankind learn not to fear death. All tyrannies and all situations of injustice exploit that fear; only those who do not fear death are free.

If we can rid ourselves of the threat of the bad dreams that gave Hamlet pause, Holbach continues, death will become a haven of peace: "To die: to sleep"; no more. Any wretch has peace within arm's reach:

Perfidious friends, do they forsake him in adversity? An unfaithful wife, does she outrage his heart? Rebellious, ungrateful children, do they afflict his old age? Has he placed his happiness exclusively on some object which it is impossible for him to procure? Chagrin, remorse, melancholy, and despair, have they disfigured to him the spectacle of the universe? In short, for whatever cause it may be, if he is not able to support his evils, let him quit a world which from thenceforth is for him only a frightful desert: let him remove himself for ever from a country he thinks no longer willing to reckon him amongst the number of her children: let him quit a house that to his mind is ready to bury him under its ruins: let him renounce a society to the happiness of which he can no longer contribute; which his own peculiar felicity alone can render dear to him. . . . Death is to the wretched the only remedy for despair; the sword is then the only friend—the only comfort that is left to the unhappy: as long as hope remains the tenant of his bosom; as long as his evils appear to him at all supportable; as long as he flatters himself with seeing them brought to a termination; as long as he finds some comfort in existence however slender, he will not consent to deprive himself of life: but when nothing any longer sustains in him the love of this existence, then to live, is to him the greatest of evils; to die, the only mode by which he can avoid the excess of despair. (137)

We are forced to conclude that the baron d'Holbach enjoyed a sanguine temperament and was not personally afflicted by any such concerns, given that he died a natural death in Paris in 1789 at the age of sixty-six. Chamfort, to the contrary, took philosophical pessimism to its logical conclusion. For him life was a trap. We are thrown into this vale of tears where "physical scourges and the calamities of human nature have made society necessary. Society has added to the woes of nature. The drawbacks of society have led to a need for government, and the government has added to the woes of society. That is the history of human nature."[10]

Life, Chamfort insists, is a long tissue of woes. "To live is a sickness . . . death is the remedy." Life's trap is diabolical because "nature, by overwhelming us with so much misery and by giving us an invincible attachment to life, seems to have acted with man like an arsonist who sets fire to our house after having posted sentinels at our door. The danger has to be grave indeed before we feel obliged to jump out the window." By inspiring in us a fear of death, our deliverance, the instinct of self-preservation thus makes us our own jailers. Society's leaders have taken that instinct, our surest guardian, and added to it the taboo of suicide: "Kings and priests, by proscribing the doctrine of suicide, have attempted to guarantee that our slavery will last. They want to keep us locked up in a dungeon with no exit."[11] Thus kept alive by our own instincts and by social prejudices, we need great courage (aided by circumstance) to dare to liberate ourselves before the appointed time. Chamfort had that courage, and he attempted suicide on 13 April 1794. Life did its best to retain its hold on him, however, and when his shot to the head only blinded him in one eye, he slit his throat, and died several weeks later.

The Years of Philosophical Suicide

Chamfort was an extreme case. As we have seen repeatedly, authentic philosophical suicides—that is, suicides motivated by a distaste for life and a sentiment of the absurdity and worthlessness of existence—were rare and dubious. Jean Meslier, a parish priest, was perhaps one of the few true cases. In a testament he wrote for the edification of his parishioners, he expressed his desire for annihilation: "After that, whatever one may think, judge, or say, and whatever anyone wants to do about it in this world, I shall not care. Let men accommodate themselves and govern themselves as they will, whether they are wise or foolish, good or evil; let them say of me or do with me what they want after my death, it will not concern me. Already I take almost no more part in what goes on in the world."[12]

Although it was never established as a matter of absolute fact that Meslier killed himself, it is highly probable that he did so, and such an act would be totally in accord with the state of mind he expressed. According to a fellow parish priest named Aubry, whose opinion was confirmed by others, Jean Meslier starved himself to death in 1729 at the age of sixty-five. Aubry states:

After spewing his bile against the religion of his fathers and having lost his sight, Meslier thought only of ending a career whose length had begun to vex him. Disgusted with life, repelled by the constraints and violences he had imposed on himself in order to live externally according to the spirit of his [clerical] state, torn by the cries of his conscience and by the fear that they might be known before his death and bring richly merited punishments down on him, he took to his bed, determined to leave it only never to return. He languished for several days, constantly refusing whatever might prolong life, and died.[13]

Memorialists, literary critics, authors, and gazetteers were all on the look-out for philosophical suicides, especially in the 1760s and 1770s. The famous *Mémoires secrets,* supposedly written (originally) by Louis Petit de Bachaumont, chronicled all the events in literary circles and fashionable society from 1762 to 1787. Among many other happenings it mentioned several voluntary deaths due to despair, moral suffering, or lassitude, which it attributed to the fashion for things English.[14] The curiosity about suicide shown by the successive authors of the *Mémoires* is in itself revealing: Behind a pro forma reprobation, we can sense an interest tinged with admiration. They were clearly intrigued.

At the date of 21 May 1762 the *Mémoires secrets* reported that in recent years many had died of "consumption," here a euphemism for suicide from despair: "Those interested in concealing these domestic misfortunes passed them off as accidents. In the last two months, one can count more than ten persons of note who were victims of a similar frenzy. This *taedium vitae* is the outcome of so-called modern philosophy, which has turned so many minds too feeble to be truly philosophical" (16:153).

On 5 May 1769 the *Mémoires* sounded the alarm again, this time with regard to the suicide of a young man who had hanged himself because his debut in a theatrical career had been a failure: "One might not have thought that this anglicism had won over even that order of citizens. Such events have been multiplying here for some time, and even without counting those not brought to the attention of the public, several occur that are hidden, out of regard for the families, and to prevent the baleful advance of the philosophical spirit contrary, in equal measure, to politics, reason, and true heroism" (4:234).

On 26 September 1770 the *Mémoires* related that a German baron, an officer in the Anhalt regiment, first shot his dog so that the animal would not grieve for him, then ran himself through with his sword, "an instrument of death more worthy of himself" than a pistol. The *Mémoires* presented him as yet another victim of the philosophic spirit: "It seems that the disgust for life that is making considerable gains in the capital was the cause of this suicide. . . . We see by this that even the officer's extravagance was planned and well thought out. One cannot account for such extraordinary cold-bloodedness. Once more, the philosophy of the day is answerable both for authorizing such dreadful crimes and for encouraging them too feelingly" (5:171).

On 5 October 1770 Monsieur Guillemin, first violinist to the king, stabbed himself "in an excess of despair over debts" (5:173). On 26 February 1772 the *Mémoires* reported the suicide of a man in the provinces who shot himself for purely philosophical reasons, leaving a note in which he "declares that not having been consulted when he was brought into the light of day, he believes himself able to deprive himself of it without asking anyone's opinion" (6:101). On 12 July 1774 the *Mémoires* reported a more classic case: Monsieur de Salis, a young officer in the Swiss Guards, strangled himself in despair when his young wife died (7:189). On 16 June 1775 the *Mémoires* noted that "two Englishmen killed themselves recently in this country, and they seemed to have come here in order to reinforce the mania that the French have taken from their land by giving us an example of it today" (8:79).

This last incident was simply an exchange of good manners, as during the same period a number of nobles from the Continent went to England to kill themselves there, in a sort of pilgrimage to the land of voluntary death. The English newspapers reported the suicide of a son of a German general in Hyde Park in 1789; in 1797 Prince Frederick, the son of the king of Corsica, shot himself in the head inside Westminster Abbey; the following year, the duke of Sorrentino did the same in a coffeehouse. In 1789 the suicide that made the biggest stir was that of a younger son of Chancellor Maupeou, who landed in England with a large sum of money, and who shot himself in Brighton, leaving a brief note that made no sense to anyone: "Je meurs innocent; J'en atteste le Ciel" (I die innocent; I swear to God).[15]

To return to France, on 16 June 1775, the same day as the suicide of the two Englishmen, Mademoiselle de Germancé attempted to poison herself with opium when her lover abandoned her. The dose was insufficient, however; she was brought around, and she later boasted about her adventure. The *Mémoires secrets* commented: "What is disturbing is that she tells all her comrades that death is nothing, that the sort [of death] she chose is very agreeable, and that just as one is falling unconscious one feels the most delicious sensations. This moral, spread among the courtesans and the debauched *petits-maîtres* of Paris, is capable of producing a thousand similar accidents" (8:79).

On 2 February 1781 the writer of the *Mémoires* was especially intrigued by the suicide of a notary for the clergy, a wealthy man with no known troubles: "People are talking about a famous suicide, of a sieur Bronod, notary, who slit his throat. Derangement was undoubtedly the cause, which is all the more astonishing because he was the wealthiest of his colleagues by his estate, his practice, and the important affairs he handled" (17:56).

Christmas 1773: "We Are Disgusted by the Universal Scene"

The most talked-of suicide of the time was undoubtedly that of two young soldiers who killed themselves in an inn at Saint-Denis on Christmas Day,

1773. The *Mémoires secrets,* of course, related the event at some length, but also all the best society in Paris talked about it for several weeks, and we find echoes of it in the correspondence of men of letters, such as Friedrich Melchior von Grimm and Voltaire. Even today their story is touching.

First the facts. On 24 December 1773 two young soldiers, one a twenty-four-year-old *maître de camp* who bore the symbolic name Humain, the other a twenty-year-old dragoon named Bourdeaux, took a room at L'Épée Royale, an inn near the basilica of St. Denis. They arrived in the post coach from Paris, and the reason for their final trip is unclear. They were certainly a homosexual couple: "Both were noted on the police registers in a hardly honorable way for their conduct or their mores," the newspapers stated. The brains of the operation was the younger one, Bourdeaux, a man who had attended Jesuit schools and had already practiced several trades. They served in the Belsunze regiment.

The pair ordered supper and rented a room. The inn personnel noted that they did not attend midnight mass. On Christmas morning they walked about the town, and at noon they had a brioche, a bottle of wine, and some paper brought up to their room. After Bourdeaux had written two long explanatory notes, they drew their pistols, and seated at the table, each one fired a shot into his mouth. On the table lay a "testament" and a letter from Bourdeaux to Monsieur de Clerac, his lieutenant in the Belsunze regiment. The letter stated, among other things:

I believe I have told you several times that my current estate displeased me. . . . Since, I have examined myself more seriously, and I have recognized that my disgust extended to everything, and that I had also had enough of all possible estates, men, the entire universe, and myself. I was forced to draw the consequences of that discovery. When you are tired of everything, you must renounce everything. This calculation is not lengthy: I made it without the help of geometry. To be brief, I am about to rid myself of the license to exist that I have possessed for nearly twenty years and that has been a burden to me for fifteen. . . . If one exists after this rough life, and if there is danger in leaving it without permission, I will try to find a minute to come tell you about it. If there is none, I advise all unhappy people—which means all men—to follow my example. . . . I owe no excuses to anyone. I am deserting: that is a crime, but I am going to punish myself so the law will be satisfied. . . . Adieu, my dear lieutenant. . . . Continue to flit from flower to flower, and continue to sip sugar from all acquaintances and from all pleasures. . . . When you receive this letter I will have ceased to be for at least twenty-four hours. With the sincerest esteem, your most affectionate servant, Bourdeaux, once the pupil of pedants, then assistant quibbler [aide-chicane], then monk, then dragoon, then nothing.

The "testament," which Bourdeaux and Humain both signed, outlined the more general reasons for their act:

No pressing reason forces us to interrupt our careers, but the pain of existing for a moment in order to cease being for eternity is what makes us agree to strip fate of that despotic act. . . . We have tried all pleasures, even those of obliging our fellows; we could still procure them, but all pleasures have a time limit, and that is their poison. We are disgusted by the universal scene. The curtain has been lowered for us, and we leave our roles to those weak enough to want to play them for yet another few hours. Disgust with life is our only reason for quitting it. . . . A few grains of [gun]powder have just broken the mainsprings of this mass of moving flesh that our prideful fellows call the king of beings. Lords of justice, our bodies are at your discretion; we scorn them too much to worry about their fate. . . . The serving maid of this inn may have our neck and pocket kerchiefs, as well as the stockings and linens I have with me. The rest of our effects will suffice to pay the costs of the inquest and the useless reports that will be drawn up about us. The écu worth 3 livres left on the table will pay for the wine we have drunk. At Saint-Denis, this Christmas Day 1773. Signed: Bourdeaux; Humain.

The affair caused an enormous stir, but reactions expressed more stupor than condemnation. The *Mémoires secrets* remarked about Bourdeaux that "from the age of five he had always been bored with life. This piece, [written] in good style and thought out philosophically, displays its author's education" (7:100). Madame du Deffand wrote to her friend Voltaire: "What do you have to say about the adventure of the two soldiers of Saint-Denis? It is worth whole folio volumes. Only Nature has the power to answer." Grimm, who reproduced the full texts of the letter and the testament in the *Correspondance littéraire,* concluded that the affair was simply one more example "of the ravages that an overly daring philosophy can cause in poorly disposed heads," but he could not conceal his interest in the case.[16] It is odd that no one at the time alluded to the two soldiers' homosexuality, which may have been the underlying cause of their act. Their love could not be expressed in a society where "sodomy" was an inadmissible crime that in flagrant or extreme cases was punishable by death. The bodies of the two young men were dragged, pierced through with a stake, and hanged, then burned and the ashes tossed on the dump heap.

It is also surprising that when Albert Bayet speaks of this episode in *Le suicide et la morale* he abruptly changes his tone. That thick book—the first genuine history of suicide and a work that is still a standard reference on the topic for the massive amounts of information it provides and the breadth of the author's views—shifts from its customary neutrality (tinged with sympathy toward what Bayet calls "la morale nuancée" and all its historical manifestations) to explode with ill-contained indignation regarding the two soldiers in Saint-Denis. Although Bayet devotes several pages to the event, he insists that it is an incident hardly worth remarking on. After discussing Robeck's suicide, he speaks of the two soldiers' death as an "utterly banal newspaper filler." It obviously infuriated him, and following extracts from Bourdeaux's letter, he states, somewhat aggressively, "If it weren't for the outcome, one would laugh." The letter and the testament are "puerile boasting," "mediocre lucubrations," or "childish reasoning." Bayet adds that Grimm's opinion seems to him "extremely indulgent" because the two young men had nothing in common with "the philosophy of their times."[17] The contrast between this treatment—an example unique in the eight hundred or so pages of a remarkable work that relates hundreds of other suicides without commentary—and Bayet's usual language shows that on that sorry Christmas Day in 1773, Bourdeaux and Humain in fact touched the nub of the problem by daring to act in concert with their thoughts. "Disgusted by the universal scene" and the spectacle of a world they found absurd, they left it in the most logical, uncomplicated manner.

This is probably what the young Marc-Antoine Calas was trying to do in 1761, but his gesture lost all its meaning because of the famous "affair" that came to be constructed around his death. When his parents discovered that their son had hanged himself, they sought to conceal the cause of death. "Do not spread the word that your brother did away with himself; save at least the honor of your miserable family," the father told his other son, Pierre, according to the latter.[18] We can see from the father's reaction how keenly suicide and its attendant ignominy were dreaded in popular milieus. When they attempted to hush up their son's death, the parents were accused of having killed him to prevent him from converting to Roman Catholicism.

More important for our purposes is the testimony of Donat Calas, Marc-Antoine's sister, because she throws light on his reasons for killing himself—on her brother's melancholy humor, his unsuccessful professional career, and his reading matter, which included Plutarch, Seneca, Montaigne, and Shakespeare. He had memorized Hamlet's soliloquy, and he must have meditated on it often. Donat Calas stated:

Our older brother Marc-Antoine Calas, the source of all our woes, was of a somber and melancholy humor. He had several skills, but not having succeeded or earned a degree in law (because he would have had to perform Catholic acts or buy certificates), not being able to become a merchant because he was not fitted for it, and seeing himself rejected in all paths to fortune, he gave himself over to a profound gloom. I often saw him reading passages on suicide by various authors, at times from

Plutarch or Seneca, at times from Montaigne. He knew by heart the translation in verse of Hamlet's soliloquy, so famous in England, and passages from a French tragi-comedy named *Sidney*.[19]

Here, as in other cases, the "philosophical" motivation for suicide clearly could not have been the only one. No one kills himself simply to imitate the ancients, or because he has memorized Hamlet's soliloquy. Hamlet himself thought it more prudent to stay alive.

Suicides among the English Aristocracy: Philosophy or Sport?

In England, as well as in France, critics and satirists showed that the philosophical reasons advanced for the aristocratic suicides were simply pretexts hiding the real reasons, which were primarily gambling debts and debauchery. In his *Full Inquiry into Suicide,* Charles Moore saw gambling, suicide, and dueling as results of the idle life led by gilded youths who were willing to kill themselves for senseless points of honor. In 1741, for example, a certain Nourse quarreled in a London casino with Lord Windsor and challenged him to a duel. When Lord Windsor refused, pointing out the social difference that separated them, Nourse cut his throat. In 1755 the gentlemen members of the Last Guinea Club swore to kill themselves after they had run through their fortunes, and they kept their word.[20] John Brown wrote, "The Roman killed himself, because he had been unfortunate in *War;* the *Englishman,* because he hath been unfortunate at Whist: the *old* Hero, because he had *disgraced* his *Country;* the *modern,* because he dare not show his head at *Arthur's* [a gaming house]."[21] The *Connoisseur* declared that the true cause of aristocratic suicides was despair "brought on by wilful extravagance and debauchery."[22] In 1774 John Herries wrote, "As the luxury and depravity of the age seem to be rising to a crisis, so *Suicide,* the offspring of hell, the dire attendant of guilt, remorse and despair, begins to infect, by its baleful influence, more unhappy votaries than ever."[23] Caleb Fleming also connected suicide with gambling, debauchery, and luxury in *A Dissertation upon the Unnatural Crime of Self-Murder,* published in London in 1773.[24] In the *World* of 16 September 1756, Edward Moore sarcastically suggested creating a "Receptacle for Suicides," a building whose apartments offered refined and noble ways of killing oneself: There would be marble baths filled with exceptionally pure spring water, daggers and poisons for actors, swords fixed to the floor for army officers, pistols charged with loaded dice for gamblers, and ropes for middle-class suicides.[25]

The list of aristocratic suicides in England during the second half of the eighteenth century is impressively long.[26] In 1798 George Hobart, earl of Buckinghamshire, listed thirty-five notables who had killed themselves since the 1750s, sixteen of them with a pistol, two with a sword, eight with a knife or razor. Hobart expressed no disapproval. In 1731 a lady of fashion given to gambling, Fanny Braddock, killed herself in Bath. In 1740 the earl of Scarborough killed himself with a pistol, as did Henry Bromley, Lord Montfort, in 1755. Montfort, a member of Parliament, had lost a fortune gambling. In 1765 Charles Paulet, duke of Bolton, killed himself; John Damer, Lord Milton's son, did the same in 1766. After running through a colossal fortune, Damer rented rooms in the Bedford Arms at Covent Garden, and at the end of an all-night party he shot himself in the head. In 1767 Thomas Davers poisoned himself, leaving a quatrain in which he complained that he no longer had the means to die like a gentleman by shooting himself with a pistol. In 1771 Jenison Shafto, who had accumulated a fortune gaming and had become a member of Parliament, lost his all and killed himself. Another member of Parliament and another great gambler, William Skrine, killed himself with a pistol in a tavern in 1783. In 1784 a young man who had run through his fortune committed suicide, with great calm according to the *Annual Register*. Captain James Battersby stabbed himself in 1785 after being arrested for dueling. In 1788 George Hesse, a friend and gambling companion of the prince of Wales, committed suicide after losing a vast amount of money in a casino. The *Times* praised him. The same year Lord Saye and Sele killed himself, followed the next year by the earl of Caithness, and in 1797 by Viscount Mountmorres.

It goes without saying that the coroners declared all these prominent persons mad—quite a paradox for suicides that claimed to be "philosophical," founded on reason and intellectual principles! The verdict of *non compos mentis* fooled no one. Often obtain by bribery, as in the case of Edward Walsingham in 1759, or by false witness, as in that of John Powell in 1783, such a verdict might also be based on a medical inquiry. It was an easy matter for prominent families to find a pliant physician. After the duke of Bolton's death in 1765, a doctor testified that the deceased had suffered from a fever "capable of depriving His Grace of his Senses."[27]

The English political world had a particularly high number of suicides: twenty-one members of Parliament killed themselves during the eighteenth century, many of them, as we have seen, for reasons extraneous to politics. The most famous victim was Lord Clive, the conqueror of India. Accused of mismanagement of the East India Company, he killed himself in 1774.

Whatever its real causes, philosophic suicide was often connected to the

Enlightenment idea that the rational man has a sovereign liberty that permits him to leave this life when it becomes burdensome. Frederick II of Prussia, a friend of the philosophes and a model for enlightened despots, carried on his person a small golden box attached to a ribbon and containing eighteen opium pills, "quite a big enough dose to send the soul to those gloomy banks whence it never returns," he wrote. Several times, when military affairs were going poorly, he expressed his intention to kill himself. After the disaster of Kunersdorf he was deeply depressed for two days: "Was it worth the pain of being born? . . . It is almost nonsense for me to go on living! . . . Oh, how much happier are the dead than the living!" After the capitulation at Maxen he wrote to d'Argens: "I am so worn out by the reverses and disasters which come upon us that I have wished a thousand times for death, and I grow more and more tired of inhabiting a worn-out body condemned to suffering." He wrote to his sister:

How can a prince survive his State, the glory of his nation and his own reputation? . . . No, no, my dear sister, your thoughts are too noble for you to give me such cowardly advice. Shall liberty, most precious of prerogatives, be less dear to the sovereigns of the eighteenth century than it was to the patricians of Rome? And where is it said that Brutus and Cato pushed generosity further than princes and kings? . . . Assuredly life is not worth the determination with which some people cling to it.[28]

Frederick II was subject to periods of depression, and it was during one of these that he declared, "The finest day in one's life is the day one leaves it." His active temperament soon got the better of his depression, however, and he warded off melancholy through hard work: "Nothing makes you feel better than serious application." He also threw himself into interminable reading projects, swallowing the thirty-six volumes of Claude Fleury's *Histoire ecclésiastique* or the sixteen volumes of Jacques-Auguste de Thou's *Histoire universelle.* People who still have the energy that such exploits require rarely kill themselves.

Romantic Suicide: The Lovers of Lyons and Rousseau

The distance between philosophical suicide and romantic suicide is shorter than it might seem. In theory, the first is motivated by intellectual reflection, the second by feeling. In reality, no one kills himself out of pure reasoning; only a machine is capable of self-destruction as the end result of calculation. Nor do people kill themselves purely for emotional reasons, unless insanity is involved. For the two soldiers at Saint-Denis, an awareness of the difficulty of existence reinforced their sense of the absurdity of the human condition. With the lovers of Lyons in 1770, certainty of an unhappy future and the intensity of their passion launched one of the most famous romantic suicides of the century.

A fencing master named Faldoni was told by his physicians that he was about to die. The young woman he loved and who loved him declared that she would not survive him. The two lovers decided to kill themselves in a romantic setting: They met in a chapel, bound their left arms together, and each held a pistol pointed at the heart, with its trigger attached to the cord that bound them together, so the guns would go off at the slightest movement. Public opinion was more touched than judgmental. The press and the entire literary world spoke of the episode; it inspired an anonymous *Histoire tragique des amours de Thérèse et de Faldoni* in 1771, a work that in turn provided the inspiration for novels by Nicolas-Germain Léonard and Pascal de Lagouthe. Delisle de Sales was admiring. Rousseau wrote of the event: "La simple piété n'y trouve qu'un forfait, / Le sentiment admire, et la raison se tait" (Simple piety sees nothing but a crime in it, sentiment admires, and reason keeps silent).

Romantic suicide, which was above all suicide for love, had a multitude of variants. The theme offered Jean-Jacques Rousseau the opportunity to write the two famous letters on suicide in *La nouvelle Héloïse* (1761). As is always the case, it is difficult to guess from the text what Rousseau's own opinions were, especially because he has one character, Saint-Preux, lay out the arguments in favor of suicide in a letter addressed to Milord Edouard, while the latter responds with arguments against suicide.

In the first of these letters, Saint-Preux declares that he is tired of living and expects nothing more from life, that all are free to put an end to existence if life is a burden and they are a charge on others, and that we have the right to sacrifice our arm to save our bodies and our bodies to save our happiness. God has given us reason, thanks to which we can discern when the moment has come to leave life; what is more, life is an accumulation of errors, torments, and vices. Does not religion teach us that the wisest way to live is to detach ourselves from the world and become dead to the senses? Here Rousseau neatly points out the ambivalence of the spirituality of annihilation. Moreover, Saint-Preux continues, when a man becomes so unhappy that his suffering is stronger than his horror of death, is that not a sign that it is time to go? The champions of traditional morality contradict themselves: They state that life is a good, but they also say that there is more courage in bearing life than in dying. Only a fool would willingly agree to bear ills that he could avoid. Is not someone who lives alone, who is of no good to anyone, and whose complaints only disturb the world, right when he leaves life? Nowhere does the Bible prohibit suicide, and the Church borrows from pagan philosophies when it claims that it does. The prohibition on killing has many exceptions: Why should suicide not be one of them, and the most logical one of all, since it involves one's own life? Must we wait until we are pushed out of life, decrepit, riddled with pain, hideous, degraded, dehumanized? Isn't it more dignified to leave like a man when death is desirable?

Milord Edouard responds: I am English, so you cannot give me any lessons on suicide. You are a believer, how can you think that God has sent you to this earth by accident, simply to exist, suffer, and die, with no aim, no moral design? You were born because you have a task to accomplish. You see only the bad parts of life, whereas in reality the good and the bad are intimately mingled. You are unhappy for the moment, but the time of consolation will come. We imagine that our ills will never end, which is totally false. We need to distinguish between ills of the body and those of the spirit: When the first are excessive and incurable, to the point of destroying our faculties and per-turbing our reason, then we cease truly to be human, and suicide is accept-able. The ills of the spirit always have a remedy, however, time chief among them. Time passes quickly; only our good actions remain. We have no right to revolt against our Creator, to change our nature, or to frustrate the end for which we were made. We also owe a debt to society and to our country.

Commentators have generally stressed the first letter and presented Rous-seau as a proponent of free suicide. The reality is probably less cut and dried. First, the novel itself proves Milord Edouard right: Saint-Preux does not commit suicide, and he is grateful to his friend for his good advice. Next, Rousseau did not kill himself, despite being strongly tempted to do so in 1761, 1763, and 1767. The story of his suicide is pure legend. The only exception that Milord Edouard seems to allow is the case Saint-Preux brings up of someone dehumanized by intolerable and incurable physical suffering. It is thus inaccurate to call Rousseau the father of romantic suicide.

Goethe, the Master of Romantic Suicide (Werther) and Philosophical Suicide (Faust)

Goethe may perhaps rightly be charged with having inspired romantic suicide. His primacy caused him problems, however. When he published *Die Leiden des jungen Werthers* (better known in English as *The Sorrows of Young Werther*) in 1774, Goethe was twenty-five years old. He had been deeply affected by the suicide of a young man he knew well, Karl Wilhelm Jerusalem, attaché of the Brunswick legation, who killed himself because he had been rejected by a married woman whom he loved. At the time, Goethe himself was in love with a married woman, Charlotte Buffe. Goethe's experience in these personal dramas (along with *Hamlet,* Richardson's *Pamela,* and *La nouvelle Héloïse*) lie behind *Werther.*

The celebrity of Goethe's novel is a good gauge of the sensibility of the time. *Werther* did not create a fashion; it expressed a climate to which it gave form. Debates on suicide had sensitized educated circles to the topic of suicide from the mid-century on. Saint-Preux's letter dates from 1761; the suicide of Thomas Chatterton, the death of the Lyons lovers, and French edition of Hume's treatise all occurred in 1770; the two soldiers killed themselves in Saint-Denis in 1773. The figure of Werther arrived on the scene just as the question of the legitimacy of voluntary death reached an emotional high point. Goethe's tale of an impossible love between a young man and a chaste wife, which ends in a touching suicide, offered in one package all the age's vague malaise and turbid emotions concerning love, death, and the irremediable human inability to communicate. Repressed sensuality, virtue, ineluctable destiny, youth, death—everything that excited people's sensibilities at the end of the ancien régime—found an outlet and a poetic, melancholic expression in Werther. The youth of Europe learned his speeches as they had learned Hamlet's:

To die? What is it? We do but dream when we talk of death. I have stood by many a death-bed, but the limits of human reason are so narrow that it cannot reach back beyond the commencement or forward beyond the conclusion of our present existence. *Now* I am still my own—still *thine,* dearest Charlotte, *thine!* and, in an instant, we are torn asunder—separated—perhaps forever? No, Charlotte, no. How is it possible, that *I* should be annihilated—that *you* should be annihilated, for do we not *exist?* Annihilation? What is it?—a word—a mere sound, that carries no meaning to my heart! Dead, Charlotte? Constrained within the dark and narrow house![29]

The Sorrows of Young Werther was translated into French in 1775; it went through fifteen printings in ten years, and several adaptations appeared as well.[30] Four translations into English appeared between 1779 and 1799, and three more before 1810. Imitations of Werther's suicide soon followed. In 1777 a young Swede named Karstens killed himself with a pistol, a copy of *Werther* lying open at his side. In the following year, Christiane von Lassberg, thinking herself abandoned by the man she loved, drowned herself with a copy of *Werther* in her pocket. An apprentice shoemaker threw himself out the window with a copy of *Werther* in his vest. In 1784 a young English-woman killed herself in her bed with a copy of *Werther* under her pillow. There were more such suicides, culminating in Karl von Hohenhauser's death in 1835. "Werther has caused more suicides than the most beautiful woman in the world," Madame de Staël wrote.

Some found the Werther mania disquieting. The book was prohibited in certain regions, and it was attacked from every side. In the single year 1775, Johann Melchior Goeze, a Protestant pastor, accused Goethe of likening suicide, an "infamous" act, to heroism; Schlettwein, a professor, called him a "public poisoner"; and Dilthey, another pastor, severely criticized him. The *Mercure de France* wrote in 1804 that "Goethe is inexcusable, and the aim of his book is visibly immoral."

This was obviously a ridiculous accusation. Goethe had written a novel, not a defense of suicide. To make him responsible for the voluntary death of impressionable young people was a charge leveled at literature as a whole. For centuries, thousands of novels had recounted suicides without kindling the moralists' ire. If the reactions to *Werther* were particularly lively, it was because many felt that suicide had become a social phenomenon, a dangerous scourge not to be treated lightly.

Concerned about the supposed effects of his work, Goethe placed a qua-train at the head of book 2 in the 1775 edition of *Werther* that ended: "Be a man, he said; do not follow my example." In 1777 Goethe paid a call on a young man who had written to say that he suffered from *mal du siècle*, attempting to reason with him, and in 1779 he declared, "God keep me from ever again finding myself in the situation of writing a *Werther*." Goethe alluded to the work on several occasions in the hope of rectifying the impression it had made. Toward the end of his life, Goethe saw things more equitably, and when Lord Bristol, the bishop of Derby, reproached him for writing a "thoroughly immoral and damnable" book, Goethe replied that politicians send millions of men to their deaths with a clear conscience.[31]

Goethe also studied philosophic suicide, the other great temptation to suicide of the eighteenth century. More, when he returned to the theme of Dr. Faustus, he gave philosophical suicide its letters of nobility and a universal dimension. His Faust, thrown into despair at his inability to attain universal knowledge and to equal God, realizes the vanity of his studies and his en-cyclopedic knowledge. Like a new Adam smitten by the mad dream of making himself master of creation, Faust stands for all humanity (but that of the Enlightenment in particular), which, refusing divine tutelage and proud of its acquisitions, thinks that it can take destiny in its own hands. Humans soon fail in this attempt, and when they discover just how weak and small they are, that awareness engenders despair and the will to destroy oneself. Faust wants to be God or nothing. His poignant soliloquy expresses human-kind's distress at comprehending its nothingness:

> I've sweated through philosophy,
> Jurisprudence, Medicine,
> Yes, and alas, Theology
> Through and through and out and in!
> Poor fool! Poor disillusioned man
> No whit more wise than you began.
> Master of Arts they call you! Doctor, too!
> These past ten years all you can do
> Is lead your pupils by the nose
> Uphill and down, past thorn and rose.
> What fires consume my heart to find
> That knowledge still evades man's mind.
> I grant you I'm wiser than fops, school-masters,
> Doctors, scribbling clerks and pastors.
> No scruples of conscience make me cavil,
> No hell appalls me, nor no devil.
> And hence—I cannot know delight!
> Cannot pretend to know what's right,
> Cannot pretend that I might learn
> To improve mankind or serve their turn.
> I've neither majesty, nor fame,
> Nor goods, nor money to my name.
> There's not a dog would tolerate
> My life.
>
>   . . .
>
> But yet I am a prisoner. Still
> Walled-up in this accursed hell!
> The paintings on the window even
> Serve to deflect the light of heaven.
> This pile of books, a dungeon wall
> Rising to the ceiling's dome!
> Worm-eaten! Dusty! And a pall
> Of smoke-stained paper charred to chrome
> Crowns all. Row after serried row
> Of glasses, instruments galore,
> Lumber, boxes by the score—
> That is your world, my friend! If you can call it so.

You think that you enquire in vain
Why cramping fears invade your breast?
Why anguish that you can't explain
Robs existence of its zest?
God, in creating man, decreed
That living Nature be his home.
But rubble, smoke and skulls impede
Your life! Ghost skeletons of bone!

    · · ·

What a show of wonders! But no more than show!
Where may I grasp eternal Nature, through?
Where are the breasts from which Life's milk first came?
Which nourished earth and heaven too?
My famished soul cries out for you!
You flow! You feed! And must I yearn in vain?

    · · ·

Anxiety then nests within our hearts,
And furtively our sufferings start
To ferment, since anxiety can display
Such different masks for her disguise. She may
Appear as hearth and home, as wife and child, as thrust
Of dagger, poison, water, fire!
You dread the darts that may misfire
And weep incessant tears for what is never lost.

    · · ·

What's this but dust?—These towering walls,
A hundred shelves confining me.
A world of moths and bric-a-brac that palls,
Crushing me oppressively.
Shall I discover what I lack
By studying a thousand books, to find
That man is stretched upon a self-made rack,
Though here and there lives one contented mind?
What, hollow death's head, do you grin and say
That you were once confused like me? Your brain
Lusting for Truth and Light, found shadows weigh
So heavy on it, you were turned insane?[32]

Two centuries after Hamlet had posed his basic question, Faust answered it. His "hollow death's head" echoes Hamlet's contemplation of Yorick's skull in the graveyard; Hamlet, too, looks at the question from every angle. To be or not to be? But what is "being" if one is not everything, does not know everything, cannot do everything? Nothing. Faust knows now that man cannot master universal knowledge or truth, so he makes his choice: not to be. Brushing aside Hamlet's fears, he chooses self-destruction, at the risk of finding hell or nothingness:

> Worm that you were! Can you deserve a place
> On heights where such Olympian pleasures run?
> Yes! You may earn it if you turn your face
> Determinedly against the sun.
> Be bold and force that door which all desire
> To slither past unwittingly. The hour
> Demands a deed to prove man dare aspire
> To dignity, undaunted by God's power.
> I will not fear the sombre cave of hell
> Where fancy figures forth her own damnation,
> But make that narrow jaw where teeth of flame repel
> My unswerving destination.
> And I shall march undaunted to the goal
> Though only void oblivion wait there for my soul.[33]

Chatterton and the Imitators of Werther and Faust

The young who committed suicide during the 1770s and 1780s followed Werther's example more than they did Faust's. After 1770 they had another example as well, this time not literary. In that year the young poet Thomas Chatterton poisoned himself at the age of seventeen in his room in the Holborn section of London. A prodigy who had begun writing verse when he was ten, Chatterton wrote poems in medieval style that were at first much admired. When he failed to gain the rapid fame to which he aspired and instead was reduced to poverty, he killed himself, and he immediately became a symbol of misunderstood genius rejected in its times.

Panegyrics were written about Chatterton in the months that followed his death. One, Herbert Croft's *Love and Madness* (1780), mythologized him. Artists depicted his death. For example, in 1775 John Flaxman produced a drawing titled *Chatterton Drinking from the Cup of Despair,* and a few years later he made a drawing for a monument to Chatterton. In 1782 a souvenir handkerchief appeared that represented Chatterton writing in his garret. The image was accompanied by a long commentary on the poet, "born to adorn the times in which he lived, yet compelled to fall a victim to pride and poverty."[34] One hopes the kerchief served to dry the floods of tears of romantic young people affected by the Sturm und Drang movement. Keats, Coleridge, Wordsworth, and Alfred de Vigny all sustained the myth in the following century. Philip Thicknesse placed a monument to Chatterton on his estate, and as late as 1856 the painter Henry Wallis produced a glacial neoclassical composition titled *The Death of Chatterton*.

Like Werther, Chatterton was not only admired but imitated. In 1789 the *Times* reported the tragic story of the beautiful young Eleanor Johnson, seventeen years of age (like Chatterton) and (like Werther) in despair over a love she thought impossible. Her beloved, Thomas Cato (an appropriate name, given the circumstances), was black. Believing herself spurned, Eleanor poisoned herself, and she left a long romantic letter to Cato much like Werther's. The jury declared her *non compos mentis,* hence not guilty, a decision that the *Times* applauded, touched by this modern version of Othello and Desdemona.[35] Following this affair, two public debates were organized in London on suicide and its relationship to unrequited love, with the overall title "Whether [suicide] proceded from 'disappointment in the tender passion.' "

Similar cases occurred in France. One young man drowned himself because the parents of his beloved rejected his suit. An abbé in love with his pupil made up his mind to kill himself. Referring to Abelard and to Julie d'Étange, the heroine of *La nouvelle Héloïse,* the man wrote, "A love as violent as it is insurmountable for an adorable girl, the fear of causing her dishonor, the need to choose between crime and death—everything has determined me to die."[36] Grimm reported several similar cases in 1784 and 1785 in his *Correspondance littéraire.*[37]

In Germany the Sturm und Drang movement had made suicide a fashionable topic among the young. Both Faust and Werther were admired as models. Henri Brunschwig tells us in his great study of Prussia in the late eighteenth century that through voluntary death, which was considered more as a liberation than as annihilation, "these dreamers aspire to find the solution of the problem of knowledge, to discover what lies behind the external world perceived by their senses."[38] In February 1792 Friedrich von Schlegel, who felt ill at ease in this world, wrote to his brother, "Why live? You can neither reply nor can you advise me to live by trying to find any other reasons to persuade me than your own sympathy. For three years suicide has been in my daily thoughts. If I had continued on the course I was pursuing at Göttingen, it would certainly have soon brought me to suicide."[39]

Although voluntary death appeared to be making progress in Prussia at the time, strictly romantic suicides were rare. All the young talked about suicide, but few actually killed themselves. Moreover, those who passed into action were in general persons who were isolated, disappointed, and unhappy in love, such as Caroline von Günderode or Heinrich von Kleist. Von Kleist was a writer and playwright who had led an adventurous life. He was the son of an army officer, and he had been a volunteer in the French army, a deserter, and a bard of German nationalism who, in 1801, had laughed at Werther's suicide. He killed himself at the age of thirty-four (in 1811), in the company of a young woman who was incurably ill.

Suicide was nonetheless a serious enough question in Prussia for Immanuel Kant to devote a passage to it in his *Grundlegun zur Metaphysik der Sitten* (*Fundamental Principles of the Metaphysics of Morals*). For Kant, the freedom to commit suicide could not in any manner be erected into a principle, for doing so would fail to satisfy the demands of the universal imperative of duty: "Act as if the maxim of thy action were to become by thy will a universal law of nature." Kant reasoned that suicide is motivated by the sentiment of self-love, and there would be a contradiction in destroying one's life in the name of a sentiment whose function is precisely to favor life. It was a powerful argument, but a decision to kill oneself lies so far outside the principles of logical contradiction that the effectiveness of reason on it is dubious. Kant states:

A man reduced to despair by a series of misfortunes feels wearied of life, but is still so far in possession of his reason that he can ask himself whether it would not be contrary to his duty to himself to take his own life. Now he inquires whether the maxim of his action could become a universal law of nature. His maxim is: From self-love I adopt it as a principle to shorten my life when its longer duration is likely to bring more evil than satisfaction. It is asked then simply whether this principle founded on self-love can become a universal law of nature. Now we see at once that a system of nature of which it should be a law to destroy life by means of the very feeling whose special nature it is to impel to the improvement of life would contradict itself, and therefore could not exist as a system of nature; hence that maxim cannot possibly exist as a universal law of nature, and consequently would be wholly inconsistent with the supreme principle of all duty.[40]

The theme of the flight of time, which steals our youth and leads us toward a dreaded old age, played an essential role in romantic reveries on suicide. Here, too, Shakespeare showed the way, linking the swiftness to time and life's absurdity in Macbeth's soliloquy:

> Tomorrow, and tomorrow, and tomorrow
> Creeps in this petty pace from day to day
> To the last syllable of recorded time;

> And all our yesterdays have lighted fools
> The way to dusty death. Out, out, brief candle!
> Life's but a walking shadow, a poor player
> That struts and frets his hour upon the stage
> And then is heard no more. It is a tale
> Told by an idiot, full of sound and fury,
> Signifying nothing.
>
> (*Macbeth,* act 5, scene 5)

The refusal to age was particularly evident in the preromantic period, and it led to the obvious conclusion that voluntary death was the only way to avoid old age, the enemy. "Since I must die, is it not just the same if I kill myself? Life is a burden to me, because I enjoy no pleasure and everything is pain for me. It weighs on me, because the men with whom I live and will probably live always have ways as distant from mine as the light of the moon differs from that of the sun." Napoleon Bonaparte wrote those lines at the age of twenty-five.[41] At about the same time, the poet Antoine-Léonard Thomas (1732–85), prefiguring Lamartine, appealed to death to spare him old age:

> Si mon cœur par mes sens devait être ammoli,
> O temps! je te dirais:—Préviens ma dernière heure,
> Hâte-toi que je meure;
> J'aime mieux n'être pas que de vivre avili.
>
> . . .
>
> O temps, suspends ton vol, respecte ma jeunesse

(If my heart were to be softened by my senses, O time! I would say to you, "Prepare my last hour, hasten my death; I would rather not be than live demeaned." O time! suspend your flight, respect my youth.)[42]

In 1806 Fichte, commenting on the *Second Faust,* speaks of his prematurely aged romantic compatriots: "When they had passed the age of thirty, it would have been better to wish them to die, for their happiness and good of the world, for from that moment on, they lived only to corrupt themselves further—themselves and their entourage."[43] To end the list, Italy had its own Werther in a character created in 1799 by Ugo Foscolo, Jacopo Ortis, who commits suicide for love and out of disillusioned nationalism.[44]

Madame de Staël and the Study of Suicide

It was a woman, Madame de Staël, who best summarized and evaluated voluntary death in the preromantic age. Born in 1766, the daughter of Jacques

Necker, Germaine Necker showed proof of genius at an early age. She was eight years old when *Werther* was published, and she was brought up in the Paris salons, where she met the entire French intellectual elite. Attracted by the idea of suicide for love, she spoke of it approvingly in *De l'influence des passions sur le bonheur des individus et des nations* (1796).

In this work Madame de Staël, a woman of both a methodical mind and a quick sensitivity, distinguishes three principal types of voluntary death. She finds suicide for love easily the most comprehensible; it is also "the least dreaded of all: How can one survive the object by whom one was loved?" Philosophical suicide, which is rarer, supposes long meditations, "profound reflections, [and] long reexaminations of oneself." Only elite souls capable of serene analysis of human life can reach the most authentic level of a distaste for existence. Not everyone who wants to be Faust can manage to do so; Faust, what is more, did not kill himself. The third sort of suicide is committed by someone guilty of a crime. For Faust, suicide is already a beginning of re-habilitation because it is a "sublime resource" not within the reach of the utterly wretched. Madame de Staël comments, "It would be difficult not to believe in some generous impulses in the man who kills himself out of re-morse." Reviewing these three types of suicide—that of the desperate lover, the pessimistic philosopher, and the repentant criminal—Madame de Staël writes, "There is something sensitive or philosophical in the act of killing oneself that is completely foreign to a depraved being."

Like Justus Lipsius, John Donne, David Hume, and Goethe, Madame de Staël came to regret her statements about voluntary death and to realize that in that domain every individual must speak for him- or herself. The remorse she felt at the thought that some may have taken her work as an apology for suicide led her, seventeen years later, to write a treatise, *Réflexions sur le suicide* (1813). This work is not a brief pleading in favor of suicide; rather, it is an essay that strives to be scientific and to treat the question of voluntary death as neutrally and exhaustively as possible. This short work can be seen as a transition point between eighteenth-century works debating the pros and cons of suicide and the psychological and sociological studies of the nineteenth century.

The first point that Madame de Staël makes in her *Réflexions sur le suicide* is that we must avoid judging those who kill themselves. They are unhappy creatures more to be pitied than hated, praised, or scorned: "Inordinate mis-ery makes people think about suicide. . . . We must not hate people who are unhappy enough to detest life, but neither should we praise the ones who give way under an overload: If they could keep going, their moral strength would be all the greater."[45]

In psychological terms, suicide always contains an element of the unreason that accompanies paroxysms of emotion:

Those who claim that suicide is an act of cowardice are wrong: This far-fetched assertion has not convinced anybody. But we do have to distinguish bravery from strength of mind. To kill oneself, one cannot be afraid of death; but there is a lack of strength in not knowing how to suffer. Some kind of anger is needed to conquer one's own will to survive, if the sacrifice is not required by religious feelings. Most people who have attempted suicide and failed do not try again, because in suicide—as in all reckless acts of the will—there is a sort of madness that quiets down when it gets too close to its own goal.[46]

Suicide can be attributed to the effect that suffering has on the human soul, most frequently with ruin or dishonor as an intermediary. The decision to kill onself is always precipitate: Dishonor is never lasting; remorse ought to incite us to live to remedy our faults; true love does not urge people to kill themselves, for that is not what the loved one would want. Physical suffering is rarely the cause of suicide because it does not inspire revolt. The most frequent cause of suicide is thus self-love.

In the second part of her *Réflexions sur le suicide,* Madame de Staël examines the relationship between suicide and the religious life: "The resignation obtained by religious faith is a sort of moral suicide, and that is why [religion] is so contrary to suicide, strictly speaking, for self-renunciation has the aim of consecrating oneself to one's fellow creatures, and suicide caused by distaste for life is but a bloody grieving for personal happiness."[47]

The casuists' suppositions are worthless because they are extremely improbable, but Hamlet's hesitation is still valid: Are we sure that death will put an end to our torments? Madame de Staël counsels prudence. As for philosophical suicide, we need to distinguish between those who kill themselves because they think it is their duty to do so, who are admirable (as is Cato, who dies to prove himself a free man), and those who kill themselves because they are prey to emotion, who are to be condemned.

The *Réflexions* ends with a sketch for a sociology of suicide by national temperament. The English are the most inclined to commit suicide because, despite appearances, they are very impetuous and sensitive to public opinion. Climate has nothing to do with it. Germans kill themselves out of "metaphysical enthusiasm." They have great qualities, but for the moment (Madame de Staël is writing in 1813) they ought to think more about liberating their land: "There should be no more morbid sentimentality or literary suicides." She criticizes the *égarement* (misconceptions) of Germans who waxed enthusiastic over the story of a man and a woman who committed suicide in a Potsdam inn after dining and singing hymns. French suicides are neither romantic nor philosophical, but rather suicides of intrepidity that have nothing to do with either melancholy or ideas. Mediterranean peoples are little inclined to kill themselves, since they have "the enjoyment of such a beautiful nature."

Madame de Staël's *Réflexions sur le suicide* moves us from morality to sociology. The shift is probably premature, given the absence of statistical data. Madame de Staël remained a romantic, imagining only noble suicides. Among the common people the daily reality of suicide was less glorious and more stable. For centuries people had killed themselves for the same reason—simple suffering—and without discourses. Such suicides aroused no enthusiasm, however, because they were not motivated by grand ideas, they failed to correspond to the canons of heroism, and they were carried out by the base means of the rope. Denesle expressed the elite's scorn for that method in 1766 when he wrote: "The rope is a sort of death of such decided shame that anyone who chooses it in despair, unless he is of the dregs of the people, would be irredeemably dishonored among people of the proper sort [honnêtes gens]. Poison, steel, or firepower are what is needed. Water is also a commoner's despair."[48]

Philosophical suicides went to the great void, romantic suicides to heaven, popular suicides to hell. The clergy held firm, but the jurists were becoming increasingly hesitant, and with Louis-Sébastien Mercier's *Tableau de Paris,* humbler suicides made a discreet entry onto the sociological scene.

ELEVEN

The Common People

The Persistence of Ordinary Suicide

Far removed from the salons, from speculations on the meaning of life, and from romantic flights, the common people continued to commit suicide. We can better appreciate how they killed themselves, for what reasons, and in what numbers by looking at country areas in eighteenth-century Brittany.[1]

A Chronicle of Suicide in Rural Brittany

13 July 1715   Brigitte Even of Spezet hanged herself out of grief over the departure of her son, who had been chosen by lot for the militia.

13 February 1720   A peddler thirty-five years old named Marquet, whose business was lagging, stabbed himself several times with a knife, then threw himself into the Loire at Nantes.

Spring 1721   Julien Deshoux attended the Lenten preaching cycle during a mission at Saulnière, in the barony of Châteaugiron. The preachers' depictions of hell drove him insane: "He fell into madness," his parish priest declared, "because of the fright the preaching caused him." He killed himself.

3 April 1725   Jacqueline Huet from Perray, near Louvigné-de-Bais, who for some time had drifted away from the Church, hanged herself.

23 January 1728   André Trumeau, forty years of age, a former merchant who had become a delinquent, hanged himself near Châteaubourg.

30 September 1728   Joseph Castille, a peasant, hanged himself from an apple tree near Domagné. Alcohol had clearly affected his mental faculties. Witnesses were unanimous: "He drank continually"; "he was perturbed." He had hallucinations, danced about in nothing but his chemise, talked to the birds, washed himself at the holy water font, and had become morbidly jealous. When he committed suicide, he had been drunk for fifteen days. Nonetheless, the verdict was culpable suicide, and his body was dragged on a hurdle.

2 February 1732 Another drunkard and a former butcher, René Saligault, hanged himself at Antrain. Drink had made him violent, and he had abandoned his wife and children. Verdict: culpable suicide.

31 October 1736 François Legay, a farmhand, hanged himself at Bain. He had just sold some sheep that did not belong to him and had spent the money. He too drank excessively and was found guilty.

20 February 1742 A peasant hanged himself at Kervignec, near Pouldavid. All his belongings had been seized for debts the day before, leaving him penniless. He was found guilty.

1 March 1743 Jean Beaubras killed himself at Fougeray for reasons unknown.

29 November 1769 A young girl of fifteen, Françoise Royer, drowned herself at Fougères. She had for some time been abused by her mother, who sent her out to beg, gave her hardly enough to eat, threw her out into the street in the middle of the night calling her a whore, and beat her with a stick. The mother showed no sorrow at her daughter's death: "It's the devil who broke her neck, but she's over seven, she isn't under my care any more. . . . There she is, the great she-devil, she was looking for trouble and she found it. . . . She's a wretch; she told me so; it's the evil spirit who whipped her."

1 February 1773 Michel Talouard, who was in intolerable pain from rheumatism and sciatica, hanged himself near Guérande.

9 May 1773 Christophe Caud, a peasant stricken with a malignant fever, hanged himself at Vergeal. He was found guilty.

Late October 1778 Jean-François Battais, twenty-one years of age and the clerk of the *procureur* of Saint-Christophe-de-Vallains, hanged himself in a wood. He too was a victim of his parents, who had turned him over to the police to be imprisoned because he had lingered too long at a wedding party. When he emerged from prison, he was stricken with shame and began to beg; his family refused to come to his aid. He asked a friend to kill him.

11 March 1784 François Grégoire, a peasant from near Lannion, hanged himself in his grain loft. Since no one could suggest a reason for his act, the verdict was culpable suicide.

4 November 1785 A court functionary in Saint-Malo, Guillaume Le Menner, killed himself with a pistol shot in bed. He too was a drunkard, but he had enough social status to have his death declared possibly accidental, and he was not condemned.

1786 Marie-Jeanne Lobel poisoned herself for unknown reasons.

7 March 1787 Yves Barguil, a known drunkard thirty years of age who had already attempted to kill himself on several occasions, hanged himself near Quimperlé. He had long declared his intention and was considered mad, as his mother had been. Alcohol aggravated his condition; his wife had hidden all the ropes and locked up the barn.

Early September 1787 Guillaume Buffe, a man forty years old who suffered terrible headaches and whose mind sometimes wandered, hanged himself at Saint-Sulpice.

22 January 1788 Vincent Cadic, a farmhand nineteen years old who couldn't bear the idea of being separated from his parents, hanged himself near Pontcroix.

Nothing had changed since the Middle Ages. Poverty and a weak physical and moral condition remained the chief causes of voluntary death among country people. One new element—alcoholism—aggravated the situation of people whose minds were already unstable. Nor had the means of death changed: hanging for men, and drowning or poison for women. Women account for five times as many suicides as men. The peak day and time for killing oneself were Tuesdays between eight and ten o'clock in the morning; the peak months, February and, to a lesser extent, September.

Suicide always caused considerable commotion in the community and prompted people to gather together. A "crowd" formed around the body of René Saligault. The first reaction of the next of kin was usually fear, and it was often difficult to conduct the inquest because the witnesses were uncooperative and intimidated by court procedures.

The predominant sentiment evoked by suicides was pity. Systematically, all the witnesses insisted on signs of madness, frequently explained by the influence of the moon. One suicide was "out of his mind [fol d'esprit] at each crescent moon"; another's head was "deranged more or less according to the variations of the moon" or "at each new moon." One witness testified about Yves Barguil that "everyone knows that at the full moon his head was more affected and more deranged than usual; his look alone made it impossible to look straight at him, and he frightened those who did look at him." All signs of madness—agitation, exhibitionism, odd behavior—were carefully reported.

The family or friends of the deceased were ready to try anything to dissimulate or excuse a suicide, sometimes with success. This was the case with Vincent Cadic: The inquest concluded that the nineteen-year-old Vincent might have strangled himself inadvertently trying to set up a swing, because if he had wanted to hang himself he would have chosen a higher branch. "It would not be physically impossible that out of awkwardness and jokingly, Vincent Cadic may have been strangled by not paying sufficient attention to the noose that he slipped around his neck; the position of the cadaver encouraged one, so to speak, to believe this was the case, because there were infinite numbers of higher branches that Cadic could have chosen if he had perhaps had the determined intention to destroy himself." When the same excuse was suggested for Christophe Caud, however, it was rejected.

Attempts to conceal a suicide at times went as far as restaging the scene, calling on accomplices, and setting up false testimony. After the suicide of Jean-François Battais, the young man's parents, who had chased him out of the parental home in agreement with his uncle, a priest, felt remorse for their part in his death. They persuaded the parish priest of Saint-Sulpice-de-Vallains to bury Battais as if he had been the victim of an accident, even a murder. The inquest revealed that when his parents discovered his body hanging in their house, they struck it with a crowbar and a stick to make the death seem murder, then rehanged the body in the woods.

Judicial procedures were well established, and they remained unchanged until the end of the ancien régime. Let us follow them in the case of Christophe Caud, the fifty-five-year-old peasant found hanged in his house in the village of Les Escures on Sunday 9 May 1773 at four o'clock in the afternoon. The authorities were advised immediately, probably through the parish priest, and on 11 May, in the presence of the *sénéchal*, the *procureur fiscal*, and other officials, the surgeons examined the cadaver, opened it, and drew up a report. Later the same day, the corpse was brought to the prison at Vitré under the guard of two police officers, where it was marked on the forehead with a stamp. The following day, 12 May, the body was embalmed to preserve it until the hearing. On 11, 13, and 21 May, witnesses were heard in the presence of the representative for the deceased, one Maître Jacques. The cadaver was present at the hearings, but the witnesses could hardly recognize it as Caud's, "given that it had fallen into putrefaction." The affair did not end until 2 September 1775, two years and four months after Caud's death, when the last interrogation was conducted by the same court-appointed lawyer, "maître Louis Eloy Jacques, curateur nommé d'office." The verdict was handed down on that day:

The bench, making its decision on the basis of the conclusions of the king's men, has declared the late Christophe Caud duly charged and proven guilty of having done away with and murdered himself with a muslin tie he had previously attached, [first] to his neck and then to a ladder that [was] kept in the storage area of his house, for reparation of which and in the public interest, orders that his memory remain extinguished and suppressed in perpetuity, that his cadaver be attached to a hurdle to be dragged through the streets and common crossings and then, at the place where the [tilting] lists used to be, to be hanged by the feet from the gallows set up there, remain there for three hours, and then be thrown into the common refuse heap; [the bench further] declares that his movable goods be acquired and confiscated to the profit of whoever holds right to them, his trial costs having previously been taken from them, and furthermore decrees [payment be made of] a fine of 3 *livres* to the profit of His Majesty, to be taken from his other possessions, and [court] costs.

This sentence was carried out several days later, and what remained of the cadaver was dragged through the streets of Rennes. We are in the age of Louis XVI, at the heart of the Enlightenment, twenty-four years after the first volume of the *Encyclopédie* had been published, fourteen years after the publication of *La nouvelle Héloïse,* eleven years after Cesare Beccaria's *On Crimes and Punishments* was first published in Italy, five years after Hume's treatise on suicide, one year after *Werther.* Nor was this the last such example: Ten years later the body of a peasant from near Lannion received similar treatment. His memory was "effaced" and his goods confiscated.

A Decline in Sentences

Contemporaries reported and historians have stated that such barbarous customs were no longer in effect at the end of the ancien régime. This assertion should be put into perspective. It was not always true in country areas. When Voltaire wrote in 1777 that the old customs are "neglected today"; when Dubois-Fontanelle declared that magistrates "close their eyes, because the punishment inflicted on a corpse deprived of feeling is useless"; and when Louis-Sébastien Mercier stated in 1783 that "those who used to be prosecuted after their death under an absurd statute are no longer carted to the scaffold," they were talking about Paris. Mercier added, "Indeed, that was a horrible and disgusting spectacle calculated to have dangerous consequences in a city teeming with pregnant women."[2]

Albert Bayet writes, "Beginning in the first half of the century, trials for suicide were already very rare; on the eve of the Revolution there were none, practically speaking." He corroborates this statement with an examination of criminal archives from some thirty *bailliages* and *prévôtés* from the Tarn to the Aisne and from Mayenne to Saône-et-Loire. He found in these records evidence of fifteen trials of cadavers from 1700 to 1760, and only three from 1760 to 1789, undeniably a small number.[3] Five of these eighteen trials took place in the most western region he studied, at courts at Laval and Craon, which would tend to show that a traditional severity remained strongest in the west of the kingdom. Brittany alone provides more trials of cadavers than the thirty *sénéchaussées* that Albert Bayet examined: twenty, as opposed to eighteen, half of which resulted in the execution of the cadaver. At the beginning of the French Revolution there was one corpse in Quimper that had been salted down awaiting execution for five or six years; some twenty others awaited trial in Saint-Malo.[4]

Some suicides did not result in a trial. In the Vermandois we can see a trend toward tolerance in four examples. In 1725 a suicide was buried in unconsecrated ground; in 1729 another was buried discreetly in the cemetery, in the evening, with no tolling of bells or singing; the same occurred in 1766; in 1782 cemetery burial seems not to have presented any problem, on the condition that the judge be notified ahead of time.[5] In Lyons the jurist Prost de Royer noted that in 1760 he had given permission for normal burial of three young women who had poisoned themselves because of disappointments in love. He told his superiors, "I dare develop my ideas on the uselessness and the dangers of such a trial." The authorities did not object.[6] The Lyons lovers (see chapter 10) were given cemetery burial. Even in Brittany, Guillaume Le Menner's lawyer declared in 1785: "Although he may have murdered himself, that is no reason to put his memory on trial."

In Paris Brissot de Warville wrote in 1781 that "formerly" suicides had been brought to trial, and in 1790 Pastoret stated that a cadaver had not been executed in that city since 1772.[7] Mercier wrote in 1782 in his *Tableau de Paris* of his delight that such "disgusting" spectacles had disappeared. Discretion had by then taken priority. He added, "The police take care to ensure that the public hears nothing of these suicides. When someone kills himself, a superintendent of police presents himself in plain clothes, draws up a report without more ado and compels the priest to bury the body hugger-mugger."[8] Siméon Prosper Hardy mentioned in his *Journal* several cases of suicide that were not followed by a trial: a poor man who hanged himself and whose wife had stolen a loaf of bread; a banker who killed himself in 1769; a secretary to the king in 1771 who killed himself with a pistol after a quarrel over money and was buried the following day in the Église de Bonne Nouvelle; a young worker in 1772 who killed himself because he had been refused a working permit. All were given religious obsequies. In the same year, Hardy mentioned a dishonest judge who had killed himself and was refused normal burial, although no penalties were inflicted on the corpse.[9] Sentenced criminals who killed themselves were still treated harshly, however. In 1768, when Simon Saladin committed suicide in a prison in Toulouse, his body was dragged, hanged, and thrown onto the refuse heap.[10] Attempted suicides were imprisoned as well.[11]

In England too, hostility to the forfeiture of suicides' goods increased. The *Gentleman's Magazine* stated in 1754, "The extreme and evident cruelty of this law has produced an almost constant evasion of it," a notion confirmed by a jurist in 1776.[12] Statistics reflect a trend toward leniency: Under the reign of George III, 97 percent of suicide trials after 1760 for which the records have been studied ended with a verdict of *non compos mentis* (not guilty by reason of mental inadequacy). This holds true for all social categories. The champions of traditional morality complained that suicides were systematically considered lunatics.[13] The least indication—even an isolated instance—in the testimony of a neighbor (for the poor) or by attestation from a physician (for the wealthy) of even vaguely perturbed behavior was considered sufficient evidence of lunacy. In 1776 one jurist stated that coroners' juries gave a verdict "without having even a shadow of presumption of proof to support them. . . . Their Judgments in general are the effect of Caprice and Partiality."[14] Often hostility reversed the reasoning process, and the fact of having attempted suicide was considered a proof of madness. All unidentified drowned persons were judged *non compos mentis,* whereas in the sixteenth century a *felo de se* verdict would have been handed up systematically. Even in cases of obvious suicide one can find verdicts of natural death: In 1762 in Norwich William Hutchon slit his throat because he could no longer endure the pain he suffered due to various chronic illnesses, including an ulcerated leg. The jury declared that he had died of natural causes due to illness.[15]

The religious factor was not taken into consideration: In contrast to sixteenth-century practice, neglecting one's religious duties was no longer a sign of the intervention of the devil. Secularization is clear in all regions of England. Coroners' juries, which tended more and more to be composed of representatives of the middle classes—hence, of persons of some education and enlightenment—no longer punished the act of suicide, concentrating instead on the individual's conduct with regard to the social group. Only the suicides of criminals, deviants, foreigners, or marginal or asocial persons were judged culpable; in other instances the juries enforced respect of the rules of inheritance, safeguarded the family's good name, and took into consideration evidence of social stability. When the royal power no longer had an active interest in condemnations, juries were free to pronounce as they saw fit, and their quite arbitrary verdicts were uniquely aimed at reinforcing social responsibility. They showed indulgence toward people mired in debt who had committed suicide, and society at large reflected their pity. Juries could even go so far as to consider repayment of debts a sign of folly, as in one case reported by the *Times* on 9 April 1790. A hanged man was discovered in a house in Bath. The *Times* reported: "From some circumstances the Jury hesitated whether or not they should bring in a verdict of lunacy, when one of them (a tailor) declared 'he must have been mad, for that yesterday the deceased paid him the amount of a bill which had been due only three months.' "[16] This argument was enough to persuade the jury that the man must indeed have been mad.

Like the French courts, the English courts were merciless toward sentenced or accused criminals who killed themselves to avoid trial or punishment. From 1760 to 1799, ten out of fifteen *felo de se* verdicts given in London concerned accused criminals. In 1783 John Powell, a paymaster accused of peculation, killed himself, and the verdict was lunacy. The *Gentleman's Magazine* remarked, "Had a criminal in Newgate, under the apprehension of an approaching trial for his life, made use of the same means to his destruction, very few juries would have hesitated to have given a contrary verdict. Suicide is too much the fashion of the present day to be considered only as an act of a lunatic."[17] On 26 January 1793 David Mendes killed himself while under suspicion of having committed two crimes; his cadaver was sentenced.[18] In December of the same year a thief hanged himself in his Newgate cell. The body was taken through the city followed by a procession that included "the Sheriffs, City Marshalls and near 50 constables." A considerable crowd thronged to see the spectacle, pressing closer when the body was thrown into a pit and a stake driven through its chest. The *Times* reported, "The concourse of people assembled on this occasion was very great."[19] Unlike the people of Paris in Sébastien Mercier's report, the London mob seems to have been fond of this sort of "horrible and disgusting spectacle." The family had no way to avoid the sentence. In 1731 the next of kin of a Shropshire shoemaker who had hanged himself and been declared *felo de se* tried to bury his body secretly in his back garden. Several days later the parish authorities had the corpse dug up and reinterred under the public highway.[20]

Another proof of a changed attitude toward suicide was the creation of associations to rehabilitate people who had attempted to kill themselves, a much larger category than successful suicides. Would-be suicides were sent to asylums, workhouses, or prisons to prevent second attempts. The Humane Society of London, founded in 1774 to rescue people from drowning, soon shifted its focus, given that most near-drownings were suicide attempts. By 1797 this philanthropic association had already saved three hundred fifty such desperate souls.[21]

A Rising Suicide Rate in the Late Eighteenth Century?

An institution like the Humane Society is also an indication of the moral, political, and religious authorities' growing concern over an increase in the number of suicides. Since the sixteenth century observers had had a vague, perhaps irrational impression that the number of voluntary deaths was rising. In the second half of the eighteenth century, figures became available. The data were still too scattered to be certain, but they justified a certain level of alarm.

In England the bills of mortality for London show that the number of suicides peaked in the years 1749, 1755, 1765, 1772, and 1778, with annual totals at times reaching as many as fifty deaths.[22] The overall curve was stable, even declining, but public opinion was impressed by the high figures for the bad years and drew disquieting conclusions. Men account for twice as many recorded suicides as women, possibly because men used more violent and effective ways to kill themselves, and they tended to have more wealth to confiscate (which may have been a contributing factor in a large number of suicide verdicts).

All social categories are represented in these statistics, but there are noticeably fewer nobles and notables, thanks to the ease with which their next of kin could obtain verdicts of accidental or natural death. One trait that is both striking in itself and indicative of ancien régime society is that children and adolescents account for a sizable proportion of suicides. In England, 33 percent of the 1,001 suicides between 1541 and 1799 whose age is known were under fourteen years of age. The age group from ten to fourteen holds the record for number of suicides (159), as opposed to 150 for the fifteen-to-nineteen age group and 121 for the twenty- to twenty-four-year-olds.[23]

The high proportion of young people who committed suicide can be in part attributed to the widespread custom of placing children and adolescents as domestic servants in another household or as apprentices, situations in which they were often mistreated or subjected to an excessively severe regimen, even to acts of savagery. The coroners' juries showed little indulgence toward this sort of suicide. The jurors themselves tended to be property owners who might have young people under their own authority, and they feared that social order might be weakened if they showed pity toward dependents. When Thomas Empson, an apprentice in Westminster, hanged himself in 1779 after his master had beaten him with a leather strap, he was declared mad, but the case was an exception. In 1778 a child tried to kill himself because his mistress had locked him up when he had failed to bring enough potatoes back from the market.[24] Girls might commit suicide when they found themselves pregnant by their masters. The press reported such cases with extreme discretion. Excessive parental severity also might lead a child to suicide. In 1729 one boy hanged himself out of fear of being beaten by his father because he had thrown a piece of glass at his brother. Another killed himself because he had lost his new hat, and his father had threatened to beat him severely if he lost it.[25]

After children and adolescents, the next largest group was old people: 18 percent of the 1,001 London suicides whose age was reported were over sixty years of age. The fate of older people, and the scorn to which society subjected them, suffices to explain their large numbers. Many were without resources and exposed to misfortunes and illness of all sorts.[26]

The most common causes of suicides in the middle and lower classes had a basic connection with the vicissitudes of a harsh, even merciless daily life. Such causes had changed little since the Middle Ages, but by this time they were better known, thanks to suicide notes, whose increasing frequency was not due solely to a higher literacy rate. Voltaire tells us that suicide notes were current in the mid-eighteenth century, and Mercier writes that in 1782 "a number of suicides have adopted the custom of previously writing a letter to the chief of police in order to avoid all difficulties after their decease. This kindness is repaid by giving them burial."[27] A note enabled a would-be suicide to inscribe that act within a logic, to give it meaning and a sequel. That way such a sacrifice might serve a purpose for the suicide's immediate entourage or for society at large if the motive had broader implications. The practice of the suicide note was an integral part of the movement to rationalize voluntary death and to take its social aspects into account.

In England suicide notes were often published in the newspapers, a custom that emphasized the theatrical aspect of some suicides to the point of exhibitionism. The more modest suicides based their notes on others they had read in the press, at times copying whole phrases, like one barely literate young woman fished out of the Thames in 1783.[28] Others borrowed from more famous examples, such as Chatterton's or Werther's notes. In all cases the note writers displayed their desire to retain control of their death in the eyes of the world and to circumvent erroneous interpretations. When the writers attempted to reach beyond death and give their act a force they themselves might not have had in real life, suicide notes expressed a will to live. Certain note writers explicitly asked that the newspapers publish their letters.

At times a suicide note could be an act of pure vengeance aimed at making life unbearable for the survivor, whom it charged with responsibility for the act. In 1750 John Stracy left a suicide note for his wife that read: "My Dear, This is to acquaint you that you are the fatal cause of this action; your behaviour to me has drove me distracted. We might have lived happily and in credit, had your conduct been like mine. I hope the man who has been the cause of it, will think of this sad catastrophe."[29] In most cases the suicide wrote a note as a simple attempt to exonerate himself and to show that he had been driven to suicide by an unjust fate. As if grasping for reassurance, the writer usually expressed belief in salvation through divine mercy: "I hope for Salvation . . . for I have wronged no body," Lewis Kennedy wrote in 1743, and a journeyman barber echoed his thought in 1758.[30] Others asserted a deist faith, even materialistic beliefs, in their notes.

Suicide notes completed the secularization of voluntary death, because they eliminated the role of the devil in suicides, and they presented the act as a rational one explicable in human terms. The reading public grew accustomed to such letters, thus absorbing the idea that suicide was an ordinary event, a news item rather than a criminal act. As an affirmation of individualism and personal liberty, but also as a means of social pressure, the suicide note was characteristic of the spirit of the Enlightenment.

What such notes tell us about why people committed suicide is that their motives remained unchanged. Conjugal discord and family problems always contributed to emotional imbalance and disarray; the wife's infidelity or marital incompatibility affected men in particular. Grief at the death of a child or a loved one, poverty, debts, shame, remorse, or humiliation because of an accusation of some sort are the reasons most frequently alleged. The newspapers often reported the suicide by hanging of a young girl seduced, made pregnant, and abandoned. Suicide for love was also a frequent occurrence among the common people, to the surprise of the newspapers and the authorities, who tended to associate romantic suicide with noble birth. The *Times* of 20 February 1790 was less than sympathetic in its report of the suicide of one love-stricken girl.[31] Often common people's suicides were mocked; stories of love in thatched huts could not be taken as seriously as ones that took place in castles. Impossible marriages of ill-suited couples from different social classes caused fatal fits of despondency, and such suicides were judged with severity, as was anything that disturbed social order and established values.

Finally, certain pernicious ancien-régime customs might lead a sensitive soul to suicide. One of these was the charivari, a boisterous disturbance that often accompanied the remarriage of a widow and that gave festive expression to public disapproval. Called "rough music" in Great Britain, such rites might, on occasion, lead to outright cruelty. On 29 March 1736 the *Caledonian Mercury* reported that a woman had killed herself for shame after being publicly and indecently beaten when she remarried.[32]

Statistics in England confirm the predominance of spring and early summer as the prime season for suicide: Out of the 12,348 cases of suicide between 1485 and 1715 that Michael MacDonald and Terence R. Murphy have studied, 43.8 percent took place between April and July. Autumn, from September through December, accounts for only 25.1 percent of voluntary deaths during the same period. The gap is somewhat smaller in an urban setting, where the rhythm of the seasons had less effect on individual and social conduct, but it is nonetheless clear: Out of 1,583 suicides that occurred in London from 1715 to 1799, 40.1 percent came in the spring and 29.8 percent in the autumn.[33]

This contrast holds true for all periods and all countries up to the present time. The early nineteenth century (the beginning of the age of statistics) amply confirms this. In Berlin 36.9 percent of the 582 suicides recorded from 1812 to 1822 took place in the spring, as against 29.2 percent in the winter; in Paris from 1817 to 1825, and out of a total of 3,184 registered suicides, the proportions are 42 percent in the spring and 26.4 percent in the winter; for France in general in 1845, out of a total of 3,092 cases, the proportions are 39 percent (spring) and 29.5 percent (winter).[34] Physiology and an as yet relatively unexplored role of biorhythms probably entered the picture as well. We also need to take into account the cultural circumstances that traditionally made spring and early summer the seasons of the festivities of renewed life, of engagements, and (in July) of marriages, joyous occasions that may have aggravated the despair of those who felt isolated, abandoned, or left out for one reason or another. Springtime, the season of love, was thus a time of great frustration; it was also a time of illnesses that attacked organisms weakened by winter and by Lenten fasting.

The suicide rate seems particularly low in the Scandinavian countries during the eighteenth century: 1.8 per 100,000 in Sweden and 1.2 per 100,000 in Finland for the period 1754–82. But it was clearly rising in those same lands by the end of the century, when Sweden shows a suicide rate of 2.9 and Finland 1.6 per 100,000 between 1783 and 1813.[35] In Germany, Johann Peder Süssmilch expressed concern over rising suicide rates in his *Die göttliche Ordnung* (1742), a work that is a precursor of later demographic studies. What was still a reflection of impressions grew more concrete in the 1780s, when the first reliable statistics became available. Henri Brunschwig (basing his assertion on statistics for Berlin) states that there were 239 suicides in that city from 1781 to 1786 (or 8 percent of all deaths), a figure that he breaks down into 136 deaths by drowning, 53 hangings, 42 deaths by gunshot, and 8 slit throats. The figures for Frankfurt-am-Main were alarming; even a small town like Kuenzelsau-am-Kocherfluss had four voluntary deaths in three years.[36] Brunschwig has shown that socioeconomic conditions in Prussia led to a rise in the suicide rate. Rapid urbanization had weakened traditional ties of family and religion, thus attacking the structure of a society in rapid change at a time of demographic growth and economic crisis. When the population grew and the overall situation became more precarious, individuals were often cast adrift just when they could no longer count on traditional solidarities. All circumstances favorable to suicide seem to have been brought together.

There are no reliable statistics for France at the end of the ancien régime, although some figures did begin to appear. Impressions all concur, however. In 1771 Grimm declared that he was living at "a time when the mania for killing oneself has become common and frequent."[37] In 1773 François-Xavier de Feller declared in his *Catéchisme philosophique* that suicides were "so frequent in this century" that they produced "an effect of incredulity."[38] In 1777 the *Mémoires philosophiques du baron de X* took up the idea, while Voltaire stated (in his entry on Cato and suicide in the *Dictionnaire philosophique*) that the French kill themselves as much as the English, especially in the city. Hardy confirmed that notion in 1772: "Examples of suicide multiply daily in our capital, where one seems to adopt, in this connection, all the character and the genius of the English nation."[39] Louis-Antoine de Caraccioli spoke of his times as "fertile in such scandals"; Fulgence Bedigis, Buzonières, and Joseph-Nicolas Camuset proclaimed in chorus that people were killing themselves much more than before, for which they blamed the philosophical spirit.

The available figures are only estimates. Some of them clearly fall short (for example, Voltaire's estimate of 50 or so voluntary deaths in Paris in 1764); others equally clearly are exaggerations (Augustin de Barruel's estimate of 1,300 suicides in Paris for the year 1781). According to Barruel, France lost

130,000 persons by suicide in fifty years.[40] Sébastien Mercier's estimate in his *Tableau de Paris* (1782) seems more reasonable: 150 suicides per year for Paris.[41] This figure corresponds to a suicide rate of 18–25 per 100,000, which is not too far from the rate for France in 1990 (21 per 100,000).

According to Mercier, the suicide rate had been rising for twenty-five years, or since about 1760. He stated that it was not intellectuals who were killing themselves but "the indigent, the wearied, those worn out by life because merely to subsist has become so difficult, nay, sometimes impossible."[42] Mercier blamed high prices, the practice of gambling, lotteries, and the tax collectors, "merciless calculators like vampires who come back to suck the dead, giving the final push on the capstan to people already under the millstone."

The situation in Paris was even bleaker than in London. In London, it was the wealthy who killed themselves; in Paris, the poor. Mercier stated that this was "because consumption attacks the opulent Englishman, and the opulent Englishman is the most capricious of men, consequently the most bored. In Paris, suicides are found in the lower classes, and the crime is committed most often in garrets or rented rooms."

If people had the impression that suicide was more frequent in England, Mercier continued, it was because it was freely discussed in the newspapers, whereas in France the authorities did their best to conceal the truth. "No public paper announces that sort of death; and a thousand years from now, those who will write history according to those papers will probably doubt what I say here, but it is only too true that suicide is more common in Paris today than in any other city of the known world."[43] Mercier also noted, as we have seen, that "the police take care to ensure that the public hears nothing of these suicides." A commissioner came discreetly to the house without his robe of office, and the parish priest was urged to inter the body without fuss. This was also why public executions were no longer held. Mercier was clairvoyant when he singled out the government's attitude toward suicide as an essential part of the picture. Suicide was treated totally differently in France and in England.

The Discussion of Suicide

In France under the absolute monarchy, the king, master of his subjects' lives, could not tolerate their disposing of life freely, thus weakening his kingdom and his authority. As God's representative on earth, it was his duty to treat severely what the Church considered a serious crime. At the same time, suicide implied that his government had failed to guarantee the well-being of his subjects. It was a disavowal, a condemnation of his reign, capable of demoralizing the population and making him unpopular. Thus the government had to work both to punish the crime and conceal it. Concealment went against all the customs of criminal law in the ancien régime, where punishment served as a dissuasive example for the population at large. When common criminals were punished publicly, it showed that order was guaranteed in the land; punishment both reassured and intimidated, and the criminal provided the public with a target for hostility. Making a public display of a suicide was a more ambiguous affair: It showed that some subjects of the kingdom were unhappy enough to prefer death to life. Moreover, since such desperate people had harmed no one else and had offered no danger to society, there was a risk that the populace might think the victim more to be pitied than censured and shift its hostility to the executioner.

Until the seventeenth century suicide was so universally condemned that repressive attitudes prevailed with little soul searching on anyone's part. In the eighteenth century the French government began to be more sensitive to a change in public opinion, which had begun to see suicides more as courageous victims than as criminals. The power structure faced difficult choices, and it adopted contradictory measures in its attempt to simultaneously prohibit suicide, punish it, and conceal it.

At first, traditional repression was reinforced. The 1736 decree reiterated an earlier decree of 1712 to state that the bodies of victims of violent death could not be interred before the proper authority, the *lieutenant criminel,* could pronounce on the manner of death. In 1737, when a prisoner committed suicide, the Parlement de Paris noted that far from extinguishing his crime, the prisoner's death had created a second crime, and it ordered the bailiff to carry out an investigation. In 1742 a new decree of the Châtelet of Paris prohibited unauthorized burials. In 1749 a decree of the Parlement de Paris commanded "that the *ordonnances, arrêts,* and *règlements* of [this] Court concerning the cadavers of persons who have murdered themselves be carried out according to their form and their tenor." This means that until the mid-eighteenth century repression remained the rule and that fear of suicide was still widespread in rural areas.

Antoine Augustin Cournot remarked in his *Souvenirs* that around 1750 "a suicide was a very rare event that threw an entire city into consternation out of terror of punishment in another life, the lugubrious decrees of temporal justice that usually ensued, and the stain it imprinted on the family."[44] In 1768 the full rigor of the law was reinstated in an *ordonnance* applying to Corsica. Here and there in France, especially in the south, resistance cropped up. In

Puy-Laurens around 1755 the cadaver of a shoemaker who had committed suicide was forcibly removed from prison by an armed band, and in Castres in the same year the assembled throng protested the execution of the cadaver of an artisan who had hanged himself. Similar happenings elsewhere encouraged governmental prudence.

In a second phase, concealment became organized, first by prohibiting the publication of all written matter in defense of suicide. The declaration of 1757, which included a threat to authors of works that attacked religion, was aimed particularly at books on suicide. Some works, such as Holbach's *Système de la nature,* were burned; in other cases passages were excised, as was one sentence in praise of Cato in Marmontel's *Belisaire.* In 1762 a work attacking the Society of Jesus, entitled *Extraits des assertions dangereuses et pernicieuses,* accused the Jesuits of publishing a book that contained a phrase tolerant of suicides. In 1770 Antoine-Louis Séguier attacked Holbach's *Système de la nature* for statements favorable to voluntary death.

The government went further in its efforts to enforce silence about suicide. The gazettes were forbidden to mention voluntary deaths, as Voltaire, Dubois-Fontanelle, and Sébastien Mercier all remind us. The French press of the latter half of the eighteenth century was as good as mute on the subject of suicide. There was something like a tacit agreement between the authorities, civil and religious, and the families of suicides: Corpses would no longer be subjected to punishment, and in exchange, families would bury their dead discreetly. Suicide was evoked only by inference. It did not exist. This ostrich policy set up ideal conditions for the perpetuation and reinforcement of the taboo on suicides.

The English attitude was diametrically opposed to the French one. Suicide was news in England. It was given full coverage in the newspapers, and it received abundant commentary, a habit that did much to secularize and normalize suicide. The extraordinary growth of the press helped create more open, more liberal ways of thinking that were very different from the ones that predominated on the Continent. In 1753 the total circulation of newspapers in England was 7.4 million; by 1790 it had risen to 15 million. Moreover, every copy of a newspaper or journal had three or four readers in the coffeehouses, public houses, and inns. Nearly every issue carried a story about a suicide (thus reinforcing the notion of an "English malady"). In 1720 the *Mercurius politicus* declared that people killed themselves more in England than in all the other countries of the world put together; in 1733 a Prussian baron, Karl Ludwig von Pöllnitz, wrote, "These Self-Murders are but too frequent here, and are committed by Persons of good Families, as well as by the Dregs of the People." In 1737 the *Gentleman's Magazine* published a letter from a foreigner who stated, "I could not, in several Weeks after my Arrival in this Metropolis of *England,* master the Astonishment it gave me, to hear of such frequent Self-Murders as happen here almost daily."[45] Montesquieu, as we have seen, was victim of the same illusion.

The newspapers did not limit themselves to a simple mention of voluntary deaths, but rather described the circumstances of the suicide, weighed its causes, and published suicide notes (even inventing them if need be). They also printed letters from readers opposed to or in favor of voluntary death, and in certain cases they gave their own editorial opinion. This made for a literature that helped remove suicide from the realm of myth and made it seem a more natural act. Although most newspapers and journals declared that in principle they were hostile to self-murder, the way in which they wrote up individual suicides, sympathizing with the victims' woes and exposing their despair, elicited pity for them.

Jurisprudence and the Exculpation of Suicide

England, the land where self-inflicted death seems to have received the most liberal treatment, was nonetheless the last to decriminalize suicide.

Jurists everywhere debated the penal aspects of suicide, and although champions of repression continued to advocate maintenance of strict sanctions, the more tolerant current of thought rapidly gained recruits. In 1760 Edward Umfreville, a judge, preached in his *Lex coronatoria* (a manual for coroners) that the *felo de se* verdict should be restricted to criminals who had killed themselves.[46] For other suicides—in particular those who killed themselves after a shock or because of an emotional strain, grief, infirm mind, or illness—the verdict of *non compos mentis* should be given. In 1764 Cesare Beccaria's famous *On Crimes and Punishments* was first published in Italian. Beccaria points out that repression of suicide is useless, ineffective, and unjust: "Although it is a crime which God punishes," he writes, suicide is in some ways comparable to emigration: It is not up to the state to take away from "its members a perpetual freedom to live elsewhere." Beccaria continues, "Suicide is a crime that seems not to admit of a punishment properly speaking, for punishment could only fall upon the innocent or upon a cold and insensible corpse. If the latter will make no more impression on the living than whipping a statue would, the former is unjust and tyrannical, for men's political liberty necessarily demands that punishments be entirely personal."[47]

In any event, we read in an anonymous English treatise published in 1776 that, because the physicians had only a corpse available for examination, there was no way of knowing whether the victim had or had not been aware of his act at the moment of committing suicide.[48] Although French jurists were still vacillating in the 1770s, they soon were nearly unanimous in demanding that penalties be mitigated or eliminated, and this movement gained further strength in the decade preceding the French Revolution. In 1742 Barthélemy-Joseph Bretonnier remarked that within the jurisdiction of the Parlement de Paris suicides were tried, their bodies were dragged on a hurdle, and their possessions were confiscated.[49] The following year François de Boutaric made a similar remark, but he added that he found it astonishing that a procedure "so brutal and so impious" still existed.[50] In 1757 François Serpillon described the same procedure, but without expressing an opinion.[51] During that same year Muyart de Vouglans was one of the last jurists to come down energetically in favor of repressive measures, the execution of cadavers, and confiscation of the possessions of a suicide. He found suicide for *taedium vitae* particularly odious because it was inspired by irreligion; it must be harshly punished as a crime against God, the sovereign, and the family.[52] Elsewhere he took sharp exception to Montesquieu for his tolerance of suicide.[53]

Guy Du Rousseaud de La Combe, who agreed in theory with the more rigorous attitudes, protested the increasingly prevalent habit of closing an official eye to suicide. He added, however, that "it is good to presume that a person of good sense cannot resolve to kill himself," and he asserted that only rarely could suicide not be excused by illness, madness, grief, or despair.[54] In 1771 Daniel Jousse noted in his *Traité de la justice criminelle de France,* after recalling the procedures for suicide, "Thus one only punishes those who kill themselves in cold blood, with full use of reason, and out of fear of punishment." He added, "In doubt one always presumes that the person who has killed himself has done so rather out of madness or grief than as a result of some crime committed."[55] Jean-Baptiste Denisart, Thomas Cottereau, Louis de Héricourt, and Pierre Guyot all simply recalled current practice.[56]

After 1780 neutrality was no longer possible. Pressures in favor of decriminalization increased. That year the Académie of Châlons-sur-Marne offered a prize for a work on the topic, "Means for Mitigating the Rigors of Penal Law." Brissot de Warville won the first prize with a vibrant plea for indulgence. The law should not punish suicide, he argued, "because one cannot become accustomed to regarding as a coward any man brave enough to confront death voluntarily. His bravery is a delirium, but it is not cowardice, and ignominy is not reserved for cowards alone. . . . We need to make happy the being who bears in his bosom the fatal germs of suicide, not punish him fruitlessly when he is no longer with us."[57] Brissot returned to the topic the following year to show that society must work to remedy the causes of suicide, not to punish the act. By implication, he held the social and political organization of the country responsible for suicides.[58]

The runner-up in the Châlons competition, Joseph-Elzéar-Dominique Bernardi, agreed with Brissot, stating that the government should act "rather to return to the source of this crime than punish it by penalties powerless [to affect] an inanimate cadaver, and whose effect is to dishonor an innocent family."[59] Bernardi also returned to the question the following year, when he declared that suicides should be considered mad.[60] In 1781 François-Michel Vermeil published a treatise demanding the complete decriminalization of suicide, a demand that Dufriche de Valazé reiterated in 1784.[61]

Brissot's *Bibliothèque philosophique,* which included pieces by many authors who later played a role in the French Revolution, offered legislative proposals energetically critical of the current laws on suicide, which it declared "of a gratuitous cruelty, invented to enrich the tax office and to dishonor families." This, it stated, was "a horrible tyranny." Everyone should enjoy total liberty: "Man is only attached to life by pleasure; when he no longer feels his existence except by pain, he is free to leave it."[62]

At least five other treatises appeared in 1789 and 1790 to demand that suicide no longer be considered a crime. All penalties were "illusory and vain," Pierre Chaussard wrote.[63] Pastoret put it more vividly, saying that dragging a dead body through the streets was a "torture for which one would hardly pardon cannibals."[64] Antoine-Joseph Thorillon added, "That ancient and hideous penalty can only make one moan over human weaknesses without correcting them." He also opposed confiscation of the suicide's goods.[65] For Georges-Victor Vasselin, suicide was perhaps a weakness or an act of cowardice, more certainly an act of madness, but in no event a crime. Someone who kills himself "in no way troubles the public peace. He does not harm mores, he threatens neither property, safety, nor his fellow citizens' honor. He may displease God, but he does not shock religion. By what right, then, or by what means are we to punish him? It is typical only of our senseless laws to outrage a citizen after his death."[66] Antoine-Gaspard Boucher d'Argis called the law against suicide "powerless and atrocious." Nicolas-Joseph Philpin de Piépape stated, "In no case should suicide be pursued, because one must presume that it is the effect of an alteration of the moral faculties or—which amounts to the same—of a violent state of the soul incompatible with freedom of thought."[67]

These theorists dealt a final blow to a moribund set of laws that had, for the most part, become a dead letter thanks to the complicity between the authorities and the suicides' families. The parish clergy in particular had long been accommodating on the matter of interment in consecrated ground. The 1712 declaration complained that many suicides enjoyed a de facto impunity, and in 1725 some officials regretted the lack of cooperation and even the opposition of many members of the lower ranks of the clergy. In all matters involving suicide it was the lay authorities that took the initiative.

The prerevolutionary *cahiers de doléance* rarely mention laws pertaining to suicide, which is an indication that by 1789 few people found them troublesome, to the point that their disappearance was not even remarked. The 1791 Penal Code says nothing about them.

By that time suicide was no longer considered a crime in most of the English colonies of North America. Forfeiture was abolished in Pennsylvania and Delaware in 1701; criminal penalties for suicide disappeared in Maryland, New Jersey, and Virginia in the 1780s.

In Europe such laws disappeared gradually. The last execution of a cadaver in Geneva probably took place in 1732. In 1735 all suicides were declared mad, and the law was officially abrogated in 1792. Punitive laws regarding suicide disappeared in Prussia in 1751. Bavaria had to wait until 1817, however, while in Austria the code promulgated in 1787 still forbade Christian burial for suicides.

The formal decriminalization of suicide came late in England. Religious penalties for suicides were not abolished until 1823, civil penalties only in 1870. Suicide was considered a crime in England until 1961. Cadavers were still subject to punishment during the first half of the nineteenth century, and arrests for attempted suicide continued through the second half of the century, with *felo de se* verdicts still being handed up until World War I.

Religious Life and Military Life: Death from Thought to Act

Two groups held a special position among the participants in the debate over suicide in the eighteenth century: Roman Catholic spiritualist authors and military writers, two milieus totally opposed by their activities, the structure of their thought, and their attitudes toward voluntary death.

As the philosophes took pains to remark, Christian spirituality encouraged a desire for death, which it sublimated by mortifications of the flesh. Doctrines of annihilation persisted into the eighteenth century, thanks to doctrines of death to the world, and they gave rise to a strange literature that mixed spiritual simplicity with an aspiration for physical death. Jacques Bridaine preached: "Die to the world, die to your parents, your friends, to all creatures, to your passions, and to yourselves; love nothing you will have to leave, and use of this life only what will be useful to prepare you to die well."[68] While Bridaine was giving this advice to his flock, Dom Jean-Paul Du Sault was proclaiming his own attachment to death: "I want, O death, to make an alliance with you. . . . I will take you for my sister, for my wife, for my friend. . . . I will make my dwelling in your house, which is the tomb. . . . I will strip myself for you, beginning now, of all I love and possess on earth."[69]

Jacques-Joseph Duguet compared Christian baptism to being laid in the tomb. The Christian should be of the living dead, and should conduct himself as if dead:

We not only die with Jesus Christ, but we are also buried with him by baptism. . . . Death, precisely as such, does not hide the traits of the face, nor the shape of the body; it does not separate us entirely from commerce with other men. . . . It does not lead us to forget one whom we continue to see; it makes the memory of his actions and his merit even more alive, and it seems that never is the willingness to praise the dead more universal as when a person has just died, and he is no longer the object of envy. Finally, death, by occupying the living with the obsequies of someone who has left them . . . makes him the object of everyone's attention. But his burial soon makes everyone lose memory of him; it separates him from the world entirely and without appeal. . . . One does not even know, some time later, whether or not he has lived . . . and it is like a study to go seek out what he was. . . . Behold the image of another burial, one that regards the soul. . . . Our life, which must be secret and hidden, like the one that Jesus Christ now has in the bosom of his father, consists in obscurity and humiliation; it can only be preserved in the tomb.[70]

Father Louis-Marie Grignon de Montfort, calculating that every day some 140,000 people die in the world, meditated on the death that awaited him: "Should I not desire such a precious moment?" This thought was tirelessly repeated in thousands of works of piety during the eighteenth century. The works of Father Ambroise de Lombez and Abbé Jean-Nicolas Grou, who denounced such morbid spirituality as dangerous, stand out as exceptions to this rule.

The monastery was often compared to a tomb. It was where one left life to bury oneself in silence and piety. In surveying the spiritual and literary aspects of the eighteenth century, Robert Favre notes that beyond their superficial opposition, contemporary spirituality and philosophy converged on a deeper level in a desire for death, hence in their suicidal tendencies. Favre states:

Is it so far from the *Préparation de la mort* to the *Réflexions sur les craintes de la mort* of baron d'Holbach, once beliefs are set aside, and only the dolorous experience of the human condition remains? The lessons of a Catholicism centered on suffering and the many philosophical consolations advising detachment from existence tended to converge on this point. Life was not worth our attachment to it; disdaining it permits us to at least tolerate it as long as it is our portion; losing it is, in the final analysis, desirable: Death opens the way to the pacification, if not full development, of our being. . . . But this is to insinuate that suicide was the great temptation of the century; of a century in which nostalgia for the sublime led to an exaltation of suicide and of the sacrifice with which many have chosen to confuse [suicide].[71]

The desire for death that the spiritualists and the philosophes shared did not lead either group to suicide. Meditation on the world and on life, no matter how pessimistic, served as an antidote to the desire for death. Like Hamlet, they got no further than the question: "To be or not to be?" But the simple fact of posing that question is already a choice for "being." To meditate is to be; to meditate on the woes and the absurdities of this life was already a way to rise above them, hence to dominate them. This was perhaps one of the great—and unexpected—lessons of the eighteenth century. To reflect on death, even to desire it, was a way of renouncing the temptation to kill oneself, because it was also a way to enjoy the essence of what it means to be human, which lies in thought about that very essence and about its ultimate purpose.

Unlike the philosophers and the clerics, few of whom killed themselves, the suicide rate among the military was particularly high. Besides the two young soldiers who committed suicide at Saint-Denis (see chapter 10), Bachaumont's *Mémoires secrets* cite the cases of an officer in the Swiss Guards and a German officer in the Anhalt regiment. In Prussia the suicide rate among the military was extremely high, and nearly half of the 239 suicides reported in Berlin from 1781 to 1786 were of military men. Suicides peaked during springtime general maneuvers. In France there were suicide clubs in the king's Swiss regiments, and military airs, such as *Sur les ramparts de Strasbourg,* bear witness to the frequency of voluntary death in the army.[72] Veterans shared that attitude: In 1772 fifteen old soldiers in the Hôtel des Invalides hanged themselves, one after the other, on the same hook.[73]

Jean-Pierre Bois, who has studied life in the Hôtel des Invalides,[74] has kindly provided information on several former soldiers who put an end to their days. On 22 May 1725 Jean La Vallée, a man fifty-five years old, born in Guyenne, who had done thirty-seven years of army service, cut his throat in the infirmary. On 18 January 1734 Louis Godefroy, fifty-five years old, born in Perche, was in great pain from a gunshot wound in the thigh that he had received during the siege of Fribourg and from rheumatism in his left shoulder; he hanged himself. On 10 July 1743 Jacques Villain, fifty-six years old, with thirty-two years of service, drowned himself in a well. On 29 July 1761 Pierre Rhémy, forty-eight years of age, born in Strasbourg, whose legs and feet had been frozen during the campaign in Bohemia, killed himself in prison. On 2 December 1780 Jacques Libersier, forty-six years of age, who suffered from a skin disease, hanged himself in the nurses' smoking room.

Nineteenth-century statistics confirm the high suicide rate among the military. When the army was camped in Boulogne in 1805, Napoleon was forced to compare suicide to desertion. During the period 1875–85, when reliable figures had become available, military men were twice as likely to kill themselves as civilians in France, three times as likely in England, four times as likely in Germany, six times as likely in Austria, seven times as likely in Russia, and nine times as likely in Italy.[75] There were two basic reasons for this high suicide rate. First, the rigors of military discipline and of military life in general, which led to frustration and inhibitions, provided the motivation. Second, a familiarity with violence and the possession of firearms provided the means. When depression struck, military men always had ways to kill themselves close to hand, and the ready availability of weapons did away with a time lag (which might have led to reflection) between the decision to kill oneself and the execution of that decision. The philosopher begins by posing the fundamental question of suicide and ends up taking pleasure in his meditation. The more he reflects, the less clear things seem; as reflection deepens, it brings doubt, hence inaction. The soldier is professionally trained to act first.

When the French Revolution broke out, debate on suicide was at its height throughout Europe. There were two major schools of thought. For the first, suicide was by that time considered by and large the consequence of an act of momentary madness committed in a state of mental shock. In this interpretation the suicide is not fully responsible for his act. For the second school, no matter what might have been the causes of suicide or the victim's degree of responsibility, penalties now seemed clearly useless and unjust. Most people thought voluntary death a baneful act, perhaps deserving of condemnation, but lying beyond all condemnation. By showing that suicide was a sociological and psychological event, the philosophes also pointed to a need to investigate its purely human causes with the aid of medicine, psychiatry, psychology, sociology, and political theory.

During the sixteenth century suicide had been an affair between the devil and the individual sinner, and a question of pure religious morality that was punished by both the civil and the religious authorities. That conception had not disappeared, but by the end of the Enlightenment it had largely given way to a secularized view that suicide was a problem that lay somewhere between society and individual psychology. Individual responsibility was diluted to become part of a complex whole in which the criminal was transformed into a victim—the victim of his own cerebral physiology, of the misfortunes that struck those close to him, of attitudes among his entourage that frustrated his loves or emotions, or of a political and social organization that led him into poverty and despair.

The law trailed behind cultural evolution. At the end of the eighteenth century, suicide was being decriminalized nearly everywhere in Europe. That process was often accompanied by a conspiracy of silence, in France in particular, where those who held political and religious responsibility slowly but vaguely came to realize that the suicide rate reflected the health of the entire social group.

From the French Revolution to the Twentieth Century, or, From Free Debate to Silence

Several lessons can be drawn from the revolutionary convulsions that covered a ten-year span and that permitted experimentation with very different political and social regimes. The first is a confirmation: Whatever its nature, power seeks to prevent and conceal suicide. The subject must dedicate his life to the king; the citizen must conserve his life for the homeland. Desertion is out of the question. The social contract requires everyone's participation in maintaining the state, which, in exchange, watches over everyone's well-being.

The Revolutionary Governments

Newspapers, manuals, and political discourses—in fact, all instruments for creating the new morality—expressed total hostility toward suicide. The newspapers hardly mentioned notorious political suicides. The suicides of ordinary people met with consistent silence, this time not by any government command. The exceptional tract that touched on the question took the traditional line. When a turnkey at the Châtelet committed suicide after he himself had been arrested, one comment was: "Any man who believes in eternity knows that only the supreme Being can be the arbiter of human life, and that it is forbidden by divine and human laws to kill or to kill oneself. Life is a gift from heaven; society alone can dispose of it."[1]

The patriotic manuals and catechisms of the new regime said much the same thing. The *Catéchisme moral républicaine* called suicide a crime, and the *Petit code de la raison humaine* forbade self-killing. In his *Principes d'une saine morale à l'usage des écoles primaires* (1795), Gerlet wrote: "There is more courage in suffering one's misfortunes than in delivering oneself from them by death. It is more magnanimous to follow Regulus than to imitate Cato." The *Journal des Théophilanthropes* advanced the traditional Christian argument of self-love, declaring that "piety does not consist in suicide."

Voluntary death among patriots, even for the good cause, was not always appreciated in the sections and popular societies. When Citizen Gaillard killed himself in Lyons in 1794 to escape the counter-revolutionaries, a lively debate arose between those who considered him a martyr to the patriotic cause and those who thought him a coward. In contrast, when counter-revolutionaries killed themselves, the patriots expressed satisfaction at seeing them die in such an "ignominious" manner.

Discussions of the death penalty also provided an occasion to express hostility to suicide. In 1791 Jérôme Pétion de Villeneuve took for granted, in a discourse he delivered before the Constituent Assembly, that it was prohibited to take one's life into one's hands. In 1796 the *Moniteur* printed a report on the death penalty, written by Joseph-Honoré Valant with the approval of the Convention, which ordered its publication.[2] In his report Valant first demonstrates that suicide is forbidden because it is contrary to nature, because someone capable of killing himself might kill others, and because an innocent person who kills himself proves he is insane. He next examines ten cases in which Justus Lipsius had condoned suicide, refuting them one by one: It is not permitted to kill oneself for the homeland, but only to brave death for it; killing oneself for a comrade is not a suicide; one must not kill oneself out of fear, or out of a feeling of uselessness, or to avoid the opprobrium of poverty (everyone knows that money does not make happiness); one must not kill oneself to flee incurable illness, because by living one can profit from the "tenderness" of other people; castration is no reason to kill oneself, as the examples of Origen and Abelard show; and, finally, one must not kill oneself to put an end to acute pain or escape the decrepitude of old age.

What this literature really shows is that when political power speaks in the name of social cohesion, it cannot admit the right to suicide. In particular, the revolutionary government could not tolerate the suicide of political prisoners, even though they were about to die anyway. There was of course a fiscal aspect to the government's stance, because a person accused of a crime who escaped paying the penalty for it also escaped confiscation of his estate. This is why the Convention reacted to the suicides of several wealthy Girondins by promulgating a decree in Brumaire Year II that stated that "the goods of any individual brought under accusation, or against whom the public prosecutor of the Revolutionary Tribunal brings an act of accusation, and who deals death to himself, will be acquired and confiscated to the profit of the Nation, in the same manner and following the same procedures as if they had been adjudicated."

There was a deeper reason for the ire of the authorities, however: The prisoner sentenced to death who killed himself deprived them of an opportunity to display their authority. How else are we to explain the letters to the minister of the interior during the Terror complaining of the deplorable conditions in the Conciergerie, where twenty-seven prisoners under death sentences attempted to "destroy" themselves, or the letters of Fouquier-Tinville announcing measures to keep prisoners destined for the guillotine from killing themselves, or the letters of one commissioner who feared that the keeper of the Conciergerie could not prevent another twenty-four prisoners who had been sentenced to death from killing themselves?[3] The republic cared deeply for its symbols, one of which was the guillotine, the instrument for the chastisement of the enemies of the people. That made it absolutely necessary for such people to die by that means, and the authorities did not hesitate to bring to it the wounded, the dying, and even the dead. Robespierre was guillotined with a smashed jaw; Soubrany, Pierre Bourbotte, and Auguste-Alexandre Darthé were half-dead when they mounted the scaffold, as was François-Noël Babeuf, who was guillotined with the knife with which he had attempted to kill himself still sticking out of his chest. Dufriche de Valazé, who killed himself before the podium of the Revolutionary Tribunal, was treated to a second, in a sense patriotic, death when his corpse was guillotined. The same thing happened to Jean-Louis Goutte and to Jean Guérin in Marseilles in March 1794.

When the revolutionary government executed cadavers, it spontaneously continued the practice of the ancien régime, involuntarily demonstrating that suicide is the supreme weapon of individual liberty in face of collective state tyranny in any guise. All forms of power and all laws were impotent before such a weapon. Killing the cadaver was the only (and derisory) response of the state. At times—for instance, after the suicides of Jean-Marie Roland, Pétion, and François Buzot—the state might also try to punish an enemy of the people who had escaped its clutches by publishing "defamatory" texts.

A Synthesis of Cato and Werther

Political convulsions and brutal reverses of the political situation, set in a climate of exacerbated violence, explain the frequency of political suicides during the French Revolution. The late eighteenth century reached out over fifteen centuries of Christianity to reestablish a link with Roman tradition, but to some extent these political suicides also reflected the literary fashion for sentimental suicide of the end of the ancien régime.[4] Roland and his fellow suicides were in a sense a synthesis of Cato and Werther—that is, of the Roman tradition and the romantic tradition—in a political mold.

How could anyone deny the continuity that existed in the literary climate in France between the end of the ancien régime and the Revolution? One of its most telling signs was a preromantic sensibility extolling suicide, particularly suicide *à deux*. Nicolas-Germain Léonard, a novelist born in Guadaloupe in 1744, provides a link between the two epochs. Touched by the story of the two lovers in Lyons, Léonard wrote an *Épître à un ami sur le dégoût de la vie* (1771), *Le tombeau des deux amants* (1773), and *Les lettres de deux amants habitants de Lyon* (1783). The three works were republished in Paris in Year VII, at the height of the Revolution. Political events did not put an end to sentimental flights, and even after 1789, writers continued to produce novels and tragedies on the theme of suicide for love: François-Guillaume Ducray-Duminil's *Coelina* and *Victor,* for example, and Louis-Jean Népomucène Lemercier's *Isule et Orovèze*.

Patriotic suicide soon overshadowed suicide for love, which seemed suspiciously aristocratic, and when the two themes were combined they might produce strange results. Thus Madame Roland contemplated suicide when she was imprisoned in October 1793, and she wrote suicide notes to her husband and to Buzot. Similarly, when Philippe-François-Joseph Lebas sensed the approach of the events of 9 Thermidor, he wrote his wife: "If it were not a crime, I would blow your brains out and kill myself; at least, we would die together." Patrice-Louis Higonnet also cites the cases of Sophie de Monnier, one of Mirabeau's mistresses, who committed suicide in 1789; of Dunel and his wife, who poisoned themselves after the failure of the insurrection of Prairial; of Boutry, who shot himself with a pistol when his wife was arrested; of one sans-culotte in the Popincourt section who killed his wife and daughter with an ax before trying to kill himself; and of Jean-Lambert Tallien and Thérésa Cabarrus, Lodoiska, and Mary Wollstonecraft.[5] In 1793 Olympe de Gouges suggested to Robespierre that they throw themselves into the Seine together to wipe away his crimes.

It was predictable, in the new political context, that revolutionary literature would return classical suicide to fashion. André Chénier wrote a *Caïus Gracchus* and a *Brutus et Cassius;* Jean-François Sobry, a *Thémistocle;* Chéron de La Bruère and Tardieu each wrote a *Caton d'Utique;* Antoine-Vincent Arnault wrote a *Lucrèce*. In her *Mémoires,* Madame Roland stated, "So long as we can see a course ahead in which we may do good and set a good example it behooves us not to abandon it. We must have the courage to persist even in misfortune. But when a term has already been set to our life-spans by our enemies, we are surely entitled to shorten the period ourselves, particularly when nobody on earth will gain anything from our battling on."[6] In her letter to Buzot, Madame Roland praised voluntary death as an affirmation of sovereign liberty: "But if relentless misfortune hunts you down, let not some mercenary hand prevail against you. Die freely as you have lived! Let your last act confirm my faith in your deathless courage!"[7]

Here too there was a continuity between the ancien régime and the Revolution. Many revolutionaries returned to ideas they themselves had advanced in their writings some years earlier. Thus Goujon, who in 1790 wrote a novel, *Damon et Phintias, ou, Les vertus de la liberté,* in which suicide figured, applied to his own case the idea that suicide could be a rejection of oppression. When he was imprisoned in the Fort du Taureau near Morlaix after the failure of the Prairial insurrection, he wrote his *Hymne à la liberté* before killing himself:

> De nos jours immolons le reste
> A nos frères, à nos amis;
> Avant que des fers ennemis
> Les chargent d'un joug trop funeste.
> Pour défendre la vérité,
> Des méchants bravons la furie.
> Mourons tous pour l'égalité,
> Sans elle il n'est plus de patrie

(Let us immolate to our brothers, to our friends, what remains of our days, before enemy arms burden them with too fatal a yoke. Let us brave the fury of evil people to defend truth. Let us all die for equality; without it there is no more homeland.)

Higonnet states: "One can also think of Goujon's death as a political transposition of an earlier vocation for suicide, a vocation formerly expressed through a sentimental literary genre and later politicized. In 1790 the other is a beloved woman; in 1795 the other can only be the Nation itself."[8]

Charles Romme presents a similar case. Jean-Paul Marat played with the idea of suicide all his life. In 1770–72, when he was in England, Marat wrote *Les Aventures du jeune comte Potowski,* a novel in which suicide is present on nearly every page; in 1774 he wrote a *Plan de législation criminelle,* reprinted in 1790, in which he defended the right to suicide; on 25 September 1792 he put a pistol to his head and declared from the podium of the Convention, "If, furious as I was, a decree of accusation had been brought against me, I would have blown my brains out." The excesses of his newspaper, *L'Ami du peuple,* were genuinely provocative, and they led to an assassination against which Marat did nothing to protect himself. I might point out that the conduct of Charlotte Corday, something of a latter-day female Brutus, was equally suicidal.

Revolutionary and Counter-revolutionary Suicides: The Return of Brutus and the Martyrs

There were impressive numbers of political suicides during the Revolution. They began with the Girondins, whose elitist spirit owed much to the philosophes, and who preferred free and voluntary death to the guillotine, which they found shameful and too vulgar for their taste. When Jean-Marie Roland was declared an outlaw, he fled to Normandy; on learning that his wife had been sentenced to death, he exclaimed, "I do not want to remain any longer on an earth soiled by crimes," and killed himself. When Condorcet was arrested as a friend of the Girondins, he poisoned himself. Étienne Clavières killed himself while reciting a couplet from Voltaire's *Orphelin de Chine:*

> Les criminels tremblants sont traînés au supplice,
> Les mortels généreux disposent de leur sort

(Criminals are dragged to punishment; but generous minds are masters of their own fate.)

Charles-Jean-Marie Barbaroux, Buzot, and Pétion declared jointly, "We have resolved to quit life and not be witnesses to the slavery that will bring desolation to our unhappy land." They then killed themselves, as did Lidon, Dufriche de Valazé, and François-Trophime Rebecquy.

Adam Lux was a special case. A native of Mainz, twenty-eight years of age, and a disciple of Jean-Jacques Rousseau, Lux was so troubled by the proscription of the Girondins that he determined to put an end to his days in a spectacular manner, by shooting himself before the tribune of the Convention. He declared to the people's representatives: "Since 2 July I have held life in horror. Was I, a disciples of Jean-Jacques Rousseau, to bear the cowardice of being a passive spectator to these men, to see liberty and virtue oppressed and crime triumphant? No!" His was to be a suicide of protest, a self-sacrifice aimed at awakening the popular conscience. In the letter that Lux sent to Margherite-Elie Guadet and to Pétion to inform them of his intentions, he explained himself in these terms:

The triumph of crime has persuaded me to make a sacrifice of my blood, and to end my innocent life by a death more useful to liberty than my life ever could be. That is the first motivation and the one that determines me. The other is to honor the memory of my master Jean-Jacques Rousseau by an act of patriotism above calumny and above all suspicion. . . . My resolve to die can only be carried out by a spirit sufficient to the task. I am of the public interest, not of any party.

Adam Lux did not carry through his plan. Stricken with enthusiasm by Charlotte Corday's assassination of Marat, he fell in love with her when he saw her going by in the wagon that took her to the scaffold. He decided to die in the same manner. He wrote a panegyric of Corday, was arrested, and was brought before the Revolutionary Tribunal, where he engaged in a short exchange with René-François Dumas on the meaning of voluntary death. Standing before the National Assembly, Dumas called Lux's idea of suicide senseless, noting, "I observe to you that when one is a good citizen one spills his blood only for his homeland and his liberty." Adam Lux replied, "The decision to destroy oneself is not senseless when it is proven that the death of just one man can bring more good to the homeland than his life, and I might add that there is a certain language of virtue that cannot be spoken with those unfamiliar with its grammar." Lux concluded, "I wanted to do it because I wanted to be free." By choosing to die by the guillotine, and by his impossible love for Charlotte Corday, Adam Lux perfected the synthesis of Cato and Werther.

In Thermidor the Montagnards also chose suicide as a way to escape the scaffold. The younger Robespierre killed himself by jumping out of a window; the older Robespierre tried to kill himself with a pistol, as did Jean-Baptiste Carrier and Georges Couthon, while Charles-Nicolas Osselin drove a nail into his chest. Lebas and the wife of the cabinetmaker Jacques-Maurice Duplay killed themselves. The last of the Montagnards were arrested after the failure of the insurrection of Prairial 1795. Romme, Ernest Duquesnoy, Goujon, Jean-Michel Duroy, Soubrany, and Pierre Bourbotte, the "martyrs of Prairial," all tried to kill themselves. The first three succeeded; the other three were guillotined. Babeuf and Darthé died on the scaffold after stabbing themselves, while Boubon threw himself off a high flight of stairs. All were aware of following illustrious Roman examples. For them, suicide was the last refuge of a free man.

People killed themselves with equal ardor in the royalist, counter-revolutionary camp. The only difference was that they called on the example of the Christian martyrs rather than on Brutus or Cato. There is a long list of people who turned themselves in or who sought death out of pure provocation.

They came from all social categories, from one daughter of workers from Feurs who trampled the tricolor *cocarde* before the Revolutionary Tribunal to the comte de Fleury, who wrote to Dumas, then president of that same tribunal, "Infamous monster . . . I declare to you that I share the sentiment of the accused. You can have me undergo the same fate." There was also one young woman, Marie-Jeanne Corrié, who cried out "Vive le roi!" as a section of sans-culottes passed by and who persisted in that sentiment, declaring that she "preferred to die than to live in unhappiness." There was also Charles Viollemier, who publicly announced he was an aristocrat "who desires nothing more than the reestablishment of the kingdom. I hope that you will try me promptly."[9] Some killed themselves directly, as did Colonel Chantereine, commander of the King's Guard; Boishardy, a Chouan; several royalists after the royal setback at Quiberon; and others, following the defeat of the Chouan army. Launay, the governor of the Bastille, the duc du Châtelet, and the comte de Sombreuil also attempted to commit suicide.

As emotion reached its height, many refractory clergy forgot the Church's prohibition of voluntary martyrdom and sought death. Aimé Guillou paid homage to them in 1821 in *Les Martyrs de la foi pendant la Révolution française*. "Those who have confessed the faith before judges, knowing they would be sentenced to death for that confession," should be considered martyrs, Guillou stated, as should "those who preferred to die rather than offend God by a lie that would have saved their lives."

Some counter-revolutionaries expressed hostility toward suicide. First among these was the king: When his knife was taken away from him, he asked, "Do you think me cowardly enough to destroy myself?" The marquis de Charette was equally offended: He declared that suicide had always been far from his principles and that he regarded it as a cowardice. Antoine-Laurent Lavoisier and Pierre-Victurien Vergniaud also refused to kill themselves.

"Altruistic" suicides also occurred on both sides. A soldier who served under Charette put on his commander's hat and was killed in his stead; a servingwoman of Madame de Lépinay's took her mistress's place on the scaffold; many wives and fiancées refused to survive their husbands or lovers. Civic and patriotic suicides were declared martyrs to liberty. There was young Joseph Bara who expired in 1793 crying, "Vive la République!"—thus updating and reversing the heroic "Vive le roi!" of the chevalier d'Assas in 1760. Edmond Richer, Pinot, Jacqueline Chataignier, and the wife of Lieutenant-Colonel Bourgeois were killed on the spot or drowned for refusing to cry "Vive la République!" Some government *représentants en mission*—Tellier at Chartres, Bayle at Toulon—killed themselves to expiate their failures, and

General Louis Blosse committed suicide at Château-Gontier at the arrival of the royalist forces.

Military men throughout history have killed themselves rather than surrender. Given an army of volunteers filled with patriotic zeal, the Revolution had many such episodes. There were the sailors of the *Vengeur* in 1794, the captain of the *Chéri* in 1798, soldiers at Bellegarde who blew themselves up with their fort, and General Jean-Baptiste Moulin, who killed himself rather than fall into the hands of the Vendéens.

One such act gave rise to official celebrations. Nicolas-Joseph Beaurepaire, the officer charged with the defense of Verdun against the Austro-Prussian army, committed suicide in 1792 rather than surrender. On 8 September of that year, the Paris Commune renamed the Section des Thermes de Julien as the Section Beaurepaire in his honor, and on 13 September the Commune decreed that an inscription commemorating his suicide be placed in the Pantheon. It read: "He preferred to deal death to himself rather than capitulate to tyrants." Delaunay seized the opportunity to lash out in the *Moniteur* at the "senseless prejudice" that called "the courage of Brutus and Cato" weakness. On 14 September Antoine-Joseph Gorsas criticized "the imbeciles who have the stupidity to reprove" suicide in the *Courrier des 83 départements*. Gorsas concluded, "When all is desperate, when one is about to flee or be taken prisoner, when death is the only way not to lose honor or liberty, when by breaking the knot of an existence useless to the state one can give a grand example, is not suicide then a virtue?"[10]

A play by Charles-Louis Lesur, *L'Apothéose de Beaurepaire,* was performed on 21 April of the same year. In it Lesur went to some length to glorify patriotic suicide, as in these verses from scene 4:

> C'est pour notre bonheur que Dieu nous mit au monde,
> C'est nier sa bonté, sa sagesse profonde
> Que croire qu'il nous fit pour être malheureux:
> Il nous donne des droits, nous respirons par eux;
> Quand l'homme en est privé, c'est un mal que la vie.
>
> . . .
>
> Ainsi, quand nous voyons la liberté ravie,
> Quand les tyrans vainqueurs nous présentent des fers,
> Dieu, de quelques forfaits punissant l'univers,
> Dit à chacun de nous: "Termine ta carrière,
> Qui n'est plus libre doit abhorrer la lumière."
>
> . . .
>
> Beaurepaire, à Verdun placé par sa patrie,
> La sert mieux par sa mort que par cent ans de vie:

Son héroïsme au loin dans le monde est vanté,
On voit ce qu'un Français fait pour la liberté.

. . .

Que des chants immortels célèbrent Beaurepaire!
Il est mort pour nous tous, il ne pouvait mieux faire.
Il donne un grand example, il produit des guerriers;
Il laisse dans nos cœurs le germe des lauriers

(It is for our happiness that God put us in this world; it is a denial of his goodness [and] his profound wisdom to believe that he made us to be unhappy: he gives us rights, we breathe by them; when man is deprived of them life becomes a burden. . . . Thus when we see liberty ravished, when conquering tyrants present us with irons, God, punishing the universe with heinous crimes, says to each of us, "End your career; anyone who is no longer free should abhor the light." . . . Beaurepaire, posted at Verdun by his homeland, served it better by his death than by a hundred years of life: His heroism is vaunted far in the world, showing what a Frenchman will do for liberty. . . . May immortal hymns celebrate Beaurepaire! He died for us all; he could do no better. He gives a grand example; he produces warriors; he leaves laurel seedlings in all our hearts.)[11]

With the outbreak of the Revolution, the fashion for classical antiquity reached its height in both art and literature. The neoclassical Pompeiian style triumphed in both aristocratic and bourgeois houses, bringing the climate of severity, virtue, and cold heroism of David's paintings, *The Death of Seneca* in particular. Cato and Brutus, who represented supreme liberty triumphing over tyrants, were part of the cultural baggage of many of the future leaders of the Revolution. The Stoics, who provided several examples of political suicide, were also much admired. Would a generation less imbued with Roman examples have furnished so many political suicides? To some extent, the suicides of Beaurepaire, Adam Lux, Roland, Robespierre, Babeuf, and others reflected a synthesis of the philosophical spirit and the romantic spirit, both of which presented voluntary death as an act of supreme liberty.

The Persistence of Common Suicide

But what about "the people" in whose name these struggles were taking place? To consider numbers first, no data confirm the usual alarmist rumors. Albert Bayet demolishes the legend of the 1,300 suicides supposed to have occurred at Versailles in 1793, a myth still repeated in some recent works.[12] On 13 August 1790 the *Journal général de la cour et de la ville* reported: "Suicides become more frequent daily; sometimes poverty, most often despair, are the true causes that engage unhappy people to put an end to their woes by shortening their days." No statistics confirm such statements, however, and the press remained as silent on the topic as it had been under the ancien régime. Not until 4 November 1796 do we learn that at Paris there were "many suicides, [the number of] which are exaggerated, and for which poverty and despair are given as motives." On 11 June 1797 the *Sentinelle* gave a first numerical estimate: Sixty suicides had occurred in Paris within the past five months, or an annual average that matches Sébastien Mercier's 1782 estimate of 144 voluntary deaths in 1797 and 147 in 1782. Nonetheless, the *Journal de l'indépendance* wrote in May 1798 that there were more suicides in Paris than in all other European capitals combined. Jean Tulard estimates that on the average 150 Parisians committed suicide each year, with a peak in 1812 of 200 voluntary deaths.[13]

Richard Cobb's remarkable study of Paris court records gives a good indication of the nature of suicides in Paris from October 1795 to September 1801.[14] There were 274 cases of sudden death that clearly involved suicide, 211 men and 63 women. Of these, only 25 deaths were from firearms, hanging, or falls from high places; 249 were drownings in the Seine. One curious instance that may not be pure coincidence was a pupil of David's who threw himself off one of the towers of the Cathedral of Notre-Dame.

Cobb's study of these 274 suicides confirms something we have already seen: People tended to kill themselves in the spring and the early summer. In fact, 45 percent of these suicides took place in the four months from April to July. Sundays, Mondays, and Fridays were the preferred days of the week for killing oneself, with 44 suicides apiece, whereas only 29 suicides occurred on a Saturday. Women committed suicide at a younger age than men, most of them between the ages of twenty and thirty, and their motivations were purely personal, unrelated to political events. The majority of the men who killed themselves did so between the ages of forty and fifty; for Richard Cobb these were the "decades of . . . maximum disappointment."[15] Younger men's motives included weariness of war and the fear of being conscripted for a new campaign. Unlike what we have seen for England, very few suicides—a dozen in all—were adolescents.

One trait that stands out is the disproportionate number of unmarried or divorced men, who account for two-thirds of male suicides. A feeling of solitude may have been the determining factor here, even when such men had a family in Paris, as they were often men who had fallen into poverty and who had stopped seeing their relatives. The social and professional composition of this group of suicides is extremely varied, but the majority were in the minor trades as porters, wagoners, day laborers, sailors, police officers, seamstresses, washerwomen, and women who did ironing. Again, there is a disproportionate number of soldiers: 23, or 8.5 percent of all suicides. Many of these were deserters or men discouraged by the idea of a new campaign in those times of perpetual war. Many suicides were in the food and clothing trades, but few were domestic servants. The wealthier social categories are less well represented: There is only one young man who had been consul general at Philadelphia, who was the son of a wealthy cloth manufacturer from Châteauroux.

The Paris statistics show that suicide was contagious in both place and time. Certain spots along the Seine were notorious for drownings: 35 cases at Passy, 15 at the Pont de Sèvres, 11 at the Quai des Invalides, and 10 at the Port de l'École, just upriver from the Louvre. In 75 percent of these cases, the suicide lived only a few minutes' walk from the river. Although one can hardly speak of epidemics, the preferred season was spring, with peaks in March 1796, March 1797, April and July 1798, and March and April 1799. Most suicides by drowning occurred between nine in the morning and noon, probably after a night spent in somber meditation, and with a thought to attracting attention to themselves. Discreet nocturnal drownings were rare. The typical case would thus be that of a forty-year-old man with few hopes in life who drowns himself at Passy, dressed in his best, toward the end of a Sunday morning in April. The court records are clear on fine dress. Some suicides, Cobb tells us, "seem actually to have dressed up for their departure, as might a highwayman for his hanging, even to the extent of including such frills as lace cuffs, gloves, a coloured necktie high on the neck, embroidered *jabot,* and top-boots over slippers."[16]

The cause of suicide was usually unknown. The fact that suicides tended to be poor does not automatically make poverty the reason for their act. Poverty was probably the motivation for mothers who threw themselves into the Seine with their children during periods of famine, as in 1794 and 1795. Richard Cobb's sampling includes only one such case, that of a forty-seven-year-old washerwoman who drowned herself with her nine-year-old daughter in 1798. In the absence of suicide notes, the motives of the rest remain unknown.

The testimony of witnesses, when it exists, is seldom very enlightening. Almost always the friends and family declare that they had no previous idea of the victim's intentions, that he or she left the house without saying anything, and that they know no more. At times they report some signs of odd behavior, but on the whole their desire to distance themselves from the act and to avoid becoming implicated is obvious. Terse, unsympathetic responses are the rule in these poor milieus. One Swiss wine merchant from Fribourg who lived on the rue Saint-Antoine came to identify his brother, whose body had been fished out of the Seine, but he refused to pay for burial.[17] Suicide was an embarrassment for the family and friends of the deceased, and it created a momentary attack of bad conscience. Discretion, already the rule under the ancien régime, was facilitated by the inertia of the civil and ecclesiastical authorities. After the promulgation of the Penal Code in 1791, suicide ceased to be a crime under civil law; the Church was undergoing too many tribulations to intervene, and a national council in 1797 said nothing about suicide.

When all forms of repression ceased, the suicide rate did not rise appreciably, as we have just seen, which can be taken as further proof that legislation has little effect on desperate individuals determined to do away with themselves. As always, the living—the victim's direct survivors—felt pity mixed with a vague sense of guilt for not having been able to make life bearable. Suicide was still felt as a blot on the family's reputation and an offense to society in general: The voluntary death of a member of either was experienced as a failure. When nineteenth-century sociologists began to investigate the social causes of suicide, they reinforced that feeling of culpability, as well as the desire to conceal suicides.

The Nineteenth Century: Suicide and Guilt

With the nineteenth century, we reach the chronological limits of the present study, to enter into a very different phase in the history of suicide. Hence I shall limit my remarks to noting trends that became established during the early decades of the century.

At that time there seems to have been a movement to destroy all the progress that the preceding three centuries had made—slowly, incompletely, and with difficulty—in the direction of interpreting suicide as a social phenomenon that deserved to be approached without prejudice, as an undeniably tragic act, but one that must be understood without a priori condemnation. From the Renaissance to the Enlightenment, suicide had slowly emerged from the ghetto of taboos and unnatural acts. Even after suicide was no longer considered a crime, it remained a topic of heated discussion, but that same debate helped to strip voluntary death of its mythical character, to secularize it, and to make it seem a more ordinary event. After the break of the French Revolution, the moral authorities (and even the political authorities), inflamed by a spirit of reaction and restoration, worked vigorously to return suicide to what they felt was its rightful place among acts that are forbidden and classified as counter to nature. But because those authorities were no longer able to coerce people into moral conformity, they moved the repression of suicide inward, shifting it to the individual conscience. Their efforts were all the more effective when—surprisingly enough—the development of the humane sciences helped, quite involuntarily, to strengthen the individual and collective guilt complex regarding suicide. The emergent science of statistics permitted measurement of the extent of the phenomenon. Psychiatry and sociology pointed out that in suicide, individual moral and mental failings play a role along with the insufficiencies and injustices of the social structure.

By this time, statistics on changes in the suicide rate had become available. Every region, every social group, and every socioeconomic context displayed a fairly stable ratio of voluntary deaths to natural deaths, a ratio that sociologists slowly managed to define.[18] To remain within the time limits of the first half of the nineteenth century, the suicide rate in 1850 varied from 3.1 per 100,000 in Italy to 25.9 per 100,000 in Denmark. England was still an anomaly, but in the other direction: From the time when reliable statistics first became available around 1800, the suicide rate in Great Britain was clearly lower than the European average, thus confirming the role of the press in creating the myth of the "English malady" in the eighteenth century.

In his *Histoire de la violence en Occident,* Jean-Claude Chesnais summarizes the practice of suicide in the nineteenth century. He demonstrates that there was a noticeable rise in suicide rates, which he attributes to the social disintegration brought on by the industrial revolution, which showed as a weakening of traditional social and religious ties; to the emancipation (consequently, the greater isolation) of the individual; to economic fluctuations; and to the poverty of the working class. Louis Chevalier also stresses the role of worker poverty in his *Classes laborieuses et classes dangereuses.*[19] I might add that for the bourgeoisie and the intellectual elite, Romanticism and the philosophical currents of despair and pessimism of Arthur Schopenhauer, Julius Bahnsen, Emil Taubert, Nicolas Hartman, Giacomo Leopardi, and Søren Kierkegaard should be included among causes of suicide.

There was no dearth of famous suicides during that tragic century: Artists, philosophers, politicians, and generals killed themselves for reasons as varied as insanity, existential anxiety, frustrated ambition, unrequited love, shame, and remorse. Among these were General Jean-Charles Pichegru, Baron Antoine-Jean Gros, Vincent van Gogh, Gérard de Nerval, General Georges Boulanger, Paul Lafargue and his wife Laura Marx, Guy de Maupassant and his brother Hervé, and Colonel Hubert-Joseph Henry. The annual mean number of suicides for the whole of France rose from 1,827 for the years

1826–30 to 2,931 during 1841–45, or a 70 percent rise. The moralists took fright, and works on suicide proliferated during the July Monarchy.

As usual, the civil authorities attempted to hide the facts from public opinion. In 1829 the *Annales d'hygiène* wrote: "The newspapers ought to refrain from reporting any suicides whatever. We have good reason to believe that such publicity has, on more than one occasion, decided people already in a desperate frame of mind to hasten the ending of their lives."[20] When Louis-Henri- Joseph, duc de Bourbon and prince de Condé, hanged himself on 27 August 1830, the *Gazette de France* refrained from mentioning how he died, the *Journal des débats* attributed his death to apoplexy, and the *Quotidienne* called it an assassination. In 1844 Louis-Gabriel Michaud wrote: "It is impossible to announce that the duc de Bourbon committed suicide, that the last of the Condés hanged himself. In pronouncing these words we would believe we were unworthily calumniating the memory of that prince." On 19 July 1870 Lucien-Anatole Prévost-Paradol killed himself. According to the *Figaro,* the *Patrie,* and the *Journal des débats,* he died of "an aneurysm"; Camille Rousset stated that Prévost-Paradol had dropped dead, "as if struck by lightning." An aneurysm was also said to be responsible for the death (by suicide) of the minister of the interior, Charles Beulé, in 1874.

At the same time the Church, which had taken a less rigid stand toward the end of the ancien régime, returned to a violent attack on voluntary death. Félicité de Lammenais sought out the harshest possible terms to lash out at "that type of murder." He called for reestablishing laws against suicide as a protection for society, stating that "anyone who thinks himself master of his own life, anyone who is ready to leave it, is by that fact and by that fact alone freed from all laws; he no longer has any other rule or brake than his will." Under the Restoration, conflicts arose between the civil authorities and the clergy when the latter once again refused cemetery burial to suicides. In 1819 Élie Decazes complained to the bishop of Quimper of "the ardor of a zeal too inclined to severity" when the bishop had refused burial to a notary from Bannalec "accused of suicide." In 1821 the parish priest of Saint-Sauveur de Recouvrance, at Brest, wrote, "As for suicides, I have refused to bury four since I have been at Recouvrance, without feeling the least regret. I have even refused church objects such as the cross, holy water basin and aspergillum, and winding sheets."[21]

Since there were no longer written rules covering the procedures to be followed, practice varied from one parish to another and one priest to another. As late as 1917, however, the new code of canon law declared that ecclesiastical burial must be refused to "those who, with full deliberation, have committed suicide."[22] Burial might be accorded, however, if doubt existed concerning the deceased person's mental faculties at the time of the act. Anyone who had attempted suicide was blocked from holy orders. In 1980 a pronouncement of the Sacred Congregation for the Doctrine of the Faith declared:

All human beings must live their lives in accordance with God's plan. Life is given to them as a possession which must bear fruit here on earth but which must wait for eternal life to achieve its full and absolute perfection.

Intentional death or suicide is just as wrong as is homicide. Such an action by a human being must be regarded as a rejection of God's supreme authority and loving plan.

In addition, suicide is often a rejection of love for oneself, a denial of the natural instinct to live and a flight from the duties of justice and charity one owes one's neighbors or various communities or human society as a whole.

At times, however, as everyone realizes, psychological factors may lessen or even completely eliminate responsibility.

Suicide must be carefully distinguished from the sacrifice of life in which men and women give their lives or endanger them for some noble cause such as the honor of God, the salvation of souls or the service of the brethren.[23]

The same document recalls the absolute interdiction of euthanasia, that is, inducing the death of a suffering person, even when his ills are incurable. It states:

Euthanasia here means an action or omission that by its nature or by intention causes death with the purpose of putting an end to all suffering. . . . We must firmly state once again that no one and nothing can, in any way, authorize the killing of an innocent human being, whether the latter be a fetus or embryo, or a child or an adult or an elderly person, or someone incurably ill or someone who is dying.

In addition, no one may ask for such a death-dealing action for oneself or for another for whom one is responsible, nor may one explicitly or implicitly consent to such an action. Nor may any authority legitimately command or permit it. For such an action is a violation of divine law, an offense against the dignity of the human person, a crime against life and an attack on the human race.[24]

To return to the nineteenth century: Lay moralists, whether they were atheists or believers, were just as hostile to the practice of suicide as the Church was. Jules Simon, Charles-Bernard Renouvier, Bazard, and Barthélemy-Prosper Enfantin all tersely expressed their disapproval. For Renouvier, if voluntary death were authorized, it would permit people to "avoid all duties toward others the moment it would be to their convenience." For Cabet, suicide was one of the "vices of the old social organization." August Comte declared that such an "antisocial practice has to be banished."

Medicine placed suicide among "shameful illnesses." As early as the beginning of the nineteenth century, Philippe Pinel helped to establish that interpretation. In his *Traité médico-philosophique sur l'aliénation mentale ou la manie,* published in Year IX (1801), he linked suicidal tendencies to a mental defect that led subjects to exaggerate disagreeable events in their lives. Pinel states, "A habitual state of illness, the grave lesion of one or several internal organs, [or] a progressive decline can further aggravate the feeling that existence is painful and hasten a voluntary death." A violent shock helps to cure a patient of suicidal tendencies. Pinel offers examples. A man of letters attracted by voluntary death was heading for the Thames to throw himself in; attacked by robbers, he took fright and defended himself; afterward he never again felt like committing suicide. A clockmaker had attempted to shoot himself; he only broke his cheekbones, but he gave himself such a fright that he was cured. Gentler treatment, however, was usually useless. Pinel relates that in 1783 he treated a worker who had "an insurmountable urge to throw himself into the Seine." Attributing this derangement to gastric troubles, Pinel prescribed "relaxing beverages" and buttermilk, but some months later the man killed himself. Thus Dr. Pinel saw repression as the best means for curing suicidal tendencies. Shifting from the domain of medical advice to moral counsel, he stated, "Energetic means of repression and an imposing apparatus of terror must second the other effects of medical treatment and diet."[25]

Early nineteenth-century medical science thus tended to see depressive melancholia and suicidal tendencies as things to feel guilty about, and physicians preferred drastic "moral methods" of treatment, as with any sort of vice. Joseph Guislain, for example, suggested using such "moral sedatives" as brutal showers, rotatory machines, restraining chairs, isolation, hunger and thirst, threats, and attacks on the patient's self-image.[26] In 1834 François Leuret's advice was "Do not employ consolations, they are useless; have no recourse to reasoning, it does not persuade; do not be sad with melancholics, your sadness sustains theirs; do not assume an air of gaiety with them, they are only hurt by it. What is required is great *sang-froid,* and when necessary, severity. Let your reason be their rule of conduct. A single string still vibrates in them, that of pain; have courage enough to pluck it."[27]

The first half of the nineteenth century in part unraveled the theoretical framework that had been worked out in the eighteenth century. Physical and natural explanations of suicide, which since Montaigne had gradually replaced supernatural ones, were now swept aside in favor of moral explanations. Johann Gaspar Spurzheim, writing in 1818, propounded a political and moral theory to replace the theory of climate that some of the philosophes had used to account for the suicidal temperament of the English. If the English were more apt to kill themselves than other nations, it was because excessive liberty was a source of imbalance and frustration. Liberty of conscience was particularly harmful. In England, Spurzheim stated, "every individual is entitled to preach to anyone who will listen to him." Hence it was impossible to know where truth lay: "Minds are disturbed in the search for truth." Liberty engendered both uncertainty and insecurity, which in turn encouraged fear, madness, and suicide.[28]

Brière de Boismont returned to the sort of sociological analysis that connected suicide with the materialistic spirit of the industrial revolution and saw it as one of the faults of that revolution. In his "De l'influence de la civilisation sur le suicide" (1855) he wrote:

One of the strongest influences we have observed is the modern melancholy, which no longer has faith, gazes complacently into a dangerous void and prides itself on a total incapacity for action. Next come the democratic idea, that is to say, the general belief that everything is easily attainable, and the cruel disappointments consequent upon it, the exaggeration of the doctrine of material interest, the disasters inseparable from unbridled competition, the frantic excitements of luxury, the consciousness of privation more deeply felt owing to the march of mind, the weakening of religious sentiment, the prevalence of doubt and materialist ideas, and the political upheavals, with their ensuing ruins.[29]

For Pinel, who wrote under the empire, it was not religious liberty that contributed to fear but, to the contrary, religious tyranny. Basically, however, Pinel reasoned in much the same way as Brière de Boismont: Suicidal madness had moral causes. Moreover, he wrote, "The sort of penchant for suicide indicated by the author of *The Spirit of the Laws,* and which is independent of the most powerful motivations for dealing death to oneself (such as loss of honor or fortune), is in no way a malady exclusive to England; it is even far from being rare in France." Pinel went on to furnish examples of "melancholy with bigotry": "A missionary, by his fiery declamations and the image of the torments of the next world, so terrorized a credulous grape farmer that the latter believed himself frankly headed for eternal flames, and he thought of nothing else but saving his family and helping them to enjoy the palms of martyrdom."[30] The treatment that Pinel suggested was to isolate the patient and keep him from all contact with religious objects.

In one manner or another, suicide was considered a form of insanity during the first half of the nineteenth century. In 1822 Fabret declared that suicide "must be considered as a delirium"; in 1828 Élias Regnault wrote that the same opinion "has become a principle in all the works dealing with madness"; in 1840 Pierre Debreyne noted that "in general" doctors thought suicidal tendencies to be a form of mental alienation; in 1845 Bourdin stated categorically that suicide "is always a malady and always an act of mental alienation."

Psychiatric theory on suicide was based above all in the writings of Étienne Esquirol, who was active under the July Monarchy. Esquirol was not always consistent. He wrote in 1838, "Man takes his own life only in delirium, and all suicides are insane," but the following year, in his *Des maladies mentales,* he attributed suicidal anxiety to moral origins:

If man has not fortified his soul, education aiding, with religious ideas, with the precepts of morality and with orderly habits and regular conduct, if he has not learned to obey the law, to fulfill his duties to society and to bear the vicissitudes of life, if he has learned to despise his fellow men, to disdain the parents who bore him and to give full rein to his desires and whims, it is certain that, other things being equal, he will be more prone than others to put an end to his life as soon as he meets with disappointment or adversity. Man needs an authority to direct his passions and govern his actions. Left to his own weakness, he falls into indifference and then into doubt; he has nothing to bolster up his courage, he is defenseless against the sufferings of life's mental anguish.[31]

On all sides, then, suicide was a taboo to be surrounded by silence. Whether it was considered an offense to God, a moral depravity typical of a mind lacking in respect for established values, a mental weakness, a scourge connected with libertarian anarchy and materialism—or with excessive bigotry—it was in all cases seen as a sickness of the mind, the conscience, and society. Hence suicide was repressed and classified with the other great social prohibitions.

Folklore, which scholars everywhere were busy collecting during this period, bears witness to a different way to reject voluntary death and to deal with the horror it inspired. In Brittany it was commonly believed that if someone put a rope around his neck, the devil would weigh down his shoulders so that he could no longer remove it. Bretons also believed that the souls of suicides wander eternally between heaven and earth, and that they can be heard moaning where the suicide took place. Moreover, the souls of drowned people call to passers-by to lure them into the water. On the other side of France, near Grenoble, those who had been hanged were thought to return to pull the living by the feet as a way to ask that masses be said for them. In the

Creuse, suicides were thought to be condemned for all eternity to turn over the stones in the riverbeds; in Poland, they were believed to become ghosts who terrorized the living. Everywhere, folklore gave a highly negative image of suicides.

Thus the nineteenth century moved to do away with the results of reflection on the subject of suicide from the Renaissance to the Enlightenment. The Renaissance had posed the question, "To be or not to be?" The seventeenth century had attempted to stifle that question and replace it with others. The eighteenth century had opened debate on the topic to show that motivations for suicide differed. The nineteenth century closed the debate. "To be or not to be?" was an importunate question; it was incongruous and shocking; it merited silence. To be sure, suicides continued to occur, as the statistics show only too well, but if it was acceptable to try to explain the origins of suicide, it was out of the question to view it as a legitimate choice. Suicide was a mental, moral, physical, and social ill. The political, religious, and moral authorities were in agreement on at least that point.

Weakness, cowardice, madness, perversion—suicide was everything except the manifestation of a human liberty, which was what the more audacious thinkers of the sixteenth through the eighteenth centuries had tried to suggest. They had been foolish enough to think that Lucretius, Cato, and Seneca perhaps deserved admiration. Such errant ideas were no longer acceptable. The parenthesis had been closed. Twentieth-century science has not challenged that attitude.

In strong contrast to the previous awkward silence, an immense specialized literature on suicide appeared during the nineteenth and twentieth centuries. Thousands of studies have now been written, as well as articles, conference papers, and books of a more general nature. The more individual suicides are treated with silence, the more talk there is about suicide in the abstract. This is a sign that voluntary death continues to disturb us. Hamlet's question is ceaselessly reborn from its ashes. The humane sciences and medicine both search for an explanation of a behavior that bewilders us but also intrigues us. Suicide inspires horror, but it remains the supreme solution to life's problems. It is within the reach of all, and no law, no power in the world, has proven strong enough to prohibit it.

Sociology, Psychoanalysis, Medicine, and Suicide

The fact remains that how and why people decide to kill themselves remains a mystery. During the past century the best the grand theories have done is to throw some light on the context of that decision. In 1897 Émile Durkheim published his monumental work, *Le suicide: Étude de sociologie,* a fully documented study based on the statistics of his time.[32] Although his conclusions have been the target of criticism since that day, the work remains a remarkably forceful explanation of suicide. For Durkheim, suicide's causes are largely social. He groups them in three categories: egoistic suicides, which affect individuals who are only minimally integrated into their familial, religious, or political groups; altruistic suicides, which concern societies that practice integration to such an excessive degree that they justify the sacrifice of the individual for the good of the group; and anomic suicides, which occur when social mechanisms break down and fail to guarantee the satisfaction of elementary needs. Durkheim's sociological theory of suicide was completed in 1930 by Maurice Halbwachs, whose *Causes du suicide* established solitude as something common to all types of suicide. Halbwachs states: "People only kill themselves following or under the influence of an unexpected event or condition, be it external or internal (in the body or in the mind), which separates or excludes them from the social milieu and which imposes on them an unbearable feeling of loneliness."[33]

Sigmund Freud gave a first explanation of suicide in 1905, as aggression turned against the self. When social pressures prevent aiming the expression of human aggressive tendencies at the detested person, who is their true object, those tendencies turn inward against the subject. In 1920, however, Freud offered another and highly contested theory: Every individual has an an instinct for death—a *destrudo,* which he opposed to the *libido,* the instinct for life and reproduction. If it is not sublimated (for example, in self-abnegation or in devotion to others), that instinct may, in certain cases, gain the upper hand. Freud's first theory is a good illustration of a phrase that Gustave Flaubert wrote to Louise Colet in 1853: "We want to die because we cannot cause others to die, and every suicide is perhaps a repressed assassination." That theory would dictate that the suicide rate ought to be higher in the more structured societies, where external violence is the most highly regimented, and it should be inversely proportional to the homicide rate.

There is, however, a third axis to an explanation of suicide, which is the individualistic, genetic, and psychological explanation that Jean Baechler expresses in *Les suicides.* For Baechler, as for Jack D. Douglas in *The Social Meaning of Suicide,* voluntary death should be studied not from statistics, but rather on the basis of individual cases.[34] Suicide is an exclusively human and personal behavior: Both animal suicides and suicide epidemics are myths. People kill themselves for reasons that are both genetic and psychological.

Genetic inheritance gives each individual a certain aggressiveness and a certain capacity to adapt to the trials of existence. Moreover, certain situations are particularly favorable to a high suicide rate: lack of integration into a group, an excessively precise moral code that goes into minute detail to suggest occasions for fault and dishonor, and extended periods of peacetime. In contrast, suicides are less numerous in times of war, which reinforces solidarity and furnishes a reason to live; among married people; and, in particular, among Roman Catholics solidly integrated into their parishes. Baechler adds that physiology too offers a partial explanation: It is probable that the higher rates of male suicide are due not only to men's better access to means for committing suicide, but also to the aggressiveness provided by the male hormone testosterone.

All of these explanations, which complete more than contradict one another, point to the complexity of suicide. The deliberate decision to put an end to one's days is the result of multiple factors, many of which are independent of the will. The final choice, however, rests with the individual. "There is nothing more mysterious than a suicide," Henry de Montherlant writes in *Le treizième César.* "When I hear someone explain the reasons for one suicide or another, I always have the impression of being sacrilegious. Only the suicide has known them and was in a position to comprehend them. I do not say, 'to make them comprehensible'; they are usually multiple, inextricable, and beyond the reach of any other person."

A Call to Debate

If it is impossible for any outside person to comprehend a suicide, it is even less possible to judge it. Nonetheless, implicit reprobation is there, now as always. The old contradictions persist unchanged: an admiration for suicides in literature, for the military suicide of soldiers who stick to their posts or for members of the Resistance who swallowed cyanide so they would not give information under torture, and, at the same time, a condemnation of all the ordinary suicides of unhappy people whose motives do not seem noble enough. The twentieth century has nonetheless seen a full harvest of celebrity suicides, modern Catos and Senecas whose exit from this life was fully dignified. They range from Stefan Zweig to Henry de Montherlant, from Roger Salengro to Pierre Bérégovoy, from Jan Palach to Cesare Pavese, from Arthur Koestler and his wife Cynthia to Bruno Bettelheim, from Marilyn Monroe to Jean Seberg, from Patrick Dewaere to Achille Zavatta, from Romain Gary to Yves Laurent, from Mike Brandt to Dalida, from Jean-Louis Bory to Yukio

Mishima, from Max Linder to Vladimir Mayakovski, and others. For all of these men and women, suicide was a free act that deserves respect. As Odile Odoul wrote regarding the death of Bruno Bettelheim on 13 March 1990: "He may have committed suicide precisely because, with the onset of old age and physical diminution, that faculty of thinking freely had declined in him. . . . It was less an act of despair than one of courage to follow his life principles to their logical conclusion."[35]

We hear echoes of Montaigne in Odoul's statement, and of Donne, Justus Lipsius, Hume, Holbach, and Rousseau—in fact, of all the writers who, from the Renaissance to the Enlightenment, tried to show that not all suicides are alike and that the act can have a noble meaning. The debate, which has been stifled since the early nineteenth century, is reappearing through these great examples. Debate also takes on a new dimension with the special problem of euthanasia. These questions are too fundamental to be ignored. Society can no more elude debate on suicide and euthanasia than it can avoid debate on genetic manipulation. Quite simply, society's own future is at stake.

Legislators do not seem to understand, it is true. This was demonstrated in France with the adoption of the law of 31 December 1987 against incitement to suicide. The immediate motivation for passage of the law was the publication of a brochure entitled *Suicide, mode d'emploi* that was considered, wrongly or rightly, to be an invitation to suicide. More revealing is the spirit of the discussion that followed. For the deputies who prepared the law, it was "medically demonstrated that candidates for suicide are pathological cases."[36] A glance at the suicides listed above should suffice to show that this interpretation is exaggerated. What is more, whoever made that statement contradicted himself by stating on the same page that the economic crisis had led to an increase in suicides among the young, which implies that socioeconomic conditions, not insanity, are a determinant cause of suicide.

Today as in the eighteenth century, moral and political leaders remain silent on the problem of suicide. In France, the law of 31 December 1987 is above all dissuasive: Its aim is to use fear of judicial procedures to hinder the free expression of opinions on voluntary death. Such procedures would seem counterproductive, as a trial would publicize the very topic that the law attempts to stifle. "Thus, out of fear of a trial, the outcome of which is never completely certain, suicide may end up becoming a taboo subject," Danielle Mayer writes in an article analyzing the implications and deeper motivation of the 1987 law.[37] Frédéric Zenati notes that "suicide spoils everyone's fun"; it perturbs social equilibrium, and it undermines the self-confidence of a society that feels guilty, or at least under accusation.[38] "Thus," Danielle Mayer concludes, "by its significance as much as by its consequences, suicide troubles society, which might be tempted, if it is not careful, to react—as if instinctively—by overuse of its favorite instrument of self-protection, which is its right to repression."

This is precisely the question that some thinkers raised during the crises of Europe's conscience in the sixteenth to eighteenth centuries. Didn't those thinkers—from Montaigne to Hume—satisfactorily prove that humankind cannot do without the question, "To be or not to be?" precisely because it forms the base of all truly human, truly worthwhile lives? Far from inciting to suicide, Hamlet's question urges the human mind to deepen its sense of life, at the risk of awakening a sense of the absurd. Is it not that very risk that provides a large part of humanity's grandeur? The absurdity of existence, however, may itself be an assumption: "Thus I draw from the absurd three consequences, which are my revolt, my freedom, and my passion," Albert Camus wrote. "By the mere activity of consciousness I transform into a rule of life what was an invitation to death—and I refuse suicide."[39]

The question of human liberty was first discussed between the sixteenth and the eighteenth centuries. When the nineteenth and twentieth centuries stifled that debate, they also censored a fundamental liberty and imposed a duty to live, which they supported by supernatural and ideological explanations. The decline of those global explanations should permit us to return to the debate that was interrupted at the end of the Enlightenment.

Envoi

Intellectual history has swung between "I know" and "What do I know?" In phases of equilibrium and stability, thought lends depth to answers; in times of crisis, it poses questions. In its quest for truth, the human mind passes from certitude to doubt, which in turn creates new and illusory certitudes. If certitudes offer security, doubts provide stimulation. There is nothing rigid about their alternation, however: The struggle is unending. During periods of crisis of conscience, the level of doubt manages to shake certitudes, which resist and use force to stifle the questions. This is because those in positions of responsibility—the political and religious leaders—are hostile to doubts. If to govern is to foresee, it is also to know. One cannot command with doubts, only with certitudes. In the name of what else could society be regulated? How, in particular, can anyone rule people who are not even sure they should remain alive? What hold can anyone have on subjects or citizens who have full liberty to leave life as they please? How can anyone inspire them with confidence if every day a certain number of them manifest their defiance and despair by preferring death to life?

The question of the individual's freedom to dispose of his or her own life reemerges when profound crises challenge traditional values. That is what began to happen in the Renaissance, for the first time since the triumph of Christianity and the installation of medieval Christendom. Hamlet's question reflects a malaise connected with the birth of modernity.

Not until contemporary times—which bring a new crisis in European conscience, when once again values that seemed certain are being over-turned—could the old question be posed again. Naturally, the philosophers of the absurd took it as their duty to reflect on it. Curiously, they rejected the solution of voluntary death, which Jean-Paul Sartre called the abandonment of all liberty and Karl Jaspers calls the "absolute action that transgresses life." Albert Camus rejected suicide. Today, although intellectuals show less inter-est in the subject than their eighteenth-century counterparts did, the debate is reappearing under the pressure of statistics. This is because the collapse of credos and ideologies places more and more individuals in a situation of despair. France, with its 12,000 suicides per year and its 120,000 attempted suicides, is not unique. Suicide kills more people in France than the highways: It claims a victim every fifty minutes, a figure that is constantly rising.

As always, those in positions of political and religious responsibility remain silent, as they must according to the law of 31 December 1987. Their reflexes have not changed through the centuries, which suggests that suicide is an accusation brought against the organization of society when society becomes incapable of guaranteeing the happiness of its members. It is time we picked up the debate where Hume, Rousseau, and Kant left off.

The period from the Renaissance to the Enlightenment showed that vol-untary death is also a class phenomenon. Elite suicide, which affected only a restricted number of individuals, obeyed conventions and rituals that were subject to the vicissitudes of fashion. Members of the elites killed themselves with noble means—sharp steel or firearms—and they did so for noble reasons: honor, debts, love. Their suicides were by and large tolerated by the authori-ties, who could afford to be indulgent, because those deaths did not challenge social order. Only rarely were the corpses and the possessions of aristocratic suicides treated with severity. Intellectuals talked about suicide but rarely committed it, even when they were in favor of liberalizing the laws pertaining to it. Philosophical suicides were extremely rare, which indicates that free debate on voluntary death, like certain forms of religious life, can act as a safety valve or provide a sort of sublimation.

Among the common people, the causes of suicide remained remarkably stable under the ancien régime. Contemporaries' impressions, diarists' reports, articles in the English press in the eighteenth century, and the few judiciary documents available are partial sources in both senses of the term, but they at least permit us to see that suicide rates remained relatively constant (a few exceptions aside), and that the immense majority of suicides were the result of excessive physical, moral, or emotional suffering.

As we have seen, ordinary, prosaic suicide was repressed ferociously, with cadavers dragged on a hurdle, hanged by the feet, burned, and then thrown on the refuse heap, or, in England, buried under the high road, pinned to the ground with a stake driven through the chest. Hell was guaranteed; worldly possessions were confiscated. Hostility to judicial savagery grew from the sixteenth to the eighteenth century. Not that suicide came to be considered a heroic, praiseworthy act, but rather the rural community stood opposed to public acts that cast opprobrium on entire families because of the fault of one of their members, and it resisted a forfeiture of goods that reduced innocent heirs to poverty. The advance of individualism that began in the Renaissance did much to personalize moral responsibility and to discourage collective punishment.

Popular suicide, almost always committed by hanging or drowning, brought shame to the family, and a suicide's next of kin worked systematically to camouflage the death as an accident or attribute it to a moment of madness. In the eighteenth century debate on elite suicide obliged the authorities to repress suicide with increased prudence and discretion. Slowly, the parish priest or pastor, the family, and the civil authorities worked in concert to conceal suicides. This helped make suicide a taboo where each party had an interest in enforcing silence.

The debate on suicide, which was born in the sixteenth century and grew steadily until the eighteenth century, put the authorities in an embarrassing position. It also incited them to move toward reducing repression in the interest of silencing a problem that was troubling the collective conscience. The philosophes demanded the decriminalization of suicide; some of them even called for a recognition of the dignity and the grandeur of certain voluntary deaths. Suicide may no longer have been considered a crime, but a reproachful silence still surrounded it in the public mind. "To be or not to be?" The question is perhaps so disturbing that it never can be raised with impunity. Even the most audacious of the humanists and the philosophes hesitated to publicize their ideas on the subject.

This study has focused on the period from the sixteenth to the eighteenth century, largely because that was a privileged time for reflection on voluntary death. The nineteenth and twentieth centuries, with their expanding interest in the humane sciences, accompanied by the colossal masses of data that make those sciences possible, deserve a volume of their own. In spite of the innumerable sociological treatises that have appeared, we cannot say that the question has made any real progress on the plane of understanding since the day of the philosophes. Today, we have all imaginable statistical information on suicide, but the basic problem has not advanced much, nor will it advance as long as society tacitly accepts the principle that life at any cost is preferable to death.

Annihilation is a yawning abyss that repels and terrifies, and those who disappear into it voluntarily are considered mad. But is not the rejection of suicide, collective or individual, dictated by an invincible and human revulsion before an imagined fate we all know will ineluctably be ours?

In spite of everything that the moral and political authorities can do, the problem of suicide is recurring today through the extreme case of euthanasia. Moral leaders continue to assert that suffering, even excruciating, incurable suffering, has a positive value; political leaders fear backsliding. This is why thousands of human beings who are dehumanized by intolerable suffering are condemned to live. In the difficult mutation that values are undergoing today, should not debate on bioethics also work to create a thanato-ethics?

NOTES

Introduction

1. Michel Vovelle, *La mort et l'Occident: De 1200 à nos jours* (Paris: Gallimard, 1983); François Lebrun, *Les hommes et la mort en Anjou aux XVIIe et XVIIIe siècles* (Paris: Mouton, 1971; Flammarion, 1975); Pierre Chaunu, *La mort à Paris: XVIe, XVIIe et XVIIIe siècles* (Paris: Fayard, 1977); Philippe Ariès, *L'homme devant la mort* (Paris: Éditions du Seuil, 1977), in English translation as *The Hour of Our Death,* trans. Helen Weever (New York: Knopf, 1981); John McManners, *Death and the Enlightenment: Changing Attitudes toward Death among Christians and Unbelievers in the Eighteenth Century* (New York: Oxford University Press, 1981).

2. Yolande Grisé, *Le suicide dans la Rome antique* (Paris: Belles Lettres, 1982; Montreal: Bellarmin, 1983); Jean-Claude Schmitt, "Le suicide au Moyen Age," *Annales ESC* 31 (1976): 3–28. Bernard Paulin, *Du couteau à la plume: Le suicide dans la littérature anglaise de la Renaissance (1580–1625)* (Lyons: Hermès; Saint-Étienne: Université de Saint-Étienne, 1977); Michael MacDonald and Terence R. Murphy, *Sleepless Souls: Suicide in Early Modern England* (New York: Oxford University Press, 1990); Albert Bayet, *Le suicide et la morale* (Paris: Félix Alcan, 1922).

3. Jean Baechler, *Les suicides* (Paris: Calmann-Lévy, 1975), in English translation, abridged, as *Suicides,* trans. Barry Cooper (New York: Basic Books, 1979).

4. Raymond Aron, foreword to Baechler, *Suicides,* xi.

5. Albert Camus, *Le mythe de Sisyphe* (Paris: Gallimard, 1942), quoted here from *The Myth of Sisyphus and Other Essays,* trans. Justin O'Brien (New York: Harcourt, Brace, 1969), 3, 5.

One. Suicide in the Middle Ages: Nuances

1. The highly fragmentary nature of the sources and their disparity hinders a thorough understanding of the practice of suicide during the Middle Ages. For judiciary documents, which offer the largest number of cases, see Edgard Boutaric, *Actes du Parlement de Paris, 1re série, de l'an 1254 à l'an 1328* (Paris: H. Plon, 1863); *Registre criminel du Châtelet de Paris, du 6 septembre au 18 mai 1389–1392,* ed. Henri Duplès-Agier, 2 vols. (Paris, 1861–64); François Des Maisons, *Nouveau recueil d'arrests et réglements du Parlement de Paris* (Paris, 1667); Arthur Auguste, comte Beugnot, *Les Olim ou registres des arrêts rendus par la Cour du roi,* 4 vols. (Paris: Imprimerie Royale, 1839–48). The records of the episcopal courts *(officialités)* also present a good number of cases, but few have been published. I might cite "Le registre de l'officialité de Cerisy," *Mémoires de la Société des Antiquaires de Normandie* 30 (1880); and "Registre des officialités de Chartres," *Bibliothèque de l'École des Chartes* (1850). Medieval customals

are more numerous and refer to precise cases. A good list of them can be found in Albert Bayet, *Le suicide et la morale* (Paris: F. Alcan, 1922). Chronicles only rarely mention suicides.

2. Jean-Claude Schmitt, "Le suicide au Moyen Age," *Annales ESC* 31 (1976): 3–28, quotation on 5.

3. Félix Bourquelot, "Recherches sur les opinions et la législation en matière de mort volontaire pendant le Moyen Age: Depuis Justinien jusqu'à Charlemagne," *Bibliothèque de l'École des Chartes* 3 (1841–42): 539–60.

4. Karen Armstrong, *Holy War* (New York: Doubleday/Anchor, 1992), 409.

5. *Les miracles de Saint Benoît,* ed. Antoine Eugène de Certain (Paris, 1858), 197.

6. *Chronique du religieux de Saint-Denis,* ed. Louis-François Bellaguet, 6 vols. (Paris, 1839–52), 5:57.

7. Ibid., 5:464.

8. Orderic Vital, *Histoire de Normandie,* in *Collection des mémoires relatifs à l'histoire de France, depuis la fondation de la monarchie française jusqu'au 13ᵉ siècle,* ed. François Pierre Guillaume Guizot, 31 vols. (Paris, 1823–35), 26:215.

9. Suger, *Vie de Louis-le-Gros,* in Guizot, ed., *Collection des mémoires,* 8:65–66; in English as *The Deeds of Louis the Fat,* ed. and trans. Richard Cusimano and John Moorhead (Washington, D.C.: Catholic University of America Press, 1992). Guillaume de Tyr, *Histoire des Croisades,* in Guizot, ed., *Collection des mémoires,* 16:12; for a modern critical edition, see Guillaume de Tyr, *Chronique,* ed. R.B.C. Huygens, 2 vols. (Turnhout: Brepols, 1986).

10. Bayet, *Le suicide et la morale,* 451–61.

11. For these examples, see ibid.

12. Chrétien de Troyes, *Yvain,* lines 3542–45, quoted here from *Yvain: The Knight of the Lion,* trans. Burton Raffel (New Haven: Yale University Press, 1987).

13. Schmitt, "Le suicide au Moyen Age," 17.

14. For a modern edition, see Prudentius, *Psychomachia,* ed. Rosemary Burton, 2 vols. (Bryn Mawr, Pa.: Thomas Library, Bryn Mawr College, 1989).

15. Bernard Paulin, *Du couteau à la plume: Le suicide dans la littérature anglaise de la Renaissance (1580–1625)* (Lyons: Hermès; Saint-Étienne: Université de Saint-Étienne, 1977), 32.

16. *Quaestiones Joannis Galli,* ed. Charles Dumoulin, in Dumoulin, *Opera,* 5 vols. (Paris, 1681), 2:599.

17. Charles de Robillard de Beaurepaire, *Précis des travaux de l'Académie de Rouen* (1892).

18. Quoted in Bayet, *Le suicide et la morale,* 471.

19. Albert d'Aix, *Histoire des faits et gestes dans les régions d'Outre-Mer depuis l'année 1095 jusqu'à l'année 1120 de Jésus-Christ,* in Guizot, ed., *Collection des mémoires,* 20:39.

20. Joseph Ha-Cohen, *La Vallée des pleurs: Chronique des souffrances d'Israël,* trans. Julien Sée (Paris, 1881). Rodulfus Glaber, *Chronique,* in Guizot, ed., *Collection des mémoires,* 6:267; for a modern edition, see *Rodulfi Glabri, Historiarum Libri Quinque;*

Rodulfus Glaber, The Five Books of the Histories, ed. and trans. John France (Oxford: Clarendon Press, 1989). We read in Guillaume de Nangis, *Chronique* (in Guizot, ed., *Collection des mémoires,* 13:344, 352), that five hundred Jews besieged by *pastoureux* (peasant Christian zealots) killed themselves in 1320, and in 1321 another forty Jews accused of poisoning fellow citizens followed their example.

21. Rodulfus Glaber, *Chronique,* 279.

22. Guillaume de Nangis, *Chronique,* 107.

23. Pierre de Vaulx-Cernay, *Histoire de la guerre des Albigeois,* in Guizot, ed., *Collection des mémoires,* 12:98.

24. Emmanuel Le Roy Ladurie, *Montaillou, village occitan de 1294 à 1324* (Paris: Gallimard, 1975), 343; in English translation as *Montaillou, the Promised Land of Error,* trans. Barbara Bray (New York: George Braziller, 1978).

25. Flavius Josephus, *The Jewish War,* trans. G. A. Williamson (Baltimore: Penguin Books, 1959), 57. This translation is the source of the quotations in the text.

Two. The Legacy of the Middle Ages: Between Madness and Despair

1. Origen, *Commentary on the Gospel according to John: Books 1–10,* trans. Ronald E. Heine (Washington, D.C.: Catholic University of America Press, 1989).

2. St. Jerome, letter 91.

3. St. Ambrose, *De officiis,* II.30; *De excessu fratris sui satyri,* II.44–46.

4. St. Augustine, *The City of God, Books I–IV,* trans. Demetrius B. Zema and Gerald G. Walsh (New York: Fathers of the Church, 1950), book 1, chap. 26, p. 61.

5. St. Augustine, *De bono conjugali,* XVI.18, quoted from "Good of Marriage" in *Treatises on Marriage and Other Subjects,* ed. Roy J. Deferrari, trans. Charles T. Wilcox et al. (New York: Fathers of the Church, 1955), 32; letter no. 228, "Augustine Gives Greetings in the Lord to His Holy Brother and Fellow Bishop, Honoratus," *Letters: Volume V (204–270),* trans. Sister Wilfred Parsons (New York: Fathers of the Church, 1956), 142–43.

6. John Duns Scotus, *Quaestiones in quatuor libros sententiarum,* dist. XV, q. 3.

7. This story can be found in Pierre de Beauvais, Guibert de Nogent, and Alfonso X, and also in a large number of sermons.

8. On the connection between suicide and despair, see Rowland Wymer, *Suicide and Despair in Jacobean Drama* (New York: St. Martin's Press, 1986); A. Sachs, "Religious Despair in Medieval Literature and Art," *Medieval Studies* 26 (1964): 231–56; Siegfried Wenzel, *The Sin of Sloth: Acedia in Medieval Thought and Literature* (Chapel Hill: University of North Carolina Press, 1967); Susan Snyder, "The Left Hand of God: Despair in Medieval and Renaissance Tradition," *Studies in the Renaissance* 12 (1965): 18–59.

9. Jean-Claude Schmitt, "Le suicide au Moyen Age," *Annales ESC* 31 (1976): 3–28, notes 80 and 81, offers several examples.

10. Civil law is perhaps the best known aspect of the question, thanks to the

publication, beginning in the seventeenth century, of customals from the various regions of France. Albert Bayet provides a long list of such compilations in *Le suicide et la morale* (Paris: Félix Alcan, 1922). For further information, see Félix Bourquelot, "Recherches sur les opinions et la législation en matière de mort volontaire pendant le Moyen Age," *Bibliothèque de l'École des Chartes* 3 (1841–42): 537–60, and 4 (1842–43): 456–75.

11. Robert Caillemer, *Confiscations et administration des successions par les pouvoirs publics au Moyen Age* (Lyons: A. Rey, 1901), 27.

12. Henry de Bracton, *On the Laws and Customs of England,* ed. and trans. Samuel E. Thorne, 4 vols. (Cambridge: Belknap Press of Harvard University Press in association with the Selden Society, 1968), 2:323, 423.

13. Schmitt, "Le suicide au Moyen Age."

14. *Registre criminel de la justice de Saint-Martin-des-Champs à Paris, au XIVe,* ed. Louis Tanon (Paris, 1877), 193, 196, 218–19, 228.

15. Barbara A. Hanawalt, *Crime and Conflict in English Communities, 1300–1348* (Cambridge, Mass.: Harvard University Press, 1979).

16. *Bedfordshire Coroners' Rolls,* ed. R. F. Hunniset, Publications of the Bedfordshire Historical Record Society 41, no. 197 (Streatley, 1961); see, for example, Michael MacDonald, introduction to John Sym, *Lifes Preservative against Self-Killing* (London: Routledge, 1988), xlvi, note 13.

17. Bayet, *Le suicide et la morale,* 444.

18. Louis-Claude Douet d'Arcq, *Choix de pièces inédites relatives au règne de Charles VI,* 2 vols. (Paris, 1863–64), 2:176.

19. "In lands of customary law, after the juridical renaissance of the twelfth century, there were efforts to revive the ancient Roman legislation. Several texts, in fact, show juridical practice unexpectedly attenuating the rigors of custom. . . . Does this mean that suicide was not punished in the Midi? I think such a statement would be seriously inaccurate. . . . I am persuaded that suicide was at times punished in the Midi. But when? Because the customals, which are above all intent on safeguarding the rights of the middle class, never speak of it, it is very probable that only the common people were convicted" (Bayet, *Le suicide et la morale,* 477).

20. Jean Boutillier, *Somme rural,* title 39, p. 273, quoted in Bayet, *Le suicide et la morale,* 478.

21. Bayet, *Le suicide et la morale,* 466.

Three. The Classical Heritage: Perfecting the Timely Exit

1. Studies of ancient suicide in practice and in theory include those of M. D. Faber, *Suicide in Greek Tragedy* (New York: Sphinx Press, 1970); John M. Rist, "Suicide," in his *Stoic Philosophy* (London: Cambridge University Press, 1969), 235–55; R. Willie, "Views on Suicide and Freedom in Stoic Philosophy and Some Related Contemporary Points of View," *Prudentia* 5 (1973).

2. Yolande Grisé, *Le suicide dans la Rome antique* (Paris: Belles Lettres, 1982; Montreal: Bellarmin, 1983), 34–53. This work provides a complete survey of Roman suicide and a copious bibliography.

3. Louis-Vincent Thomas, *L'anthropologie de la mort* (Paris: Payot, 1975, 1980).

4. Grisé, *Le suicide dans la Rome antique,* 136–41.

5. "Seneca to His Friend Lucilius," *Seneca's Letters to Lucilius,* trans. E. Phillips Barker, 2 vols. (Oxford: Clarendon Press, 1932), no. 24, 1:82.

6. Grisé, *Le suicide dans la Rome antique,* 70.

7. Seneca quoted in ibid., 71–72.

8. *Seneca's Letters to Lucilius,* letter no. 58, 1:189–91.

9. See J. Kany, "Le suicide politique à Rome et en particulier chez Tacite," thèse de troisième cycle, Université de Rheims, 1970.

10. *Seneca's Letters to Lucilius,* letter 24, 1:81.

11. Albert Bayet, *Le suicide et la morale* (Paris: Félix Alcan, 1922); Gaston Garrisson, "Le suicide en droit romain et en droit français," thèse d'État, Université de Toulouse, 1883, published as *Le suicide dans l'antiquité et dans les temps modernes* (Paris: A. Rousseau, 1885), chap. 3.

12. Tacitus, *Annals* VI.29, quoted from *The Complete Works of Tacitus,* ed. Moses Hadas, trans. Alfred John Church and William Jackson Brodribb (New York: Modern Library / Random House, 1942), 211–12.

13. Marcus Aurelius, V.29, quoted from *The Meditations of Marcus Aurelius Antoninus,* ed. R. B. Rutherford, trans. A.S.L. Farquharson (Oxford: Oxford University Press, 1989), 42.

Four. The Early Renaissance: Rediscovery of the Enigma of Suicide

1. Henri Estienne, *Introduction au Traité de la conformité des merveilles anciennes avec les modernes* (1566), 399; Michel de Montaigne, *Journal de voyage en Italie,* ed. Fausta Garavini (Paris: Gallimard, 1983).

2. Félix Bourquelot, "Recherches sur les opinions et la législation en matière de mort volontaire pendant le Moyen Age: Depuis Justinien jusqu'à Charlemagne," *Bibliothèque de l'École des Chartes* 3 (1841–42): 539–60; 4 (1842–43): 242–66.

3. William Edward Hartpole Lecky, *History of European Morals from Augustus to Charlemagne,* 2 vols. (London, 1877; New York: D. Appleton, 1921; reprint, New York: Arno Press, 1975), 2:55.

4. James J. O'Dea, *Suicide: Studies on Its Philosophy, Causes and Prevention* (New York: G. P. Putnam's Sons, 1882), 91.

5. Gaston Garrisson, "Le suicide en droit romain et en droit français," thèse d'État, Université de Toulouse, 1883; published as *Le suicide dans l'antiquité et dans les temps modernes* (Paris: A. Rousseau, 1885).

6. Ruth Shonle Cavan, *Suicide: A Study of Personal Disorganization* (Chicago: University of Chicago Press, 1928).

7. Albert Desjardins, *Les sentiments moraux au XVIe siècle* (Paris, 1887). Émile Durkheim, *Le suicide: Étude de sociologie* (Paris: Félix Alcan, 1897); in English translation as *Suicide: A Study in Sociology,* ed. George Simpson, trans. John A. Spaulding and George Simpson (Glencoe, Ill.: Free Press, 1951). Henry Romilly Fedden, *Suicide: A Social and Historical Study* (London: P. Davies, 1938; reprint, New York: B. Blom, 1972); Samuel Ernest Sprott, *The English Debate on Suicide from Donne to Hume* (Lasalle, Ill.: Open Court, 1961).

8. Robert Mandrou, *Introduction à la France moderne, 1500–1640: Essai de psychologie historique* (Paris: A. Michel, 1961, 1974), 315–16, quoted here from *Introduction to Modern France, 1500–1640: An Essay in Historical Psychology,* trans. R. E. Hallmark (New York: Harper and Row, 1977), 231.

9. Jean Delumeau, *La civilisation de la Renaissance* (Paris: Arthaud, 1967), 345.

10. *Journal d'un bourgeois de Paris sous le règne de François Premier (1515–1536),* ed. Ludovic Lalanne (Paris, 1854), 327, 436.

11. Pierre de L'Estoile, *Journal de Pierre de L'Estoile,* vols. 45–49 of *Collection complète des mémoires relatifs à l'histoire de France, depuis le règne de Philippe-Auguste jusqu'au commencement du XVIIe siècle,* ed. Claude Bernard Petitot, 52 vols. (Paris, 1819–26), entries for 18 July 1576, 45:136, and 18 April 1584, 45:274–75, quoted here from *The Paris of Henry of Navarre as Seen by Pierre de l'Estoile: Selections from His Mémoires-Journaux,* ed. and trans. Nancy Lyman Roelker (Cambridge, Mass.: Harvard University Press, 1958), 100–101. L'Estoile continues the second entry to state, "On the same day the physician Malmédy . . . committed suicide by cutting his throat in despair over the crushing debts he had (thanks to the tax farms he had taken from the king and to the large guarantees and pledges he had made for a number of persons)."

12. This case is mentioned in *Recueil des actes, titres et mémoires concernant les affaires du clergé de France,* 14 vols. (Paris, 1716–52), 7:508.

13. Henri Estienne, *Apologie pour Hérodote (Satire de la société au XVIe siècle par Henri Estienne,* ed. P. Ristelhuber, 2 vols. (Paris, 1879), vol. 2. Estienne believed that ecclesiastical suicides were the result of pride, as in the case of a hermit named Héron who was persuaded by the devil to throw himself into a well because he thought his merits would save him.

14. Michael MacDonald and Terence R. Murphy, *Sleepless Souls: Suicide in Early Modern England* (New York: Oxford University Press, 1990). This study combines a wealth of documentary information with remarkably prudent judgments, making it a valuable reference for all studies on suicide from the sixteenth to the eighteenth century.

15. Ibid., table 1.1, "Suicide Verdicts Returned to King's Bench, 1485–1659," 29. For the following, see ibid., 24–25.

16. S. J. Stevenson, "The Rise of Suicide Verdicts in South-East England: The Legal Process, 1530–1590," *Continuity and Change* 2, no. 1 (1987): 37–76, especially 63–65.

17. MacDonald and Murphy, *Sleepless Souls,* 58.

18. Markus Schär, *Seelennöte der Untertanen: Selbstmord, Melancholie und Religion im alten Zürich, 1500–1800* (Zurich: Chronos-Verlag, 1985); L. Haeberli, "Le suicide à Genève au XVIIIe siècle," in *Pour une histoire quantitative* (Geneva, 1975).

19. Christine Martineau-Genieys, *Le thème de la mort dans la poésie française de 1450 à 1550* (Paris: H. Champion, 1978).

20. Bernard Paulin, *Du couteau à la plume: Le suicide dans la littérature anglaise de la Renaissance (1580–1625)* (Saint-Étienne: Université de Saint-Étienne; Lyon: Hermès, 1977).

21. Pierre de La Primaudaye, *Académie française,* 3d ed. (Paris, 1580), 368, 140, quoted here from *The French Academie: Fully Discoursed and Finished in Foure Bookes* (London, 1618), 119, 120.

22. Paulin, *Du couteau à la plume,* 105; title given here from Samuel Ernest Sprott, *The English Debate on Suicide: From Donne to Hume* (Lasalle, Ill.: Open Court, 1961), 15–16, which credits John Harrington's papers, British Museum, Add. MSS 27, 632.

23. Thomas More, *Utopia,* ed. Edward Surtz and J. H. Hexter, vol. 4 of *The Complete Works of St. Thomas More* (New Haven: Yale University Press, 1965), 187.

24. Ibid.

25. Antonio de Guevara, *Horologium principum,* in French translation as *L'Horloge des princes,* trans. Nicole Herberay (Paris, 1588), 305.

26. François Villon, "Le Grand Testament," XLVII, quoted here from *Complete Poems of François Villon,* trans. Beram Saklatvala, Everyman's Library (New York: Dutton, 1968), 44–45.

27. Villon, "Grand Testament," XLIV; *Complete Poems,* 42–43.

28. *Œuvres du bienheureux Jean d'Avila,* ed. Jacques-Paul Migne (Paris, 1863), 438.

29. See Alberto Tenenti, *La vie et la mort à travers l'art du XVe siècle* (Paris: A. Colin, 1952), 97–120.

30. Hervé Martin, *Le métier de prédicateur à la fin du Moyen Age: 1350–1520* (Paris: Éditions du Cerf, 1988), 259.

31. Francisco de Vitoria, *Sentencios morales* (Barcelona: Ediciones de Fe, 1939), no. 558.

32. *Catechism of the Council of Trent, Issued by Order of Pope Pius V,* trans. with notes by John A. McHugh and Charles J. Callan (South Bend, Ind.: Marian Publications, 1976; Rockford, Ill.: Tan Books, 1982), 423.

33. Martín de Azpilcueta (Navarrus), *Enchiridion, sive Manuale confessariorum et poenitentium* (Antwerp, 1581), chap. 15.

34. Martin Luther, *Mémoires,* ed. and trans. Jules Michelet (1854), Le Temps retrouvé 27 (Paris: Mercure de France, 1990), 272–73, quoted here from *The Life of Luther Written by Himself,* collected and arranged by Jules Michelet, trans. William Hazlitt (London: David Bogue, 1846), 320.

35. Théodore Agrippa d'Aubigné, *Sa vie à ses enfants,* in *Œuvres complètes,* ed. Eugène Réaume and François de Caussade, 6 vols. (Paris, 1873–92), 1:12; available in English as *His Life, To His Children,* trans. John Nothnagle (Lincoln: University of

Nebraska Press, 1989). Aubigné relates that he attempted suicide in 1563, at the age of eleven, when he was living in poverty in Lyons, but was saved by a miracle.

36. Henri Estienne, *L'Introduction au "Traité de la conformité des merveilles anciennes avec les modernes," ou, Traité préparatif pour l'Apologie pour Hérodote,* ed. P. Ristelhuber (Paris, 1879), 1:chap. 18, quoted from *A World of Wonders; or, An Introduction to a Treatise touching the Conformitie of ancient and moderne Wonders: or, A Preparative Treatise to the Apologie for Herodotus* (London, 1607), book 1, chap. 18, "Of Murthers committed at this day," 158.

37. For the situation in England at this time, see Paulin, *Du couteau à la plume,* 32–39, 50–52.

38. Edmond Bicknoll, *A Svvord agaynst Swearyng* (London, 1579).

39. Hugh Latimer, *The Works of Hugh Latimer,* ed. George Elwes Corrie, 2 vols. (Cambridge: Cambridge University Press, 1844–45), 1:435, quoted here from MacDonald and Murphy, *Sleepless Souls,* 34.

40. Andrew Boorde, *The Breviary of Helthe, for all maner of syckenesses and diseases the whiche may be in man, or woman* (London, 1547).

41. John Foxe, *The Acts and Monuments of John Foxe,* ed. Josiah Pratt, 8 vols. (London, 1877), 8:670, quoted here from MacDonald and Murphy, *Sleepless Souls,* 61.

42. *A True and Summarie reporte of the declaration of some part of the Earle of Northumberlands treasons* (1585), quoted here from MacDonald and Murphy, *Sleepless Souls,* 64.

43. Albert Bayet, *Le suicide et la morale* (Paris: F. Alcan, 1922), 447–48.

44. *Encyclopédie mthodique, ou par ordre de matières: par une société de gens de lettres, de savans et d'artistes,* 200 vols. (Paris and Liège, 1782–1832), *Jurisprudence,* vol. 7 (1787), s.v. "suicide."

45. Jean Bacquet, *Œuvres,* ed. Claude de Ferrière (Paris, 1688), 7:17; Anne Robert, *Quatre livres des arrests et choses jugées par la cour, mis en français* (Paris, 1611).

46. Michel Foucault, *Histoire de la folie à l'âge classique* (Paris: Gallimard, 1972), 26, quoted here from *Madness and Civilization: A History of Insanity in the Age of Reason,* trans. Richard Howard (New York: Vintage Books, 1965, 1973), 15–16.

47. Erasmus, *In Praise of Folly,* trans. Hoyt Hopewell Hudson (Princeton: Princeton University Press, 1941), 41. This translation is the source of the quotations in the text.

48. Paulin, *Du couteau à la plume,* 241.

49. Christopher Marlowe, *Doctor Faustus,* scene 5, lines 200–205; in *The Complete Works of Christopher Marlowe,* ed. Roma Gill, 4 vols. (Oxford: Clarendon Press, 1987), 2:21.

50. Marlowe, *Doctor Faustus,* scene 12, lines 37–39; *Complete Works,* ed. Gill, 2:40–41.

51. Pierre de Bourdeille, seigneur de Brantôme, *Œuvres complètes,* 11 vols. (Paris, 1864–82), 4:135–38.

52. Henry Thomas Buckle, *Introduction to the History of Civilization in England,* rev. ed. (London: G. Routledge and Sons; New York: E. P. Dutton, 1904), 707.

53. Denis Crouzet, *Les guerres de Dieu: La violence au temps des troubles de religion (vers 1525–vers 1610)*, 2 vols. (Seyssel: Champ Vallon, 1990).

54. Benvenuto Cellini, *La Vita*, consulted in French as *Mémoires*, ed. Giuliano Maggiora, trans. Léopold Leclanché (Paris: Club français du livre, 1955), 260, quoted here and below from *Autobiography*, trans. George Bull (London: Penguin Books, 1956), 217–18.

Five. To Be or Not to Be: The First Crisis of Conscience in Europe

1. Bernard Paulin, *Du couteau à la plume: Le suicide dans la littérature anglaise de la Renaissance (1580–1625)* (Saint-Étienne: Université de Saint-Étienne; Lyon: Hermès, 1977).

2. Sir Philip Sidney, *The Countess of Pembroke's Arcadia (The Old Arcadia)*, ed. Jean Robertson (Oxford: Clarendon Press, 1973).

3. Michel de Montaigne, *Essais*, 1:chap. 14, quoted here from *The Complete Essays of Montaigne*, trans. Donald M. Frame (Stanford: Stanford University Press, 1943), 36.

4. Montaigne, *Essais*, 1:chap. 14; *Complete Essays*, 251–52.

5. Montaigne, *Essais*, 2:chap. 3; *Complete Essays*, 254–55.

6. Montaigne, *Complete Essays*, 256, 257.

7. Ibid., 255, 262.

8. Pierre Charron, *De la sagesse, livres trois* (Bordeaux, 1601), II.11.18, quoted here from *On Wisdome*, trans. Samson Lenard (London, 1651), 364.

9. Pierre de Dampmartin, *La Fortune de la cour* (1585; Liège, 1713), 345.

10. Justus Lipsius, *Manuductio ad stoicam philosophiam* (Antwerp, 1604).

11. Caspar Scioppius (Kaspar Schoppe), *Elementa philosophiae stoicae moralis* (Mainz, 1606).

12. Francis Bacon, "History Natural and Experimental, or, of the Prolongation of Life" (1638) (*Instauratio*, part 3), in *The Works of Francis Bacon*, 3 vols. (Philadelphia, 1852), 3:467–518, quotation on 511.

13. John Donne, *Biathanatos*, ed. Michael Rudick and M. Pabst Battin, Garland English Texts (New York: Garland, 1982), xcvii, 4. This edition is the source of the quotations in the text.

14. Jean Duvergier de Hauranne, *La question royalle et sa decision* (Paris, 1609), 3, 4.

15. Henri Bremond, *Histoire littéraire du sentiment religieux en France depuis la fin des Guerres de Religion jusqu'à nos jours*, 11 vols. (Paris: Bloud et Gay, 1923), 4:50.

16. Abbé de Saint-Cyran (Jean Duvergier de Hauranne), *Maximes saintes et chres-tiennes tirées des lettres de Messire Jean Du Vergier de Hauranne, abbé de Saint-Cyran*, 2d ed. (Paris, 1653), 76, 77. Somewhat later Saint-Cyran adds, "The fastest way to get out of our afflictions is to take pleasure in remaining in them as long as it may please God to so ordain."

17. Timothy Bright, *A Treatise of Melancholie* (London, 1586); Jean Fernel, *Physiologia* (1607), 121.

18. Johann Weyer, *De praestigiis daemonum* (1563), quoted here from Michel Foucault, *Madness and Civilization: A History of Insanity in the Age of Reason,* trans. Richard Howard (New York: Vintage Books, 1965, 1973), 117–18.

19. Philip Barrough, *The Methode of Phisicke* (London, 1596), 46, quoted here from Michael MacDonald and Terence R. Murphy, *Sleepless Souls: Suicide in Early Modern England* (New York: Oxford University Press, 1990), 102. Pierre de La Primaudaye, *Académie française,* 3d ed. (Paris, 1580); in English translation as *The French Academie: Fully Discoursed and Finished in Foure Bookes* (London, 1618).

20. Felix Plater, *Praxeos medicae opus . . . in tres tomi* (Basel, 1609).

21. For a study of melancholia in England in this period, see Lawrence Babb, *The Elizabethan Malady: A Study of Melancholia in English Literature from 1580 to 1642* (East Lansing: Michigan State College Press, 1951).

22. Robert Burton, *The Anatomy of Melancholy,* ed. Thomas C. Faulkner, Nicholas K. Kiessling, and Rhonda L. Blair, 3 vols. (Oxford: Clarendon Press, 1989–94), 1:6. This edition is the source of the quotations in the text. For systematic studies of this work, see Jean Robert Simon, *Robert Burton et l'Anatomie de la mélancholie* (Paris: Didier, 1964); H. R. Trevor-Roper, "Robert Burton and the *Anatomy of Melancholy,*" in *Renaissance Essays* (London, 1961; Chicago: University of Chicago Press, 1985).

23. *Encyclopédie méthodique,* entry "Mélancholie"; quoted in Foucault, *Histoire de la folie à l'âge classique* (Paris: Gallimard, 1972), 387, a study that remains a prime reference for questions of insanity.

24. Zacatus Lusitanus, *Praxis medica* (1637); Foucault, *Madness and Civilization,* 188.

25. Albert Bayet, *Le suicide et la morale* (Paris: Félix Alcan, 1922), 521.

26. On the authors discussed in the following, see ibid., 521–26.

27. Ollenix du Mont-Sacré (Nicolas de Montreux), *Œuvre de la chasteté* (Paris, 1595), 78.

28. Gilbert Saulnier Du Verdier, *Le temple des sacrifices* (Paris, 1620), 172.

29. On suicide in French tragedy of the time, see Bayet, *Le suicide et la morale,* 527–30.

30. Antoine de Montchrestien, *La Carthaginoise,* act 3.

31. Ibid.

32. Robert Garnier, *Phèdre,* final scene.

33. Robert Garnier, *Marc Antoine,* act 3.

34. Ollenix du Mont-Sacré (Nicolas de Montreux), *Cléopâtre,* act 1.

35. Jean de La Taille, *Saül le furieux,* act 5.

36. Paulin, *Du couteau à la plume,* 533.

37. Ibid., 340.

38. G. Wilson Knight, *The Imperial Theme* (London: Methuen, 1965), chap. 9.

39. Jan Kott, *Shakespeare, notre contemporain* (Verviers: Julliard, 1962), in English translation as *Shakespeare, Our Contemporary,* trans. Boleslaw Taborski (Garden City, N.Y.: Doubleday, 1964), 100–109. This work was also published as *Szkice o sekspirze* (Warsaw: Panstwowe Wydawnictwo Naukowe, 1964).

40. MacDonald and Murphy, *Sleepless Souls,* table 1.1, "Suicide Verdicts Returned to King's Bench, 1485–1659," 29.

41. P.E.H. Hair, "A Note on the Incidence of Tudor Suicide," *Local Population Studies* 5 (1970): 36–43.

42. Samuel Ernest Sprott, *The English Debate on Suicide: From Donne to Hume* (Lasalle, Ill.: Open Court, 1961).

43. Michael Zell, "Suicide in Pre-Industrial England," *Social History* 11 (1986): 303–17, especially 309–10.

44. J. A. Sharpe, *Early Modern England: A Social History, 1550–1760* (London and Baltimore: E. Arnold, 1987).

45. MacDonald and Murphy, *Sleepless Souls,* 241–43.

46. Paul S. Seaver, *Wallington's World: A Puritan Artisan in Seventeenth-Century London* (Stanford: Stanford University Press, 1985), 204, quoted here from MacDonald and Murphy, *Sleepless Souls,* 33.

47. Nehemiah Wallington, "Memorial", quoted from MacDonald and Murphy, *Sleepless Souls,* 50.

48. John Dee, *The Private Diary of Dr. John Dee,* ed. James Orchard Halliwell (London: Camden Society, 1842).

49. MacDonald and Murphy, *Sleepless Souls,* 51, 53.

50. For the persons discussed in this paragraph, see ibid., 263–65, 291–92, 296.

51. George Trosse, *The Life of the Reverend Mr. George Trosse,* ed. A. W. Brink (Montreal: McGill-Queen's University Press, 1974).

52. For a discussion of the relationship between Puritanism and suicide, see, for example, Howard I. Kushner, *Self-Destruction in the Promised Land: A Psychocultural Biology of American Suicide* (New Brunswick: Rutgers University Press, 1989).

53. William Gouge, introduction, "To the Christian Reader," in John Sym, *Lifes Preservative Against Self-Killing* (London, 1637), unpaginated; facsimile reprint, ed. Michael MacDonald (New York: Routledge, 1988).

54. Pierre de L'Estoile, *Journal de Pierre de L'Estoile,* in *Collection complète des mémoires relatifs à l'histoire de France, depuis le règne de Philippe-Auguste jusqu'au commencement du XVIIe siècle,* ed. Claude Bernard Petitot, 52 vols. (Paris, 1819–26), vols. 45–49, 47:309.

55. Nicolas Rémy, *Daemonolatreiae* (Lyons, 1595); available in English translation as *Demonolotry,* ed. Montague Summers, trans. E. A. Ashwin (London: J. Rodker, 1930).

56. Sir Walter Raleigh, *Sir Walter Raleigh: Selections from his Historie of the World, his Letters, etc.,* ed. G. E. Hadow (Oxford: Clarendon Press, 1917).

Six. The Seventeenth Century: Reaction and Repression

1. On the French casuists, see Albert Bayet, *Le suicide et la morale* (Paris: Félix Alcan, 1922), 542–46.

2. Tommaso de Vio, Cardinal Cajetan, *Commentaria super tractatum de ente et essentia sanctissimi doctoris Thome de Aquino* (Venice, 1506), II.2, q. cxxiv.

3. Martin de Azpilcueta, known as Navarrus, *Enchiridion, sive, Manuale confessariorum et poenitentium* (Antwerp, 1581), chap. 15.

4. Louis Lopez, *Instructor conscientiae* (Lyons, 1587), chap. 64.

5. Jean Benedicti, *La Somme des pechez, et le remède d'iceux* (Paris, 1595), II.4.

6. Francisco de Toledo, *De instructione sacerdotum* (1599), published in French translation as *La Somme des cas de conscience, ou L'instruction des prestres* (Lyons, 1649), chap. 6; Sayrus (Robert Sayr, in religion Gregorius), *Compendii clavis regiae pars prima* (Venice, 1621).

7. Leonardus Lessius (Leonardo Lessio), *De justitia et jure caeterisque virtutibus cardinalibus* (Paris, 1606), II.9.6.

8. Comitolus (Paolo Comitoli), *Responsa moralia in VII libros digesta* (Rouen, 1709), book 4, q. 10.

9. Francisco Suárez, *Tractatus de legibus, ac Deo legislatore* (Antwerp, 1613), book 5, chap. 7.

10. Michael Rothardus, *Crux saulitica duabus pertractata quaestionibus* (Frankfurt, 1615).

11. Filliucius (Vincenzo Filliucci), *Moralium quaestionum de christianis officiis in casibus conscientiae, tomi duo* (Lyons, 1626), tract. 29, chap. 4. On Filliucci and the moralists who repeated his cases, see also Bayet, *Le suicide et la morale,* 588–90.

12. Martino Bonacina, *Opera omnia,* 3 vols. (1629), 2:673; Tomas Hurtado, *Resolutiones orthodoxo-morales* (Cologne, 1655); Hermann Busenbaum, *Medulla theologiae moralis* (Paris, 1657).

13. Juan Caramuel (Juan Caramuel Lobkowitz), *Theologia moralis fundamentalis* (Frankfurt, 1652), chap.6, fund. 55, para. 13.

14. Antoninus (Antonino) Diana, *Resolutiones morales,* 12th ed., 5 vols. (Antwerp, 1645–57), pars 3, tract. 5, resol. 7.

15. Valerii Reginaldus (Valère Regnault), *Theologia practica et moralis* (Cologne, 1653), XXI.4.

16. Antonio Escobar y Mendoza, *Liber theologiae moralis* (Lyons, 1644).

17. François Le Poulchre, seigneur de La Motte-Messené, *Le Passe-temps,* quoted from Bernard Paulin, *Du couteau à la plume: Le suicide dans la littérature anglaise de la Renaissance (1580–1625)* (Saint-Étienne: Université de Saint-Étienne; Lyon: Hermès, 1977), 41; Jean-Baptiste Chassignet, *Le mespris de la vie et consolation contre la mort: Choix de sonnets* (1594), ed. Armand Müller (Geneva: Droz, 1953), 13.

18. Nicolas Coëffeteau, *Tableau des passions humaines, de leurs causes et de leurs effects* (Paris, 1620), 434.

19. Armand Jean du Plessis, duc de Richelieu and cardinal, *Instruction du chrestien* (Paris, 1626), 208, quoted here from *A Christian Instruction Composed longe a goe, by that most Eminent Cardinall Armand Iohn de Plessis Cardnall of Richeliev,* trans. Thomas Carre, 3d ed. (Paris, 1662), 250.

20. Father Coissard, *Sommaire de la doctrine chrétienne* (Lyons, 1618), 326.

21. Jacques Du Boscq, *L'honneste femme* (Paris, 1632); *La femme héroïque, ou Les héroïnes, comparées avec les héros en toute sorte de vertus,* 2 vols. (Paris, 1645).

22. Pierre Le Moyne, *La gallerie des femmes fortes* (Paris, 1663), 1:225.

23. René de Cerisiers, *Le philosophe françois* (Rouen, 1651).

24. Urbain Chevreau, *Le tableau de la fortune* (Paris, 1648), 2:280; Jean-Louis Guez de Balzac, *Les entretiens de feu monsieur de Balzac* (Paris, 1657), 332, available in a modern edition, ed. Bernard Beugnot (Paris: Didier, 1972).

25. François Hédelin, abbé d'Aubignac, *Macarise, ou La reine des Isles fortunées, Histoire allégorique contenant la philosophie morale des stoïques, sous le voile de plusieurs aventures agréables, en forme de roman* (Paris, 1664), 15.

26. For this aspect of Camus, see René Godenne, "Les Spectacles d'horreur de J.-P. Camus," *XVIIIᵉ siècle* 92 (1971): 25–36.

27. Henri Bremond, *Histoire littéraire du sentiment religieux en France depuis la fin des Guerres de Religion jusqu'à nos jours,* 11 vols. (Paris: Bloud et Gay, 1923), vol. 1, *L'humanisme dévot, 1580–1660.* The first two volumes of this work are available in English as *A Literary History of Religious Thought in France from the Wars of Religion Down to Our Own Times,* 3 vols. (London: Society for Promoting Christian Knowledge; New York: Macmillan, 1928–36), vol. 1, *Devout Humanism,* trans. K. L. Montgomery.

28. Jean-Pierre Camus, *Les spectacles d'horreur, où se découvrent plusieurs tragiques effets de notre siècle* (Paris, 1630), 312.

29. William Fulke, *A Defense of the Sincere and True Translations of the Holie Scriptures in the English Tong* (London, 1633). I am indebted to Bernard Paulin, *Du couteau à la plume,* 52–65, for the discussion that follows.

30. John Case, *Speculum moralium quaestionum in universam Ethicen Aristotelis* (Oxford, 1585), quoted here from Samuel Ernest Sprott, *The English Debate on Suicide: From Donne to Hume* (Lasalle, Ind.: Open Court, 1961), 8.

31. Timothy Bright, *A Treatise of Melancholie* (London, 1586).

32. Henry Smith, *A Preparative to Marriage,* rev. ed. (London, 1591); Richard Hooker, *Of the Laws of Ecclesiastical Polity* (London, 1593), available in a modern edition (Folger Library) as vol. 1 of *Works,* 5 vols. (Cambridge, Mass.: Belknap Press of Harvard University Press, 1977–90).

33. John King, *Lectures upon Ionas delivered at York in the Yeare of our Lorde 1594* (Oxford, 1597); Anthony Copley, *A Fig for Fortune* (London, 1596).

34. William Whitaker, *A Disputation on Holy Scripture, Against the Papists, especially Bellarmine and Stapleton,* trans. William Fitzgerald (Cambridge: Cambridge University Press, 1849), 95.

35. George Abbot, *An Exposition upon the Prophet Ionah* (London, 1600).

36. William Perkins, *The Whole Treatise of the Cases of Conscience,* ed. Thomas Pickering (London, 1608).

37. Andrew Willet, *An Harmonie upon the First Book of Samuel* (Cambridge, 1607).

38. George Strode, *The Anatomie of Mortalitie* (London, 1618).

39. John Wing, *The Crowne Conjugall or, the Spouse Royall* (Middleburgh, 1620); George Hakewill, *King Davids Vow for Reformation of Himselfe* (London, 1621).

40. John Abernethy, *A Christian and Heavenly Treatise* (London, 1623).

41. Nathaniel Carpenter, *Achitophel, or, The Picture of a Wicked Politician* (London, 1629).

42. Richard Capel, *Tentations, Their Nature, Danger, Cure* (London, 1633).

43. Peter Barker, *A Learned and Familiar Exposition upon the Ten Commandments* (London, 1633); William Gouge, *Of Domesticall Duties, Eight Treatises,* 3d ed. (London, 1634).

44. John Downame, *The Christian Warfare against the Deuill, World and Flesh,* 4th ed. (London, 1633–34).

45. Richard Younge, *The Drunkard's Character, or, A True Drunkard with such Sinnes as Raigne in Him* (London, 1638).

46. Lancelot Andrewes, *The Morall Law Expounded* (London, 1642); Henry Hammond, *A Practicall Catechisme* (London, 1645); William Fenner, *Wilfull Impenitency the Grossest Self-Murder* (London, 1648); Thomas Fuller, *A Comment on the Eleven First Verses of the Fourth Chapter of S. Matthew's Gospel concerning Christ's Temptations* (London, 1652); Edward Phillips, *The New World of English Words, or, A General Dictionary* (London, 1658); Jeremy Taylor, *Ductor dubitantium or the Rule of Conscience* (London, 1660); Thomas Philipot, *Self-Homicide-Murther, or, Some Antidotes and Arguments Gleaned out of the Treasures of our Modern Casuists and Divines against that Horrid and Reigning Sin of Self-Murther* (London, 1674).

47. Sir William Denny, *Pelicanicidium, or, The Christian Adviser against Self-Murder* (London, 1653).

48. Ibid., A5r–v, quoted in Sprott, *The English Debate on Suicide,* 31–32.

49. Thomas Browne, *Religio medici* (1635), ed. James Winny (Cambridge: Cambridge University Press, 1963); Browne, *Hydriotaphia, urne-Buriall, or a Discourse of the sepulchrall urnes lately found in Norfolk* (London, 1658); Browne, "A Letter to a Friend upon Occasion of the Death of his Intimate Friend," in *The Works of Sir Thomas Browne,* ed. Geoffrey Keynes, 6 vols. (London: Faber and Gwyer; New York: W. E. Rudge, 1928–31).

50. Browne, *Religio medici,* part 1, sec. 26, quoted from Browne, *Selected Writings,* ed. Sir Geoffrey Keynes (Chicago: University of Chicago Press, 1968), 33.

51. Browne, *Urne-Buriall,* in Keynes, ed., *Selected Writings,* 146.

52. Thomas Browne, "Dr. Browne to His Son Thomas at Plymouth," February 1667, in Keynes, ed., *Selected Writings,* 409.

53. Richard Greenham, *The Works of the Reverent and Faithfull Servant of Jesus Christ M. Richard Greenham* (London, 1599), quoted here from Michael MacDonald and Terence R. Murphy, *Sleepless Souls: Suicide in Early Modern England* (New York: Oxford University Press, 1990), 34.

54. Richard Gilpin, *Daemonologia sacra, or, A Treatise on Satan's Temptations* (Lon-

don, 1677), part 3, 108–16, quoted here from MacDonald and Murphy, *Sleepless Souls,* 34 n.66.

55. Hannah Allen, *Satan His Methods and Malice Baffled . . . Reciting the Great Advantage the Devil Made of Her Deep Melancholy and the Triumphant Victories, Rich and Sovereign Graces God Gave Her Over All His Stratagems and Devices* (London, 1683), quoted here from MacDonald and Murphy, *Sleepless Souls,* 51.

56. Henry Walker, *Spirituall Experiences of Sundry Beleevers* (London, 1652).

57. John Bunyan, *Grace Abounding for the Chief of Sinners and The Pilgrim's Progress,* ed. Roger Sharrock (London and New York: Oxford University Press, 1966), 232, quoted here from MacDonald and Murphy, *Sleepless Souls,* 37–38.

58. *A Sad and Dreadful Account of the Self-Murther of Robert Long, alias Baker* (London, 1685), quoted here from MacDonald and Murphy, *Sleepless Souls,* 41.

59. Jean-Baptiste Massillon, "Sur le petit nombre des élus," in *Sermons,* 9 vols. (Paris, 1747–51), 2:279. On the topic of the elect, see Georges Minois, *Histoire des enfers* (Paris: Fayard, 1991), 284–88.

60. Nicolas Malebranche, *Recherche de la vérité* (1674).

61. John Sym, *Lifes Preservative against Self-Killing, or, An Useful Treatise Concerning Life and Self-Murder* (London, 1637), quoted here from the facsimile edition (without the subtitle), ed. Michael MacDonald (New York: Routledge, 1988), 236.

62. Ibid., 323, 293.

63. For a discussion of many of the French figures in the following paragraphs, see Bayet, *Le suicide et la morale,* 600–603.

64. Jean Duret, *Traicté des peines et amandes* (Lyons, 1573); Barthélemy de Chasseneux, *Commentarii in consuetudinus ducatus Burgondiae* (Lyons, 1517).

65. Jean de Coras, *Arrest mémorable du parlement de Tholose contenant une histoire prodigieuse* (Paris, 1572).

66. Pierre Ayrault, *Des procez, faicts au cadaver aux cendres, a la memoire, aux bestes brutes, choses inanimées, et aux contumax* (Angers, 1591), 3–4.

67. Charondas (Louis Le Caron), *Somme rural, ou le Grand Coustumier général de pratique civil et canon, avec annotations* (Paris, 1603).

68. Gomezio de Amescua, *Tractatus de potestate in se ipsum* (Palermo, 1604); Erasmus Ungepauer, *Disputatio de autocheira singularis, homicidium suiipsius jurecivili licitum esse demonstrans* (Iena, 1609).

69. Anne Robert, *Quatre livres des arrests et choses jugées par la Cour, mis en français* (Paris, 1611), book 1, chap. 12.

70. Joost Damhouder, *Praxis criminalium rerum* (Venice, 1555).

71. Claude Lebrun de La Rochette, *Le procès civil et criminel* (Rouen, 1629).

72. Antoine Despeisses, *Œuvres,* 3 vols. (Lyons, 1660), vol. 2, part 3; 1:705–7.

73. René Choppin, *Œuvres,* 5 vols. (Paris, 1661–63), 1:177.

74. François Des Maisons, *Nouveau recueil d'arrests et règlements du Parlement de Paris* (Paris, 1667).

75. Cardin Le Bret, sieur de Flacourt, *Œuvres* (Paris, 1689), 349.

76. Paul Challine, seigneur de Saint-Luperce, *Maximes générales du droit français* (Paris, 1665), 31. For a discussion of Challine and some of the figures who follow, see Bayet, *Le suicide et la morale,* 602–3.

77. Laurent Bouchel, *La bibliothèque, ou Trésor du droit français,* 2 vols. (Paris, 1615).

78. Guy Coquille, *Les Œuvres de Maistre Guy Coquille,* 2 vols. (Paris, 1665), 2:35, 171.

79. Scipion Dupérier, *Œuvres de Scipion Du Périer,* new ed., ed. M. de La Touloubre, 3 vols. (Avignon, 1759), vol. 3, *Dissertationes,* no. 5, p. 4.

80. Thomas Willis, *Opera omnia* (Lyons, 1682), 2:255, quoted here from Michel Foucault, *Madness and Civilization: A History of Insanity in the Age of Reason,* trans. Richard Howard (New York: Pantheon/Random House, 1965), 131.

81. Willis, *Opera omnia,* quoted here from Foucault, *Madness and Civilization,* 121, 122.

82. Michel Foucault, *Histoire de la folie à l'âge classique* (Paris: Gallimard, 1972), 108–9.

83. See ibid., 329; Foucault, *Madness and Civilization,* 162–63.

84. Jean Deprun, *La philosophie de l'inquiétude en France au XVIIIᵉ siècle* (Paris: J. Vrin, 1979).

85. Des Maisons, *Nouveau recueil d'arrêts,* 123ff.

86. Le Bret, *Œuvres,* 349, quoted in Bayet, *Le suicide et la morale,* 602.

87. Jean Imbert and Georges Levasseur, *Le pouvoir, les juges et les bourreaux: Vingt-cinq siècles de répression* (Paris: Hachette, 1972), 202.

88. Hyacinthe de Boniface, *Arrests notables de la cour du Parlement de Provence,* 2 vols. (Paris, 1670), vol. 2, part 3; see also Bayet, *Le suicide et la morale,* 604–5.

89. For the articles of the Ordonnance criminelle of 1670, see Bayet, *Le suicide et la morale,* 605.

90. Ibid., 607.

91. Ibid.

92. Madame de Sévigné (Marie de Rabutin-Chantal, marquise de Sévigné), *Correspondance,* ed. Roger Duchêne, Bibliothèque de la Pléiade, 3 vols. (Paris: Gallimard, 1972–78), 1:236 (26 April 1671), quoted here from *The Letters of Madame de Sévigné,* introduction by A. Edward Newton, 7 vols. (Philadelphia: J. P. Horn, 1927), 1:166–67.

93. Simon d'Olive du Mesnil, *Questions notables du droit, décidées par divers arrêts de la Cour de Parlement de Toulouse* (Toulouse, 1682), book 4, chap. 40.

94. *Recueil des actes, titres et mémoires concernant les affaires du clergé de France,* 14 vols. (Paris, 1716–52), vol. 7 (1719), 508.

95. MacDonald and Murphy, *Sleepless Souls,* table 4.4, "Social Status of Suicides, 1485–1714," 127–28.

96. Ibid., 126–27.

97. Mary Freer Keeler, *The Long Parliament, 1640–1641: A Biographical Study of Its Members* (Philadelphia: American Philosophical Society, 1954), 224.

98. Samuel Pepys, *The Diary of Samuel Pepys,* ed. Robert Latham, William Matthews et al., 11 vols (Berkeley: University of California Press, 1970–83), 21 January 1668, 9:32–33.

99. G. Colman and B. Thornton, *Connoisseur* (London, 1755), no. 50: 298, quoted here from MacDonald and Murphy, *Sleepless Souls,* 126.

Seven. Substitutes for Suicide in the Seventeenth Century

1. *A Petition unto his Excellencie, Sir Thomas Fairfax, Occasioned by the Publishing of the Late Remonstrance* (London, 1647); Sir William Denny, *Pelicanicidium, or, The Christian Adviser against Self-Murder* (London, 1653).

2. Jacques and Michel Dupâquier, *Histoire de la démographie: La statistique de la population des origines à 1914* (Paris: Perrin, 1985), 67–71.

3. John Graunt, *Natural and Political Observations Mentioned in a Following Index, and Made upon the Bills of Mortality* (London, 1662), in *The Economic Writings of Sir William Petty,* ed. Charles Henry Hull, 2 vols. (New York: A. M. Kelley, 1963), 2:355, 360.

4. Isaac Watts, *A Defense Against the Temptation of Self-Murder, wherein the Criminal Nature and Guilt of it are Display'd* (London, 1726), iv.

5. Michael MacDonald and Terence R. Murphy, *Sleepless Souls: Suicide in Early Modern England* (New York: Oxford University Press, 1990), table 1.1, "Suicide Verdicts Returned to King's Bench, 1485–1659," 29.

6. Ibid., 80 and 80 n.8.

7. Essex Record Office, D/P 30/28/9; MacDonald and Murphy, *Sleepless Souls,* 83.

8. John March, *Amicus reipublicae: The Common-Wealths Friend* (London, 1651), 109, quoted here from MacDonald and Murphy, *Sleepless Souls,* 84.

9. For Bourne and Sindercome, see MacDonald and Murphy, *Sleepless Souls,* 284.

10. Claude Mignot in *Encyclopaedia Universalis,* s.v. "Borromini."

11. W. G. Hoskins, "Harvest Fluctuations in English Economic History, 1620–1759," *Agricultural History Review* 16 (1968): 15–31.

12. Michel Devèze, *L'Espagne de Philippe IV (1621–1665): Siècle d'or et de misère,* 2 vols. (Paris: SEDES, 1970), 2:318.

13. Daniel Defoe, *A Journal of the Plague Year: Being Observations or Memorials of the most Remarkable Occurrences, as well Publick as Private, which happened in London during the last Great Visitation in 1665* (Oxford: Basil Blackwell, 1928), 212–13. This edition is the source of the quotations in the text.

14. Sir James George Frazer, *The Golden Bough,* 3d ed., 12 vols. (New York: Macmillan, 1935), vol. 4, part 3, *The Dying God,* 42–45.

15. François Billacois, *Le duel dans la société française des XVIᵉ–XVIIᵉ siècles: Essai de psycholosociologie historique* (Paris: École des Hautes Études en Sciences Sociales, 1986), 389, quoted here from Billacois, *The Duel: Its Rise and Fall in Early Modern France,* ed. Trista Selous (New Haven: Yale University Press, 1990), 232.

16. Albert Bayet, *Le suicide et la morale* (Paris: Félix Alcan, 1922), 559–65.

17. Alexandre Hardy, *Scédase, ou L'hospitalité violée*, final scene.

18. Jean de Mairet, *La Silvanire, ou La morte-vive*, act 2, scene 4.

19. Théophile de Viau, *Pyrame et Thisbé*, act 5, scene 1.

20. Mairet, *La Silvanire*, act 5, scene 1.

21. Jacques Benserade, *Corésus et Callirhoé*, act 4, scene 4.

22. Jacques Pradon, *Statira*, act 5.

23. Mademoiselle de Scudéry, *Ibrahim, ou, L'illustre Bassa*, 4 vols. (Rouen, 1665), 4:423.

24. Pierre d'Ortique de Vaumorière, *L'inceste innocent* (1638), 285.

25. Bayet, *Le suicide et la morale*, 565–72. Bayet cites cases of suicide taken from the works of Beaulieu, Boisrobert, Daudiguier, Des Fontaines, Desmarets, Du Bail, Du Pelletier, Du Perier, Durand, Du Verdier, Gerzan, Gombaud, Gomberville, La Calprenède, Madame de La Fayette, Lannel, La Serre, La Tour-Hotman, Mailly, Mareschal, Merille, Mézerai, Molière d'Essertines, Montagathe, Préchac, Rémy, Rosset, Saint-Real, Mademoiselle de Scudéry, Segrais, Sorel, Tristan, Turpin, d'Urfé, and Vaumorière.

26. Thomas Hobbes, *Leviathan*, chap. 14, "Of the First and Second Natural Laws, and of Contracts," in *The English Works of Thomas Hobbes of Malmesbury*, 11 vols. (London, 1839; 2d reprint, Aalen: Scientia Verlag, 1966), 3:116–17.

27. René Descartes, letter to Christian Huygens, October 1639, in Descartes, *Œuvres et lettres*, ed. André Bridoux, Bibliothèque de la Pléiade (Paris: Gallimard, 1952), 1058.

28. It should be noted that Descartes approved wholeheartedly of risking one's life to save a friend, for one's country, or for the sovereign.

29. Descartes, *Œuvres et lettres*, 1222.

30. Pierre Gassendi, *Syntagma philosophica*, in Gassendi, *Opera omnia*, 6 vols. (Lyons, 1658–75), 2:672.

31. François La Mothe Le Vayer, *La promenade: Dialogue entre Tubertus Ocella, et Marcus Bibulus* (Paris, 1662), 4.1.

32. Sir Thomas Browne, *Religio medici*, part 1, sec. 44, quoted here from *Selected Writings*, ed. Geoffrey Keynes (Chicago: University of Chicago Press, 1968), 50.

33. Walter Charleton, ed., *Epicurus's Morals: Collected and Faithfully Englished* (London, 1656), quoted here from MacDonald and Murphy, *Sleepless Souls*, 88–89.

34. George Mackenzie, *Religio Stoici* (Edinburgh, 1665), 84–85; MacDonald and Murphy, *Sleepless Souls*, 93.

35. *Questions traitées ès conférences du Bureau d'Adresses*, 2:639, *conférence* of 19 November 1635.

36. Pasquier Quesnel, *Le bonheur de la mort chrétienne* (Paris, 1687).

37. Pierre de Bérulle, *Œuvres complètes*, ed. Jacques-Paul Migne (Paris, 1856), 914, 1182.

38. Ibid., 1296, 960.

39. Henri Bremond, *Histoire littéraire du sentiment religieux en France depuis la fin des Guerres de Religion jusqu'à nos jours,* 11 vols. (Paris: Bloud et Gay, 1923), vol. 3, part 2, p. 85.

40. Ibid., p. 136.

41. Alexandre Piny, *L'état de pur amour, ou Conduite pour bientôt arriver à la perfection* (Paris, 1676).

42. Marie de l'Incarnation, *Lettres,* 2:145, quoted in Bremond, *Histoire littéraire,* 6:114.

43. On François de Sales, Jeanne de Chantal, and Madeleine de Saint-Joseph, see Bremond, *Histoire littéraire,* 1:67–72, 58–100, 176, 260; 2:238–52, 301.

44. Anne de Jésus, *Mémoire,* 1:778, quoted in Bremond, *Histoire littéraire,* 2:306; quoted here from Bremond, *A Literary History of Religious Thought in France from the Wars of Religion Down to Our Own Times,* 2 vols. (New York: Macmillan, 1928–30), vol. 2, *The Coming of Mysticism (1590–1620),* trans. K. L. Montgomery, 226. The Carmelites had an extremely simple way of uncovering heresy: As Anne de Jésus declared, "Nearly all the inhabitants were heretics; that could be seen by their faces— truly they looked like lost souls."

45. Jean Deprun, *La philosophie de l'inquiétude en France au XVIII* siècle (Paris, J. Vrin, 1979).

46. Pierre Nicole, *Traité de l'oraison* (Paris, 1679).

47. François Garasse, *Apologie du pere Francois Garassus, de la compagnie de Iesus, pour son Liure contre les Atheistes & Libertins de nostre siècle* (Paris, 1624), 45.

48. Pierre de Besse, *Le Démocrite chrétien, c'est à dire Le mespris et mocquerie des vanites du monde* (Paris, 1615), 2.

49. Étienne Binet, *Des attraits tout-puissants de l'amour de Jésus-Christ et du Paradis de ce monde* (Paris, 1631), 677, quoted here from Bremond, *A Literary History,* 1:112. Father Surin wrote in his spiritual canticles: "Ce m'est tout un que je vive ou que je meure, / Il me suffit que l'amour me demeure" (It is the same to me whether I live or die; it is enough for me that love remain with me).

50. Étienne Binet, *Consolation et resjouissance pour les malades et personnes affligées* (Paris, 1620), quoted here from Bremond, *A Literary History,* 2:246.

51. Étienne Binet, *Essay des merveilles de nature et des plus nobles artifices* (Rouen, 1621), quoted here from Bremond, *A Literary History,* 1:211.

52. On pious humanism and science, see Georges Minois, *L'Église et la science: Histoire d'un malentendu de Saint Augustin à Galilée,* 2 vols. (Paris: Fayard, 1990–91), 2:48–52.

53. Louis Richeome, *L'adieu de l'âme dévote laissant le corps* (Lyon, 1590), 50.

54. François de Sales, *An Introduction to a Devout Life,* trans. Allan Ross (London: Burns Oates and Washbourne, 1937), 259.

55. François de Sales, *Treatise on the Love of God,* ed. and trans. John K. Ryan, 2 vols. (Rockford, Ill.: Tan Books, 1975), 2:259; François de Sales, *An Introduction to a Devout Life,* 261.

56. François de Sales, *Treatise on the Love of God*, 2:226–27.

57. François de Sales, *Introduction to the Devout Life*, 261.

58. François de Sales, *Treatise on the Love of God*, 226–27.

59. Ibid., 41.

60. Nicolas Malebranche, *Traité de morale* (Rotterdam, 1684), quoted here from *Treatise on Ethics (1684)*, trans. Craig Walton, International Archives of the History of Ideas 133 (Dordrecht: Kluwer Academic Publishers, 1993), 222.

61. Antoine Arnauld, *De la nécessité de la foi en Jésus-Christ pour être sauvé*, in *Œuvres de Messire Antoine Arnauld*, 43 vols. (Brussels: Culture et Civilisation, 1964–67), 10:360, 139.

62. Pierre Nicole, *Essais de morale*, 2 vols. (Amsterdam, 1672), 1:chap. 13, quoted here from *Moral Essays, Contain'd in several Treatises on Many Important Duties* (London, 1677), 1:53–55.

63. Blaise Pascal, *Pensées*, in *Œuvres complètes*, ed. Jacques Chevalier, Bibliothèque de la Pléiade (Paris: Gallimard, 1954), 1104, quoted here from *Pascal's Pensées*, trans. H. F. Steward (New York: Pantheon Books, 1950), 365.

64. Lucien Goldmann, *Le Dieu caché: Étude sur la vision tragique dans les Pensées de Pascal et dans le théâtre de Racine* (Paris, Gallimard, 1959, 1971); in English translation as *The Hidden God: A Study of Tragic Vision in the Pensées of Pascal and the Tragedies of Racine*, trans. Philip Thody (New York: Humanities Press, 1964).

65. Goldmann, *Le Dieu caché*, 241, quoted here from *The Hidden God*, 215.

66. Goldmann, *Le Dieu caché*, 421; *The Hidden God*, 376, 377.

67. Some have remarked that Jansenism did not necessarily contribute to despair, at least concerning the fate of humankind in the next world, because although it asserted that the elect were very few, it required everyone to believe that they themselves were of that number: "All men in the world are obliged to believe," Pascal writes, "that they are of the small number of the elect whom God wants to save" (*Écrits sur la grâce*, in *Œuvres complètes*, 967). In 1732 Father Gilles Vauge stated that the fear of offending God is a sign of predestination, thus a good reason to hope: "That fear, which can be found even among the just and in the most perfect saints, is one of the means by which God is accustomed to carry out the decree of his predestination; and far from weakening the confidence that each of us is obliged to have to be of the number of the elect, it must, to the contrary, augment it, since it is one of the great means of our salvation and is the state in which God wants us to be in order to attain it" (*Traité de l'espérance chrétienne* [Paris, 1732], 218).

Eight. The Birth of the English Malady, 1680–1720

1. Voltaire, "De Caton, du suicide," in *Dictionnaire philosophique*, quoted here from "Cato: On Suicide, and the Abbé St. Cyran's Book Legitimating Suicide," in *A Philosophical Dictionary*, in *The Works of Voltaire*, trans. William F. Fleming, 42 vols. (Paris, London, New York, and Chicago: E. R. Dumont, 1901), 7:23. For the hostile

observer, see Michael MacDonald and Terence R. Murphy, *Sleepless Souls: Suicide in Early Modern England* (New York: Oxford University Press, 1990), 152.

2. *The Early Essays and Romances of Sir William Temple,* ed. G.C.M. Smith (Oxford: Clarendon Press, 1930), 193, quoted here from MacDonald and Murphy, *Sleepless Souls,* 277. For the other cases cited in this paragraph, see MacDonald and Murphy, *Sleepless Souls,* 70–75, 67–68, 125, 41, 70.

3. John Smith, *The Judgment of God upon Atheism and Infidelity* (London, 1704). For Smith and the suicides described in this paragraph, see MacDonald and Murphy, *Sleepless Souls,* 250, 277, 269, 310, 69.

4. John Evelyn, *The Diary of John Evelyn,* ed. E. S. de Beer (Oxford: Clarendon Press, 1955), 505–6, quoted here from MacDonald and Murphy, *Sleepless Souls,* 310.

5. George Cheyne, *The English Malady, or, A Treatise of Nervous Diseases of All Kinds,* 3d ed. (London, 1734), iii, quoted here from MacDonald and Murphy, *Sleepless Souls,* 307.

6. John Sena, "The English Malady: The Idea of Melancholy from 1700 to 1760," Ph.D. diss., Princeton University, 1967, 44. See also MacDonald and Murphy, *Sleepless Souls,* 312.

7. Edward Phillips, *The New World of English Words, or, A General Dictionary* (London, 1658), preface, C2r–v.

8. *Le Pour et le Contre, ouvrage périodique d'un goût nouveau,* 20 vols. (Paris, 1733–40), vol. 4 (1734). For a modern edition, see *Le Pour et le Contre: Nos. 1–60,* ed. Steve Larkin, 2 vols. (Oxford: Voltaire Foundation at the Taylor Institution, 1993).

9. *Le Pour et le Contre* (Paris, 1733–40), 4:56.

10. Ibid., 4:64. Prévost states, "He [Cheyne] says it is because they only burn peat [charbon de terre], or because the beef that makes up their usual nourishment is never more than half roasted, or because, having given themselves overly much to pleasures of the senses, God permits the enemy of salvation to deceive their reason. The proofs of these alternatives make up the matter of a thick book, which has merited him a number of pleasantries on the part of London scoffers."

11. David Daube, "The Linguistics of Suicide," *Philosophy and Public Affairs* 1, no. 4 (1972): 387–437.

12. See MacDonald and Murphy, *Sleepless Souls,* fig. 7.2, "Suicides in the London Bills of Mortality, 1660–1799," 246.

13. William Congreve, *The Complete Works,* ed. Montague Summers, 4 vols. (Soho: Nonesuch Press, 1923), 3:206; Evelyn, *The Diary of John Evelyn,* 593; both quoted here from MacDonald and Murphy, *Sleepless Souls,* 239.

14. James Runcieman Sutherland, *The Restoration Newspaper and Its Development* (Cambridge: Cambridge University Press, 1986); Jeremy Black, *The English Press in the Eighteenth Century* (Philadelphia: University of Pennsylvania Press, 1987).

15. Roland Bartel, "Suicide in Eighteenth Century England: The Myth of a Reputation," *Huntington Library Quarterly* 23 (1960): 145–58.

16. *Lettres de la princesse Palatine (1672–1722)* (Paris: Mercure de France, 1981), 129–30, 176.

17. Ibid., 175, quoted here from *The Letters of Madame: Elizabeth-Charlotte of Bavaria,* trans. Gertrude Scott Stevenson (New York: Appleton, 1924), 184.

18. *Correspondance complète de Madame la duchesse d'Orléans, née princesse Palatine,* ed. Brunet, 2 vols. (Paris, 1886), 2:269, letter of 21 September 1720.

19. Bernard Lamy, *Démonstration ou preuves évidentes de la vérité de la religion et la sainteté de la morale chrétienne* (Paris, 1705), 150.

20. For the statistics and the incidents that follow, see MacDonald and Murphy, *Sleepless Souls,* 218, 268.

21. *Weekly Journal,* 14 January 1721.

22. Marcel Lachiver, *Les années de misère: La famine au temps du Grand Roi, 1680– 1720* (Paris: Fayard, 1991).

23. *Weekly Journal,* 18 May 1717; see MacDonald and Murphy, *Sleepless Souls,* 272.

24. *Strange and Bloody News of a Most Horrible Murder* (London, 1684); MacDonald and Murphy, *Sleepless Souls,* 295 (for the previous incidents, see 264, 289, 266).

25. William Ramesey, *The Gentleman's Companion, or, A Character of True Nobility and Gentility* (London, 1672), 240–41, quoted here from MacDonald and Murphy, *Sleepless Souls,* 145.

26. Charles Moore, *A Full Inquiry into the Subject of Suicide,* 2 vols. in 1 (London, 1790), 1:359, quoted here from MacDonald and Murphy, *Sleepless Souls,* 185.

27. See MacDonald and Murphy, *Sleepless Souls,* 185.

28. *Gentleman's Magazine* 7 (1737): 315, quoted here from MacDonald and Murphy, *Sleepless Souls,* 181.

29. William Withers, *Some Thoughts Concerning Suicide, or Self-Killing: With General Directions for the more Easie Dispatch of that Affair* (London, 1711), 3, quoted here from MacDonald and Murphy, *Sleepless Souls,* 187.

30. Moore, *Full Inquiry into Suicide,* 2:68, quoted here from MacDonald and Murphy, *Sleepless Souls,* 200.

31. Benjamin Dennis and Thomas Plant, *The Mischief of Persecution Exemplified* (London, 1688).

32. For Charles Gildon, see MacDonald and Murphy, *Sleepless Souls,* 150–51.

33. Thomas Philipot, *Self-Homicide-Murther, or, Some Antidotes and Arguments Gleaned out of the Treasures of our Modern Casuists and Divines against that Horrid and Reigning Sin of Self-Murther* (London, 1674); Charles Leslie, *A Short and Easie Method with the Deists* (London, 1699); MacDonald and Murphy, *Sleepless Souls,* 152.

34. John Adams, *An Essay concerning Self-Murther* (London, 1700); on this, see MacDonald and Murphy, *Sleepless Souls,* 164–68.

35. Richard Cumberland, *De legibus naturae* (London, 1672).

36. *Self-Murder and Duelling the Effects of Cowardice and Atheism* (London, 1728), 5–6.

37. Samuel Clarke, *A Discourse Concerning the Unchangeable Obligations of Natural Religion* (London, 1706), 101–2, quoted here from MacDonald and Murphy, *Sleepless Souls,* 153.

38. George Berkeley, *Alciphron, or, The Minute Philosopher,* in *The Works of George Berkeley, Bishop of Cloyne,* ed. A. A. Luce and T. E. Jessop, 9 vols. (London: T. Nelson, 1948–57), 3:92; John Prince, *Self-Murder Asserted to be a Very Heinous Crime* (London, 1709).

39. Thomas Hearne, *Remarks and Collections of Thomas Hearne,* 11 vols. (Oxford: Clarendon Press, 1885–1921), vol. 1, ed. C. E. Doble (1885), 73.

40. Charles Gildon, *The Deist's Manual, or, A Rational Enquiry into the Christian Religion* (London, 1705), sigs. A7v–B2v, quoted here from MacDonald and Murphy, *Sleepless Souls,* 153.

41. On Gilpin and the other figures discussed in this paragraph, see MacDonald and Murphy, *Sleepless Souls,* 34, 207, 201, 53, 203–4.

42. Prince, *Self-Murder Asserted to be a Very Heinous Crime,* 18, quoted here from MacDonald and Murphy, *Sleepless Souls,* 207.

43. Thomas Aldridge, *The Prevalency of Prayer* (London, 1717), 34–36; MacDonald and Murphy, *Sleepless Souls,* 208.

44. Isaac Watts, *A Defense Against the Temptation of Self-Murder, wherein the Criminal Nature and Guilt of it are Display'd* (London, 1726).

45. Charles Wheatly, *A Rational Illustration of the Book of Common Prayer* (London: 1715).

46. MacDonald and Murphy, *Sleepless Souls,* 122, 124.

47. Ibid., 113–14.

48. Daniel Defoe, in *Defoe's Review,* ed. Arthur Wellesley Secord (New York: Columbia University Press, 1938), no. 60 (30 September 1704), 255.

49. MacDonald and Murphy, *Sleepless Souls,* 250.

50. Antoine Bruneau, *Observations et maximes sur les matières criminelles* (Paris, 1715), 223.

51. Philippe Bornier, *Conférences et ordonnances de Louis XIV avec les anciennes ordonnances du royaume,* 2 vols. (Paris, 1719), 2:340.

52. Michel Foucault, *Histoire de la folie à l'âge classique* (Paris: Gallimard, 1972), 402.

53. Thomas Willis, *Opera omnia,* 2 vols. (Lyons, 1681), 2:238, quoted here from Michel Foucault, *Madness and Civilization: A History of Insanity in the Age of Reason,* trans. Richard Howard (New York: Pantheon/Random House, 1965), 121, 122.

54. Charles de Marguetel de Saint-Denis, seigneur de Saint-Évremond, *Œuvres,* 2:135, quoted in Albert Bayet, *Le Suicide et la morale* (Paris: Félix Alcan, 1922), 575.

55. Dirk Van der Cruysse, *La mort dans les "Mémoires" de Saint-Simon: Clio au jardin de Thanatos* (Paris: A.-G. Nizet, 1981).

56. Louis de Rouvroy, duc de Saint-Simon, *Mémoires,* ed. Yves Coirault, Bibliothèque de la Pléiade, 8 vols. (Paris: Gallimard, 1983–88), 1:602 (Belcastel), 2:703 (Péchot). This edition is the source of the quotations in the text.

57. Edmond Jean François Barbier, *Chronique de la régence et du règne de Louis XV, 1718–1763, ou Journal de Barbier,* 5 vols. (Paris, 1857–85), 1:128–29.

58. *Mémoires du marquis de Sourches sur le règne de Louis XIV,* ed. Gabriel-Jules Cosnac and Arthur Bertrand, 13 vols. (Paris, 1882–93), 1:215.

59. Gédéon Tallemant des Réaux, *Œuvres: Les Historiettes de Tallemant des Réaux,* 3d rev. ed., ed. Louis Jean Nicolas Monmerqué and Paulin Paris, 6 vols. (Paris, 1862), 5:336, 3:305, 5:336, 6:164, 2:113.

60. Mathieu Marais, *Journal et mémoires de Mathieu Marais, avocat au parlement de Paris sur la régence et le règne de Louis XV (1715–1737),* ed. Mathurin de Lescure, 4 vols. (Paris, 1863–68), 2:164.

61. Jean Baptiste Morvan, abbé de Bellegarde, *Lettres curieuses de littérature et de morale* (Paris, 1702), 377; César Vichard, abbé de Saint-Réal, *Réflexions sur la mort,* in *Œuvres,* 2:213–14. See also Bayet, *Le suicide et la morale,* 581.

62. Tallemant des Réaux, *Œuvres,* 5:377, 3:305.

63. Marais, *Journal et Mémoires,* 2:430–31.

64. This case is mentioned in François Lebrun, *Les hommes et la mort en Anjou aux XVIIe et XVIIIe siècles* (Paris: Mouton, 1971; Flammarion, 1975), 302.

65. *Quelques procès criminels des XVIIe et XVIIIe siècles,* edited under the direction of Jean Imbert (Paris: Presses Universitaires de France, 1964), 129–38.

66. Louis Racine, *Mémoires sur la vie de Jean Racine,* in *Œuvres de Jean Racine,* ed. Paul Mesnard, 9 vols. (Paris: Hachette, 1865–73), 1:261.

67. Ibid., 6:473.

68. Guy Patin, *Lettres choisies du feu Monsieur Guy Patin* (Paris, 1685).

69. Princess Palatine, *Correspondance complète,* letter of 15 January 1699; see also *The Letters of Madame,* 173–74.

70. Madame de Sévigné, *Correspondance,* ed. Roger Duchêne, Bibliothèque de la Pléiade, 3 vols. (Paris: Gallimard, 1972–78), 3:767, quoted here from *The Letters of Madame de Sévigné,* introduction by A. Edward Newton, 7 vols. (Philadelphia: J. P. Horn, 1927), 7:92–93.

71. Sévigné, *Correspondance,* 3:1135.

72. See *Seneca's Letters to Lucilius,* trans. E. Phillips Barker, 2 vols. (Oxford: Clarendon Press, 1932), letter 58, 2:189: "The man who awaits his doom inertly is all but afraid, just as the man who swigs off the bottle and drains even the lees is over-given to his liquor."

73. Tallemant des Réaux, *Œuvres,* 1:370.

74. Marais, *Journal et Mémoires,* 275, 289.

75. Saint-Simon, *Mémoires,* 3:970, 6:507.

76. On the suicides of prisoners discussed in this paragraph, see Bayet, *Le suicide et la morale,* 608.

77. Pontchartrain quoted from Georges Minois, *Le confesseur du roi: Les directeurs de conscience sous la monarchie française* (Paris: Fayard, 1988), 436.

78. *Correspondance administrative sous le règne de Louis XIV,* ed. Georg Bernhard Depping, 4 vols. (Paris, 1850–55), 2:616.

79. *Correspondance des contrôleurs généraux des Finances avec les intendants des provinces,* 3 vols. (Paris, 1874–97), 1:1517.

80. *Correspondance administrative,* 2:720.

81. *Correspondance des contrôleurs généraux des Finances,* 2:551.

82. François-André Isambert, *Recueil général des anciennes lois françaises depuis l'an 420 jusqu'à la révolution de 1789,* 29 vols. (Paris and Berlin: Leprieur, 1822), 20:575.

83. Lebrun, *Les hommes et la mort en Anjou,* 305.

84. Jean Pontas, *Dictionnaire des cas de conscience,* ed. Jacques-Paul Migne, 2 vols. (Paris, 1847).

85. Jean Deprun, *La philosophie de l'inquiétude en France au XVIIIᵉ siècle* (Paris: J. Vrin, 1979).

86. Claude-François Milley, quoted in Jean Bremond, *Le courant mystique au XVIIIᵉ siècle: L'abandon dans les lettres du père Milley* (Paris: Lethielleux, 1943).

87. Jean Meslier, "Mémoire des pensées et des sentiments de Jean Meslier," in vols. 2 and 3 of *Œuvres complètes,* ed. Roland Desné, Jean Deprun, and Albert Soboul, 3 vols. (Paris: Anthropos, 1970–72), 3:176–77.

88. Pierre Maine de Biran, *Journal intime de Maine de Biran,* ed. Amable de La Valette-Monbrun, 2 vols. (Paris: Plon, 1927–31), 122.

89. Paul Hazard, *La crise de la conscience européenne* (Paris: Fayard, 1961), 400, quoted here from *The European Mind, the Critical Years, 1680–1715,* trans. J. Lewis May (Cleveland: World, 1963), 425–26.

90. Jacques-Bénigne Bossuet, *Troisième Écrit sur les maximes des saints* in *Œuvres complètes de Bossuet,* 12 vols. (Besançon, 1836), 10:286.

91. Jacques-Bénigne Bossuet, *Pensées chrétiennes et morales sur divers sujets* (London: L. B. Hill, 1920), XXIX.

92. Louis Tronson, *Examens particuliers sur divers sujets propres aux ecclésiastiques et à toutes personnes qui veulent s'avancer dans la perfection* (1690) (Paris, 1823). Similar advice can be found in the anonymous *De l'éducation des ecclésiastiques dans les séminaires* (Paris, 1699).

93. Matthieu Beuvelet, *Instructions sur le Manuel par forme de demandes et responses familières pour servir à ceux qui dans les séminaires se préparent à l'administration des sacremens,* 2 vols. (Paris, 1659).

Nine. The Debate on Suicide in the Enlightenment: From Morality to Medicine

1. *Times* (London), 1789, quoted here from Michael MacDonald and Terence R. Murphy, *Sleepless Souls: Suicide in Early Modern England* (New York: Oxford University Press, 1990), 172.

2. The treatises mentioned in the following paragraphs are the following: Jean-Baptiste Gaultier, *Les Lettres persanes, convaincues d'impiété* (Paris, 1751); Chevalier de

C[hampdevaux], *L'honneur considéré en lui-même et relativement au duel* (Paris, 1752); Gabriel Gauchat, *Lettres critiques, ou, Analyse et réfutation de divers écrits modernes contre la religion,* 19 vols. (Paris, 1756); Claude Dupin, *Observations sur un livre intitulé "De l'Esprit des lois",* 3 vols. (Paris, 1757–58); *La religion vengée* (Paris, 1757); Louis-Antoine de Caraccioli, *La grandeur d'âme* (Frankfurt, 1761); Jean-Georges Lefranc de Pompignan, *Instruction pastorale de monseigneur l'évêque de Puy, sur la prétendue philosophie des incrédules modernes* (Le Puy, 1763); Jean-Henri-Samuel Formey, *Principes de morale, déduits de l'usage des facultés de l'entendement humain,* 2 vols. (Paris, 1762); Lacroix, *Traité de morale, ou, Devoirs de l'homme envers Dieu, envers la société et envers lui-même* (Paris, 1767); Flexier de Reval (François-Xavier de Feller), *Catéchisme philosophique, ou, Recueil d'observations propres à défendre la religion chrétienne contre ses ennemis,* 2d ed. (Paris, 1777); Simon Hervieux de La Boissière, *Les contradictions du livre intitulé De la philosophie de la nature* (Paris, n.d.); Augustin Barruel, *Les Helviennes, ou, Lettres provinciales philosophiques* (1781), 6th ed., 4 vols. (Paris, 1823); *La petite encyclopédie, ou, Dictionnaire des philosophes,* ed. Abraham Joseph de Chaumeix (Antwerp, 1772); Joseph-Nicolas Camuset, *Principes contre l'incrédulité, à l'occasion du "Système de la nature"* (Paris, 1771); J. de Castillon (Giovanni Francesco Mauro Melchior Salvemini da Castiglione), *Observations sur le livre intitulé "Système de la nature"* (Paris, 1771); Audierne, *Instructions militaires* (Rennes, 1772); Jean Dumas, *Traité du suicide, ou, Du meurtre volontaire de soi-même* (Amsterdam, 1773); Charles-Louis Richard, *Défense de la religion, de la morale, de la vertu, de la politique et de la société* (Paris, 1775); Richard, *Exposition de la doctrine des philosophes modernes* (Lille, 1785); *Dictionnaire universel françois et latin, vulgairement appelé Dictionnaire de Trévoux,* new ed., 8 vols. (Paris, 1771). For a discussion of these works, see Albert Bayet, *Le suicide et la morale* (Paris: Félix Alcan, 1922), 619–25.

3. *Encyclopédie méthodique, ou par ordre de matières: Par une société de gens de lettres, de savans et d'artistes,* 200 vols. (Paris and Liège, 1782–1832), *Jurisprudence,* vol. 7 (1787), s.v. "suicide."

4. Ibid., *Théologie,* vol. 3 (1790), s.v. "suicide."

5. Paul-Henri Thiery, baron d'Holbach, *Système de la nature,* chap. 14, quoted here from *The System of Nature, or, Laws of the Moral and Physical World,* trans. H. D. Robinson (Boston, 1889), 137n.

6. Alfonso de' Liguori, "Instruction pratique pour les confesseurs," in *Œuvres complètes de Saint Alphonse Marie de Liguori,* 31 vols. (Paris, 1834–43), 23:426–27.

7. Richard Steele, *Tracts and Pamphlets,* ed. Rae Blanchard (New York: Octagon Books, 1967); see MacDonald and Murphy, *Sleepless Souls,* 203.

8. On Henley, see MacDonald and Murphy, *Sleepless Souls,* 204.

9. George Berkeley, *Alciphron, or, The Minute Philosopher,* in *The Works of George Berkeley, Bishop of Cloyne,* ed. A. A. Luce and T. E. Jessop, 9 vols. (London: T. Nelson, 1948–57), 3:92, quoted here from MacDonald and Murphy, *Sleepless Souls,* 205.

10. Edward Umfreville, *Lex coronatoria, or, The Office and Duty of Coroners* (London, 1760); see MacDonald and Murphy, *Sleepless Souls,* 205–6.

11. Isaac Watts, *A Defense Against the Temptation to Self-Murder* (London, 1726), 75; see MacDonald and Murphy, *Sleepless Souls,* 207.

12. Francis Ayscough, *A Discourse Against Self-Murder* (London, 1755), 15, 17; see MacDonald and Murphy, *Sleepless Souls,* 207.

13. These cases are reported in MacDonald and Murphy, *Sleepless Souls,* 211–12.

14. *Arminian Magazine* 4 (1784): 356, quoted here from MacDonald and Murphy, *Sleepless Souls,* 208.

15. See MacDonald and Murphy, *Sleepless Souls,* 209–10.

16. Ibid., 201–2.

17. Ibid., 200–203.

18. Alexander Crichton, *An Inquiry into the Nature and Origin of Mental Derangement,* 2 vols. (London, 1798), 2:57–58; William Pargeter, *Observations on Maniacal Disorders* (Reading, 1792), 35–36; see MacDonald and Murphy, *Sleepless Souls,* 203.

19. Holbach, *Système de la nature,* quoted here from *The System of Nature,* trans. Robinson (Boston, 1889), 138.

20. On Robeck, see MacDonald and Murphy, *Sleepless Souls,* 147.

21. *Correspondance littéraire, philosophique et critique par Grimm, Diderot, Reynal, etc.,* ed. Maurice Tourneux, 16 vols. (Paris, 1877–82), 5:286.

22. Alberto Radicati, count of Passerano, *Recueil de pièces curieuses sur les matières les plus intéressantes* (Rotterdam, 1736), part 1, 15.

23. On the subject of dueling, see Robert Favre, *La mort au siècle des Lumières* (Lyons: Presses Universitaires de Lyon, 1978), 298–300.

24. Pierre Sylvain Maréchal, *Dictionnaire des athées anciens et modernes* (Paris, Year VIII [1800]), xx.

25. Julien Offroy de La Mettrie, *Système d'Épicure,* in *Œuvres philosophiques,* 3 vols. (Berlin, 1796), 2:257.

26. Bayet, *Le suicide et la morale,* 636–40, 644. Bayet discusses seventeenth-century drama on pp. 641–44.

27. Voltaire, *Mérope,* act 2, scene 7, quoted in English here from *The Works of Voltaire,* trans. William F. Fleming, 42 vols. (Paris: E. R. Du Mont, 1901), 15:56.

28. Pierre Carlet de Chamblain de Marivaux, *Annibal,* act 5, scene 9.

29. Prosper Jolyot de Crébillon, *Catalina,* act 5, scene 6.

30. Decaux (Gilles de Caux, sieur de Montlebert), *Marius,* act 5, scene 4.

31. Jean-Baptiste Sauvé, called de Lanoue, *Mahomet Second,* act 2, scenes 4, 7.

32. Voltaire, *L'Orphelin de la Chine,* act 5, scene 1, quoted here from *The Works of Voltaire,* 5:233.

33. Voltaire, *Alzire, ou, Les Américains,* act 5, scene 3, quoted here from *The Works of Voltaire,* 17:54.

34. See Favre, *La mort au siècle des Lumières,* 439.

35. Ibid., 430.

36. Ibid., 426.

37. Matthieu-François-Xavier Bichat, *Recherches physiologiques sur la vie et la mort* (Paris, 1800); in English translation as *Physiological Researches on Life and Death* (London, 1815); Pierre-Jean-Georges Cabanis, *Rapports du physique et du moral de l'homme,* 2 vols. (Paris, 1802); in English translation as *On the Relations between the Physical and Moral Aspects of Man,* ed. George Mora, trans. Margaret Duggan Saidi (Baltimore: Johns Hopkins University Press, 1981).

38. Favre, *La mort au siècle des Lumières,* 428–29.

39. Madame de Staël, *Lettres à Narbonne,* ed. Georges Solovieff (Paris: Gallimard, 1960), letter 15, p. 92.

40. Denis Diderot, *Lettres à Sophie Volland,* ed. Jean Varloot, Folio 1547 (Paris: Gallimard, 1994).

41. Antoine-François Prévost, known as Prévost d'Exiles, in *Le Pour et le Contre, ouvrage périodique d'un goût nouveau,* 20 vols. (Paris, 1733–40), vol. 4 (1734), 64.

42. Charles-Louis de Secondat, baron de la Brède et de Montesquieu, *Les lettres persanes,* quoted here from *The Persian Letters,* trans. George R. Healy, Library of Liberal Arts (Indianapolis: Bobbs-Merrill, 1964), 129–30.

43. Montesquieu, *The Persian Letters,* 117–18.

44. Montesquieu, *Considérations sur les causes de la grandeur des Romains et de leur décadence,* chap. 12, quoted from *Considerations on the Causes of the Greatness of the Romans and Their Decline,* ed. and trans. David Lowenthal (Ithaca: Cornell University Press, 1968), 117.

45. Montesquieu, *Considérations sur les causes,* 117–18.

46. Montesquieu, *De l'esprit des lois,* part 3, book 14, chap. 12, quoted here from *The Spirit of the Laws,* trans. Thomas Nugent, 2 vols. (London: G. Bell and Sons, 1914), 1:249.

47. Ibid.

48. Voltaire, marginal note on *Les lois de Minos.*

49. Voltaire, *Précis du siècle de Louis XV.*

50. Voltaire, letter to Mme. du Deffand, 22 February 1769, in *Correspondence,* ed. Theodore Besterman, 107 vols. (Geneva: Institut et Musée Voltaire, 1953–65), 103:no. 14519.

51. Voltaire, "Du Caton, du suicide," in *Dictionnaire philosophique,* quoted here from "Cato: On Suicide, and the Abbé St. Cyran's Book Legitimating Suicide," in *A Philosophical Dictionary,* in *The Works of Voltaire,* 7:21, 22.

52. Voltaire, "Cato: On Suicide," 24. For the Smiths and Lord Scarborough, see ibid., 24–25.

53. Ibid., 26.

54. Ibid., 27.

55. Voltaire, *Candide, or The Optimist,* in *The Works of Voltaire,* 1:105.

56. Voltaire, "Cato: On Suicide," 20.

57. Ibid., 26, 20, 29, 26.

58. Ibid., 23.

59. Voltaire, letter to Mme. du Deffand of 3 March 1754, quoted here from *The Selected Letters of Voltaire*, ed. and trans. Richard A. Brooks (New York: New York University Press, 1973), 170–71.

60. Voltaire, *Lettres à Monsieur de Voltaire sur la Nouvelle Héloïse*, in Voltaire, *Mélanges*, ed. Jacques Van den Heuvel, Bibliothèque de la Pléiade (Paris: Gallimard, 1961), 395–408, quotation 404–5.

61. Voltaire, "Cato: On Suicide," 23, 24, 21.

62. Voltaire, letter to Mme. du Deffand of 21 October 1770, in *Correspondence*, ed. Besterman, 77:34–36. Besterman identifies "Crawford" as John Craufurd of Auchinames.

63. Voltaire, letter to David Louis de Constant Rebecque, seigneur Hermenches, 9 August 1775, in ibid., 9:148–49.

64. Voltaire, "Cato: On Suicide," 27.

65. Voltaire, *The Huron*, in *The Works of Voltaire*, 3:160.

66. Voltaire, note to act 4 of *Olympie*.

67. Voltaire, "Sur les Pensées de Monsieur Pascal," in *Lettres philosophiques*, quoted from "On the Pensees of M. Pascal," in *Philosophical Letters*, trans. Ernest Dilworth, Library of Liberal Arts (Indianapolis and New York: Bobbs-Merrill, 1961), 135–36.

68. Voltaire, "Cato: On Suicide," 32–33.

69. Ibid., 33.

70. Voltaire, *Prix de la justice et de l'humanité*, art. 5, "Du suicide." For a similar passage, see "Cato: On Suicide," 33.

71. For example, Voltaire writes in a letter to Joseph Michel Antoine Servan dated 27 September 1769 that a foreigner "wearied with life (often for very good reason) may decide to separate his soul from his body, and in order to console his son, his possessions are given to the king, who almost always gives half to the first Opéra girl who asks for it through one of her lovers; the other half belongs to the gentlemen of the tax office."

72. Denis Diderot, *Essai sur les règnes de Claude et de Néron*, in *Œuvres complètes*, ed. J. Assézat and Maurice Tourneux, 20 vols. (Paris: Garnier, 1875–77), 3:244.

73. Jean Le Rond d'Alembert, *Éléments de philosophie*, in *Œuvres*, 5 vols. (Paris, 1821–22), 1:227.

74. Ibid.

75. Julien Offroy de La Mettrie, *Anti-Sénèque, ou, Discours sur le bonheur*, in *Œuvres philosophiques*, 3 vols. (Berlin, 1796), 2:186.

76. Julien Offroy de La Mettrie, *Système d'Épicure*, in *Œuvres philosophiques*, 2:37.

77. Jean-Baptiste de Boyer, marquis d'Argens, *Lettres juives, ou, Correspondance philosophique, historique et critique*, 6 vols. (The Hague, 1738), 4:no. 145, quoted here from *The Jewish Spy: Being a Philosophical, Historical and Critical Correspondence*, 4 vols. (London, 1740), 4:195, 197.

78. Johann Bernhard Merian, "Sur la crainte de la mort, sur le mépris de la mort, sur le suicide," in *Histoire de l'Académie royale des sciences et belles-lettres* (Berlin, 1770).

79. Delisle de Sales (Jean-Claude Izouard), *Mémoire adressé aux législateurs par la veuve d'un citoyen puni pour crime de suicide*, in *De la philosophie de la nature*, 3d ed., 6 vols. (London, 1777), 117–20.

80. Claude-Adrien Helvétius, *De l'esprit* in *Œuvres complètes de M. Helvétius*, 5 vols. (London, 1781), 1:132, quoted here from *De L'Esprit; or, Essays on the Mind and its Several Faculties*, Research and Source Works Series 515; Philosophy Monograph Series 33 (London, 1810; photographic reprint, New York: Burt Franklin, 1970), 92.

81. René-Louis de Voyer de Paulmy, marquis d'Argenson, *Essais dans le goût de ceux de Montaigne* (Amsterdam, 1785), 48.

82. Pierre-Louis Moreau de Maupertuis, *Essai de philosophie morale* (Berlin, 1749), chap. 5.

83. Bayet, *Le suicide et la morale*, 650–51.

84. Joseph-Gaspard Dubois-Fontanelle, *Théâtre et Œuvres philosophiques*, 3 vols. (London and Paris, 1785), 2:125.

85. Jean-François Marmontel, *Morale* and *Des mœurs*, in *Œuvres complètes*, 19 vols. (Paris, 1818–20), 17:268, 379.

86. Eustache Le Noble, *L'école du monde*, 6 vols. (Paris, 1702), 6:141.

87. Jean-Baptiste-René Robinet, *Dictionnaire universel des sciences, morale, économique, politique et diplomatique*, 30 vols. (London, 1777–83), s.v. "suicide."

88. Denesle, *Les préjugés du public sur l'honneur*, 3 vols. (Paris, 1766), 3:425.

89. Feucher d'Artaize, *Prisme moral, ou, Quelques pensées sur divers sujets* (Paris, 1809).

90. See Richard Mead, *A Treatise Concerning the Influence of the Sun and the Moon upon Human Bodies, and the Diseases Thereby Produced*, translated from Latin by Thomas Stack (London, 1748).

91. Giuseppe Toaldo, *Della vera influenza degli astri, delle stagioni, e mutazioni di tempo: Saggio meteorologico* (Padua, 1770), translated into French by Joseph Daquin as *Essai météorologique sur la véritable influence des astres, des saisons et changemens de tems* (Chambéry, 1784); Joseph Daquin, *La philosophie de la folie, ou, Essai philosophique sur le traitement des personnes attaquées de folie* (Paris, 1792).

92. *Encyclopédie méthodique, Médecine*, vol. 8, s.v. "Manie, vésanies, aliénation mentale, ou dérangemens des fonctions intellectuelles (Nosologie médecine pratique)," signed "Pinel."

93. Jean-François Dufour, *Essai sur les opérations de l'entendement humain et sur les maladies qui les dérangent* (Amsterdam and Paris, 1770).

94. Quoted here from Michel Foucault, *Madness and Civilization: A History of Insanity in the Age of Reason*, trans. Richard Howard (New York: Pantheon/Random House, 1965), 295 n.8.

95. Georges-Louis Leclerc de Buffon, *Natural History, General and Particular*, trans. William Smellie, 2d ed., 9 vols. (London, 1785), 3:264.

96. Ibid., 3:267, 270.

97. Sir Richard Blackmore, *Treatise of the Spleen and Vapours, or, Hypochondriacal*

and Hysterical Affections (London, 1725); Robert Whytt, *Observations on the Nature, Causes, and Cure of those Disorders which have been Commonly Called Nervous, Hypochondriac, or Hysteric,* 2d ed. (Edinburgh, 1765); in French translation as *Traité des maladies nerveuses* (Paris, 1777), 2:132. Blackmore and Whytt are quoted here from Foucault, *Madness and Civilization,* 137.

98. Whytt is quoted here from Foucault, *Madness and Civilization,* 165–66.

99. François Doublet and Jean Colombier, "Instructions sur la manière de traiter les insensés," *Journal de médecine,* August 1785. See Foucault, *Madness and Civilization,* 164 (for Doublet), 165–66 (for Muzell and Raulin).

100. Johann Karl Wilhelm Möhsen, *Geschichte der Wissenschaften in der Mark Brandenburg* (Berlin and Leipzig, 1781).

101. *Encyclopédie méthodique, Médecine,* vol. 9, s.v. "Mélancholie (Médecine clinique)," signed "M. Pinel," quoted here from Foucault, *Madness and Civilization,* 215.

102. Philippe Pinel, *Traité médico-philosophique sur l'aliénation mentale ou la manie* (Paris, Year IX [1801]), 458, quoted here from Foucault, *Madness and Civilization,* 255.

103. See Georges Minois, *Histoire des enfers* (Paris: Fayard, 1991), 294–99.

104. MacDonald and Murphy, *Sleepless Souls,* 233.

105. William Black, *A Dissertation on Insanity,* 2d ed. (London, 1811), 13–14; MacDonald and Murphy, *Sleepless Souls,* 233.

106. Adam Smith, *The Theory of Moral Sentiments,* ed. D. D. Raphael and A. L. Macfie (Oxford: Clarendon Press, 1976), 287, quoted here from MacDonald and Murphy, *Sleepless Souls,* 198.

107. William Rowley, *A Treatise on Female, Nervous, Hysterical, Hypochondriacal, Bilious, Convulsive Diseases . . . With Thoughts on Madness, Suicide, &c.* (London, 1788), quoted here from MacDonald and Murphy, *Sleepless Souls,* 198.

108. Favre, *La mort au siècle des Lumières,* 469.

Ten. The Elite: From Philosophical Suicide to Romantic Suicide

1. Alberto Radicati, conte di Passerano, *A Philosophical Dissertation upon Death: Composed for the Consolation of the Unhappy* (London, 1732), quoted here from Samuel Ernest Sprott, *The English Debate on Suicide from Donne to Hume* (Lasalle, Ind.: Open Court, 1961), 108.

2. Richard and Bridget Smith's letter is given at length in Paul Rapin de Thoyras, *L'histoire d'Angleterre,* 16 vols. (The Hague, 1749), 14:386–88. The portion of it given here but not quoted from Sprott, *The English Debate on Suicide,* 103, is enclosed in square brackets.

3. David Hume, *Essays on Suicide and the Immortality of the Soul* (London, 1783), ed. John Vladimir Price, facsimile ed., Key Texts (Bristol: Thoemmes Press, 1992). This edition is the source of the passages quoted in the text.

4. See Tom L. Beauchamp, "An Analysis of Hume's Essay 'On Suicide'," *Review of Metaphysics* 30, no. 1 (1976–77): 73–95.

5. John Vladimir Price, introduction to Hume, *Essays on Suicide and the Immortality of the Soul,* xii–xiv.

6. Hume, *Essays on Suicide,* 48, "Anti-Suicide."

7. David Hume, *The Letters of David Hume,* ed. J.Y.T. Greig, 2 vols. (Oxford: Clarendon Press, 1932; New York: Garland, 1983), 1:452.

8. Ibid., 1:97.

9. Paul Henri Thiery, baron d'Holbach, *Système de la nature,* quoted here from *The System of Nature,* trans. H. D. Robinson (Boston, 1889), 139.

10. Sébastien-Roch-Nicolas Chamfort, *Maximes et pensées,* in *Œuvres complètes,* ed. Pierre René Auguis, 5 vols. (Chaumerot, 1824–25), 1:354.

11. Ibid., no. 484.

12. Jean Meslier, "Mémoire des pensées et des sentiments de Jean Meslier," in *Œuvres complètes,* ed. Roland Desné, Jean Deprun, and Albert Soboul, 3 vols. (Paris: Anthropos, 1970–72), 3:176–77.

13. "Note du Curé Aubry (1783)," in Meslier, *Œuvres complètes,* 3:397.

14. *Mémoires secrets pour servir à l'histoire de la République des Lettres en France depuis 1762 jusqu'à nos jours,* 36 vols. (London, 1783–89). This collection of curious anecdotes, attributed to Louis Petit de Bachaumont (1690–1771), was continued from 1762 to 1771 by Pidansat de Mairobert (who, incidentally, committed suicide), then, until 1787, by Mouffle d'Angerville. Bachaumont was initially continuing the tradition of *nouvelles à la main.*

15. *Times* (London), 19 September–6 October 1789. For the instances in this paragraph, see Michael MacDonald and Terence R. Murphy, *Sleepless Souls: Suicide in Early Modern England* (New York: Oxford University Press, 1990), 277–78.

16. Friedrich Melchior Grimm, *Correspondance littéraire, philosophique et critique par Grimm, Diderot, Reynal, etc.,* ed. Maurice Tourneux, 16 vols. (Paris: Garnier, 1877–82), 10:341ff.

17. Albert Bayet, *Le suicide et la morale* (Paris: Félix Alcan, 1922), 681–82.

18. "L'Affaire Calas: Pièces originales concernant la mort des sieurs Calas et le jugement rendu à Toulouse," in Voltaire, *Mélanges,* ed. Jacques Van den Heuvel, Bibliothèque de la Pléiade (Paris: Gallimard, 1961), 547.

19. Ibid., 539.

20. *Connoisseur* 1 (London, 1755): 295–96; see MacDonald and Murphy, *Sleepless Souls,* 278, 279 (Nourse).

21. John Brown, *An Estimate of the Manners and Principles of the Times* (London, 1757), 95, quoted here from MacDonald and Murphy, *Sleepless Souls,* 188.

22. *Connoisseur* 1 (London, 1755): 299–300, quoted here from MacDonald and Murphy, *Sleepless Souls,* 188.

23. John Herries, *An Address to the Public, on the Frequent and Enormous Crime of Suicide* (London, 1774), 6, quoted here from MacDonald and Murphy, *Sleepless Souls,* 189.

24. See MacDonald and Murphy, *Sleepless Souls,* 189.

25. *World,* 16 September 1756, 1161–62; MacDonald and Murphy, *Sleepless Souls,* 187–88.

26. For the instances that follow, see MacDonald and Murphy, *Sleepless Souls,* 185, 189, 277, 279, 275, 280, 186, 280, 279, 184, 189, 277.

27. Ibid., 128; for the immediately preceding examples, see ibid., 128–29, 281.

28. Frederick II of Prussia, in Pierre Gaxotte, *Frédéric II* (Paris: Fayard, 1938, 1972), 361, quoted here from *Frederick the Great,* trans. R. A. Bell (London: G. Bell and Sons, 1941), 359–60.

29. Johann Wolfgang von Goethe, *Die Leiden des jungen Werthers* (1774), quoted here from *George Ticknor's The Sorrows of Young Werther,* ed. Frank G. Ryder (Chapel Hill: University of North Carolina Press, 1952), 87–88.

30. Fernand Baldensperger, *Goethe en France: Étude de littérature comparée* (Paris: Hachette, 1902), 18.

31. Orie W. Long, "English Translations of Goethe's Werther," *Journal of English and German Philology* 14 (1915): 169–203.

32. Johann Wolfgang von Goethe, *Faust: The Tragedy, Part One,* trans. John Prudhoe (Manchester: Manchester University Press; New York: Barnes and Noble, 1974), 15–24.

33. Ibid., 25.

34. E.H.W. Meyerstein, *A Life of Thomas Chatterton,* 2 vols. (London: Ingpen and Grant, 1930), 475–76, plate facing p. 476.

35. *Times* (London), no. 1268 (28 September 1789), 3; see also MacDonald and Murphy, *Sleepless Souls,* 195–96.

36. Quoted in Bayet, *Le suicide et la morale,* 683.

37. Grimm, *Correspondance littéraire,* 9:231.

38. Henri Brunschwig, *La crise de l'état prussien à la fin du XVIIIe siècle et la genèse de la mentalité romantique* (Paris: Presses Universitaires de France, 1947), 267, quoted here from Brunschwig, *Enlightenment and Romanticism in Eighteenth-Century Prussia,* trans. Frank Jellinek (Chicago: University of Chicago Press, 1974), 220.

39. Schlegel quoted in *Enlightenment and Romanticism.*

40. Immanuel Kant, *Fundamental Principles of the Metaphysics of Morals,* trans. Thomas K. Abbott, Library of Liberal Arts (Indianapolis: Bobbs-Merrill, 1949), 38, 39.

41. Jacques Godechot, *L'Europe et l'Amérique à l'époque napoléonienne (1800–1815)* (Paris: Presses Universitaires de France, 1967), 68.

42. Antoine-Léonard Thomas, *Ode sur le temps* (Paris, 1762), lines 93–96, 103.

43. Fichte quoted in Jean-Pierre Bois, *Les vieux, de Montaigne aux premiers retraités* (Paris: Fayard, 1989), 271.

44. Ugo Foscolo, *Le ultime lettere di Jacopo Ortis* (1799), vol. 4 of *Edizione nazionale delle opere di Ugo Foscolo,* ed. Giovanni Gambarin, 21 vols. (Florence: Le Monnier, 1933–55).

45. Madame de Staël, *Réflexions sur le suicide,* in *Œuvres complètes* (Paris, 1861),

3:179, quoted here from "Reflections on Suicide," in *An Extraordinary Woman: Selected Writings of Germaine de Staël*, trans. Vivian Folkenflik (New York: Columbia University Press, 1987), 348–58, quotation on 348.

46. Staël, *Réflexions sur le suicide*, 185; "Reflections on Suicide," 352–53.

47. Staël, *Réflexions sur le suicide*, 185.

48. Denesle, *Les préjugés du public sur l'honneur* (Paris, 1766), 459; see Bayet, *Le suicide et la morale*, 684.

Eleven. The Common People: The Persistence of Ordinary Suicide

1. For the information on eighteenth-century Brittany that follows, I have made use of Guy Barreau, "Les suicides en Bretagne au XVIIIᵉ siècle," *mémoire de maîtrise*, Université de Rennes, 1971.

2. See Albert Bayet, *Le suicide et la morale* (Paris: Félix Alcan, 1922), 668–69; Louis-Sébastien Mercier, *Tableau de Paris*, 8 vols. (Amsterdam, 1783), 3:chap. 258, 176, quoted here from Louis Chevalier, *Laboring Classes and Dangerous Classes in Paris during the First Half of the Nineteenth Century*, trans. Frank Jellinek (New York: H. Fertig, 1973), 281.

3. Bayet, *Le suicide et la morale*, 667, 671–72.

4. Armand Corre and Paul Aubry, *Documents de criminologie rétrospective (Bretagne, XVIIᵉ–XVIIIᵉ siècle)* (Paris, 1895), 378.

5. Amédée Combier, *Les justices subalternes de Vermandois* (Amiens, 1885), 43, 134, 140.

6. Antoine-François Prost de Royer, ed., *Dictionnaire de jurisprudence et des arrêts, ou nouvelle édition du Dictionnaire de Brillon*, 7 vols. (Lyons, 1781–88).

7. Jacques-Pierre Brissot de Warville, *Théorie des lois criminelles*, 2 vols. (Paris, 1781); Claude Emmanuel Joseph Pierre, marquis de Pastoret, *Des lois pénales* (Paris, 1790).

8. Mercier, *Tableau de Paris*, 3:chap. 258, 176, quoted here from Chevalier, *Laboring Classes*, 281.

9. Siméon Prosper Hardy, *"Mes Loisirs": Journal d'événements tels qu'ils parviennent à ma connaissance (1764–1789)*, ed. Maurice Tourneux and Maurice Vitrac (Paris: A. Picard et fils, 1912), 1:80, 160, 306, 323, 325.

10. Jean Imbert and Georges Levasseur, *Le pouvoir, les juges et les bourreaux: Vingt-cinq siècles de répression* (Paris: Hachette, 1972), 203.

11. *Lettres de Monsieur de Marville, lieutenant général de police au Ministre Maurepas (1742–1747)*, ed. A. de Boislisle, 3 vols. (Paris: H. Champion, 1896–1905).

12. *Gentleman's Magazine* 24 (1754): 507; *Considerations on Some of the Laws Relating to the Office of a Coroner* (Newcastle and London, 1776), 53–54, quoted here from Michael MacDonald and Terence R. Murphy, *Sleepless Souls: Suicide in Early Modern England* (New York: Oxford University Press, 1990), 121.

13. Two examples of traditional attitudes are Isaac Watts, *A Defense against the*

Temptation of Self-Murder (London, 1726), and Francis Ayscough, *Duelling and Suicide Repugnant to Revelation, Reason and Common Sense* (London, 1774).

14. *Considerations on Some of the Laws Relating to the Office of a Coroner* (London, 1776), 45–46, quoted here from MacDonald and Murphy, *Sleepless Souls,* 126.

15. MacDonald and Murphy, *Sleepless Souls,* 238.

16. *Times* (London), no. 1651 (9 April 1790), 2, quoted here from MacDonald and Murphy, *Sleepless Souls,* 142.

17. *Gentleman's Magazine* 52 (1783): pt. 1, 539, quoted here from MacDonald and Murphy, *Sleepless Souls,* 136 and 136 n.74.

18. *Times* (London), no. 2518 (28 January 1793), 4; MacDonald and Murphy, *Sleepless Souls,* 136–37.

19. *Times* (London), no. 2855 (10 December 1793), 3; no. 2858 (13 December 1793), 3; both quoted here from MacDonald and Murphy, *Sleepless Souls,* 138.

20. *Fog's Weekly Journal,* 20 March 1731; MacDonald and Murphy, *Sleepless Souls,* 213.

21. George Gregory, *A Sermon on Suicide, Preached . . . at the Anniversary of the Royal Humane Society,* 2d ed. (London, 1797); MacDonald and Murphy, *Sleepless Souls,* 350.

22. See MacDonald and Murphy, *Sleepless Souls,* figure 7.2, "Suicides in the London Bills of Mortality, 1660–1799," 246.

23. MacDonald and Murphy, *Sleepless Souls,* table 7.2, "Age Structure of Reported Suicides," 251.

24. *Annual Register* 21 (1778): 172; MacDonald and Murphy, *Sleepless Souls,* 255.

25. *Fog's Weekly Journal* 41 (5 July 1729); *Weekly Miscellany* 264 (13 January 1737–38); MacDonald and Murphy, *Sleepless Souls,* 253.

26. On this topic, see Georges Minois, *Histoire de la vieillesse en Occident de l'Antiquité à la Renaissance* (Paris: Fayard, 1987); in English translation as *History of Old Age from Antiquity to the Renaissance,* trans. Sarah Hanbury Tenison (Chicago: University of Chicago Press, 1987); Jean-Pierre Bois, *Les vieux, de Montaigne aux premiers retraités* (Paris: Fayard, 1989).

27. Mercier, *Tableau de Paris,* 3:chap. 258, 177.

28. See MacDonald and Murphy, *Sleepless Souls,* 325–26.

29. *Gentlemen's Magazine* 20 (1750): 473, quoted here from MacDonald and Murphy, *Sleepless Souls,* 328.

30. *Gentleman's Magazine* 13 (1743): 543–44, quoted here from MacDonald and Murphy, *Sleepless Souls,* 331; *Annual Register* 1 (1758), 99.

31. See MacDonald and Murphy, *Sleepless Souls,* 293.

32. E. P. Thompson, "Rough Music: Le Charivari anglais," *Annales ESC* 27, no. 2 (1972): 285–312.

33. MacDonald and Murphy, *Sleepless Souls,* table 9.1, "Seasonality of Suicide," 313.

34. Louis Chevalier, *Classes laborieuses et classes dangereuses à Paris pendant la première moitié du XIXe siècle* (Paris: Plon, 1958; Hachette, 1984); in English translation as *Laboring Classes and Dangerous Classes in Paris* (see note 2 above).

35. These figures are drawn from Jean-Claude Chesnais, *Histoire de la violence en Occident de 1800 à nos jours* (Paris: R. Laffont, 1981).

36. Henri Brunschwig, *La crise de l'état prussien à la fin du XVIIIe siècle et la genèse de la mentalité romantique* (Paris: Presses Universitaires de France, 1947), 267–68, 221.

37. Friedrich Melchior Grimm, *Correspondance littéraire, philosophique et critique par Grimm, Diderot, Reynal, etc.*, ed. Maurice Tourneux, 16 vols. (Paris: Garnier, 1877–82), 9:231.

38. Flexier de Reval (François-Xavier de Feller), *Catéchisme philosophique, ou, Recueil d'observations propres à défendre la religion chrétienne contre ses ennemis* (Paris, 1773), 139.

39. Hardy, *"Mes Loisirs,"* 323 (for the year 1772).

40. Augustin Barruel, *Les Helviennes, ou, Lettres provinciales philosophiques* (1781), 6th ed., 4 vols. (Paris, 1823), 1781), 4:272.

41. Mercier, *Tableau de Paris*, 3:chap. 258, 176.

42. Ibid., 3:chap. 258, 175, quoted here from Chevalier, *Laboring Classes*, 281.

43. Mercier, *Tableau de Paris*, 3:chap. 258, 177.

44. Antoine Augustin Cournot, *Souvenirs (1760–1860)*, introduction by E. P. Bottinelli (Paris: Hachette, 1913), 20.

45. *Gentleman's Magazine* 7 (1737): 289–90, quoted here from MacDonald and Murphy, *Sleepless Souls*, 308. For newspaper circulation, the *Mercurius politicus*, and Baron von Pöllnitz, see MacDonald and Murphy, *Sleepless Souls*, 303, 309, 308.

46. Edward Umfreville, *Lex coronatoria; or, The Office and Duty of Coroner* (London, 1761); see MacDonald and Murphy, *Sleepless Souls*, 205–6.

47. Cesare Beccaria, *On Crimes and Punishments*, ed. and trans. David Young (Indianapolis: Hackett, 1986), 60–61.

48. *Considerations on Some of the Laws Relating to the Office of a Coroner*, 44; MacDonald and Murphy, *Sleepless Souls*, 142.

49. Barthélemy-Joseph Bretonnier, *Recueil par ordre alphabétique des principales questions de droit qui se jugent diversement dans les différents tribunaux du royaume* (1718; Paris, 1742), 182.

50. François de Boutaric, *Explication de l'ordonnance de Louis XIV . . . sur les matières criminelles*, 2 vols. (Toulouse, 1743), 2:262.

51. François Serpillon, *Code criminel, ou, Commentaire sur l'ordonnance de 1670*, 4 vols. (Lyons, 1757), 3:960.

52. Pierre-François Muyart de Vouglans, *Institutes au droit criminel* (Paris, 1757).

53. Pierre-François Muyart de Vouglans, *Lettre sur le système de l'auteur de "L'esprit des lois,"* touchant la modération des peines (Brussels, 1785).

54. Guy Du Rousseaud de La Combe, *Traité des matières criminelles*, 6th ed., 3 vols.

(Paris, 1769), 3:422. For a discussion of many of the legal theorists in the following paragraphs, see Bayet, *Le suicide et la morale,* 622–26.

55. Daniel Jousse, *Traité de la justice criminelle de France,* 4 vols. (Paris, 1771), vol. 4, part 4.

56. Jean-Baptiste Denisart, *Collection de décisions nouvelles et . . . de notions relatives à la jurisprudence actuelle,* 3 vols. (Paris, 1763–64); Thomas-Jules-Armand Cottereau, *Le droit général de la France, et le droit particulier à la Touraine et au Lodunois* (Tours, 1778); Louis de Héricourt, *Supplément aux lois civiles de Domat* (Paris, 1787); Pierre-Jean-Jacques-Guillaume Guyot, *Répertoire universel et raisonné de jurisprudence civile, criminelle, canonique et bénéficiale,* 17 vols. (Paris, 1784–85).

57. Jacques-Pierre Brissot de Warville, in *Les moyens d'adoucir les rigueurs des lois pénales en France,* Discours couronnés par l'Académie de Châlons-sur-Marne (Châlons-sur-Marne, 1781), first discourse, p. 60.

58. Brissot de Warville, *Théorie des lois criminelles,* 343.

59. Joseph-Elzéar-Dominique Bernardi, in *Les moyens d'adoucir les rigueurs des lois pénales en France,* second discourse, p. 110.

60. Joseph-Elzéar-Dominique de Bernardi, *Principes des lois criminelles* (Paris, 1781).

61. François-Michel Vermeil, *Essai sur les réformes à faire dans notre législation criminelle* (Paris, 1781); Charles-Eléonor Dufriche de Valazé, *Lois pénales* (Paris, 1784).

62. *Bibliothèque philosophique du législateur, du politique, du jurisconsulte,* 10 vols. (Berlin and Paris, 1782–85), 5:401, 184.

63. Piere-Jean-Baptiste Chaussard, *Théorie des lois criminelles* (Auxerre, 1789).

64. Pastoret, *Des lois pénales.*

65. Antoine-Joseph Thorillon, *Idées sur les lois criminelles* (Paris, 1788).

66. Georges-Victor Vasselin, *Théorie des peines capitales, ou Abus et dangers de la peine de mort et des tourmens* (Paris, 1790).

67. Nicolas-Joseph Philpin de Piépape, *Suite des observations sur les lois criminelles de la France* (Paris, 1790).

68. Jacques Bridaine, *Sermons,* 2d ed., 7 vols. (Avignon, 1827), 1:210.

69. Jean-Paul Du Sault, *Le religieux mourant, ou, Préparation à la mort pour les personnes religieuses* (Avignon, 1751), 15–16.

70. Jacques-Joseph Duguet, *Le Tombeau de Jésus-Christ; ou, Explication du mystère de la sépulture, suivant la concorde* (Paris, 1731).

71. Robert Favre, *La mort au siècle des Lumières* (Lyons: Presses Universitaires de Lyon, 1978), 464–66.

72. Numa Tetaz, *Le suicide* (Geneva: Éditions Labor et Fides, 1971).

73. Chevalier, *Classes laborieuses et classes dangereuses,* 467 n.1; *Laboring Classes,* 471 n.15.

74. Jean-Pierre Bois, *Les anciens soldats dans la société française au XVIIIe siècle* (Paris: Economica, 1990).

75. Chesnais, *Histoire de la violence,* 305.

Epilogue. From the French Revolution to the Twentieth Century,
or, From Free Debate to Silence

1. Quoted in Albert Bayet, *Le suicide et la morale* (Paris: Félix Alcan, 1922), 691. Bayet devotes an entire chapter to suicide under the French Revolution, pp. 687–725.

2. Joseph-Honoré Valant, "De la garantie sociale considérée dans son opposition avec la peine de mort," *Le Moniteur* 7 (1796): 548. See Bayet, *Le suicide et la morale,* 693 and, for the examples just given, 692.

3. Alexandre Tuetey, *Répertoire général des sources manuscrites de l'histoire de Paris pendant la Révolution française,* 11 vols. (Paris: Imprimerie nouvelle, 1890–1914), 7:no. 1892, 8:nos. 1774, 2867.

4. Patrice-Louis Higonnet, "Du suicide sentimental au suicide politique," in *La Révolution et la mort: Actes du Colloque international organisé à Toulouse, 9–10 mars 1989,* ed. Elisabeth Liris and Jean-Maurice Biziere (Toulouse: Presses Universitaires de Mirail-Toulouse), 137–50.

5. Ibid., 140–41.

6. Madame Roland, quoted here from "Final Thoughts," in *The Memoirs of Madame Roland: A Heroine of the French Revolution,* ed. and trans. Evelyn Shuckburgh (Mount Kisco, N.Y.: Moyer Bell, 1989), 253.

7. Ibid., 255.

8. Higonnet, "Du suicide sentimental," 145.

9. For these instances, see Bayet, *Le suicide et la morale,* 718–19.

10. On Beaurepaire, see ibid., 710–12.

11. See also ibid., 711–12.

12. Jean-Claude Chesnais, *Histoire de la violence en Occident de 1800 à nos jours* (Paris: R. Laffont, 1981), 241.

13. Jean Tulard, table, "Les suicides à Paris sous l'Empire," in *Nouvelle histoire de Paris, le Consulat et l'Empire 1800–1815* (Paris: Association pour la Publication d'une Histoire de Paris, distributed by Hachette, 1970), 332.

14. Richard Cobb, *Death in Paris: The Records of the Basse-Geôle de la Seine, October 1795–September 1801, Vendémiaire Year IV–Fructidor Year IX* (New York: Oxford University Press, 1978); consulted in French as *La mort est dans Paris: Enquête sur le suicide, le meurtre, et autres morts subites à Paris au lendemain de la Terreur* (Paris: Chemin Vert, 1985).

15. Cobb, *Death in Paris,* 9.

16. Ibid., 23.

17. Ibid., 64–65.

18. Pierre Moron, *Le suicide,* Que Sais-je? 1569 (Paris: Presses Universitaires de France, 1975).

19. Louis Chevalier, *Classes laborieuses et classes dangereuses à Paris pendant la première moitié du XIXe siècle* (Paris: Plon, 1958; Hachette, 1984); in English translation as *Laboring Classes and Dangerous Classes in Paris during the First Half of the Nineteenth Century,* trans. Frank Jellinek (New York: H. Fertig, 1974).

20. *Annales d'hygiène* (1829), quoted here from Chevalier, *Laboring Classes,* 283.

21. See Yves Le Gallo, *Clergé, religion et société en Basse-Bretagne de la fin de l'Ancien Régime à 1840,* 2 vols. (Paris: Éditions Ouvrières, 1991), 2:735.

22. John A. Abbo and Jerome D. Hannan, *The Sacred Canons: A Concise Presentation of the Current Disciplinary Norms of the Church,* 2d rev. ed., 2 vols. (St. Louis: Herder, 1960), 2:495.

23. Quoted here from "Euthanasia: Declaration of the Sacred Congregation for the Doctrine of the Faith (May 5, 1980)," *The Pope Speaks* 25, no. 4 (1980): 291.

24. Ibid., 292.

25. Philippe Pinel, *Traité médico-philosophique sur l'aliénation mentale ou la manie* (Paris, An IX [1801]), 188, 241–42.

26. See Michel Foucault, *Histoire de la folie à l'âge classique* (Paris: Gallimard, 1972), 346 n.2.

27. François Leuret, *Fragments psychologiques sur la folie* (Paris, 1834), 321, quoted here from Michel Foucault, *Madness and Civilization: A History of Insanity in the Age of Reason,* trans. Richard Howard (New York: Pantheon/Random House, 1965), 182.

28. Johann Gaspar Spurzheim, *Observations on the Deranged Manifestations of the Mind, or Insanity* (London, 1817); consulted in French as *Observations sur la folie* (Paris, 1818); quoted here from Foucault, *Madness and Civilization,* 213.

29. Alexandre-Jacques-François Brière de Boismont, "De l'influence de la civilisation sur le suicide," *Annales d'hygiène* (1855), quoted here from Chevalier, *Laboring Classes,* 474n.27.

30. Pinel, *Traité médico-philosophique,* 146, 72.

31. Étienne Esquirol, *Maladies mentales* (1839), quoted here from Chevalier, *Laboring Classes,* 289.

32. Émile Durkheim, *Le suicide: Étude de sociologie* (Paris: Félix Alcan, 1897); in English translation as *Suicide: A Study in Sociology,* ed. George Simpson, trans. John A. Spaulding and George Simpson (Glencoe, Ill.: Free Press, 1951).

33. Maurice Halbwachs, *Les causes du suicide* (Paris: Félix Alcan, 1930), quoted here from *The Causes of Suicide,* trans. Harold Goldblatt (New York: Free Press, 1978), 10.

34. Jean Baechler, *Les suicides* (Paris: Calmann-Lévy, 1975), in English translation (abridged) as *Suicides,* trans. Barry Cooper (New York: Basic Books, 1979); Jack D. Douglas, *The Social Meaning of Suicide* (Princeton: Princeton University Press, 1967).

35. Odile Odoul, "Bruno Bettelheim est mort," in *Agora,* special issue, *Autour du suicide* (June 1990): 89.

36. Rapport Dailly, doc. Sénat, 1982–83, no. 359, p. 9.

37. Danielle Mayer, "En quoi le suicide intéresse-t-il le droit?" *Agora,* special issue, *Autour du suicide* (June 1990): 29–36.

38. Frédéric Zenati, "Commentaire de la loi du 31 décembre 1987 tendant à réprimer la provocation au suicide," *Revue trimestrielle de droit civil* (1988): 427–28.

39. Quoted here from Albert Camus, *The Myth of Sisyphus and Other Essays,* trans. Justin O'Brien (New York: Alfred A. Knopf, 1969), 64.

BIBLIOGRAPHY

In spite of recent advances in the historical study of suicide, only a small number of works exclusively dedicated to the topic are as yet available, and the better part of the relevant documentation is dispersed in works on death, criminal law, psychology, medicine, psychiatry, sociology, literature, theology, and demography, too numerous to mention here.

"Autour du suicide." Special issue of *Agora* (June 1990).

Baechler, Jean. *Les suicides.* Paris: Calmann-Lévy, 1975. In English translation, abridged, as *Suicides,* translated by Barry Cooper (New York: Basic Books, 1979).

Barreau, Guy. "Les suicides en Bretagne au XVIIIᵉ siècle." Mémoire de maîtrise, Université de Rennes, 1971.

Bartel, Roland. "Suicide in Eighteenth-Century England: The Myth of a Reputation." *Huntington Library Quarterly* 23, no. 1 (1960): 145–58.

Bayet, Albert. *Le suicide et la morale.* Paris: Félix Alcan, 1922.

Beauchamp, Tom L. An Analaysis of Hume's Essay 'On Suicide.' " *Review of Metaphysics* 30, no. 1, issue 117 (1976–77): 73–95.

Bellefont, Laurence-Gigault. "Du désir de mort." In Laurence-Gigault de Bellefont, *Les œuvres spirituelles de Madame de Bellefont* (Paris, 1688).

Bourquelot, Félix. "Recherches sur les opinions et la législation en matière de mort volontaire pendant le Moyen Age: Depuis Justinien jusqu'à Charlemagne." *Bibliotèque de l'École des Chartes* 3 (1841–42): 537–60.

Burton, Robert. *The Anatomy of Melancholy.* 3 vols. Oxford: Clarendon Press, 1989–94.

Cavan, Ruth Shonle. *Suicide: A Study of Personal Disorganization.* Chicago: University of Chicago Press, 1928.

Cobb, Richard. *Death in Paris: The Records of the Basse-Geôle de la Seine, October 1795–September 1801, Vendémiaire Year IV–Fructidor Year IX.* New York: Oxford University Press, 1978.

Crocker, Lester G. "The Discussion of Suicide in the Eighteenth Century." *Journal of the History of Ideas* 13, no. 1 (1952): 47–72.

Dabadie, F. *Les suicides illustres.* Paris, 1859.

Daffner, H. "Der Selbstmord bei Shakespeare." *Shakespeare Jahrbuch* (1928).

Daube, David. "The Linguistics of Suicide." *Philosophy and Public Affairs* 1, no. 4 (1972): 387–437.

Delcourt, Marie. "Le suicide par vengeance dans la Grèce ancienne." *Revue d'histoire des religions* 99 (1939).

Denny, Sir William. *Pelicanicidium, or, The Christian Adviser against Self-Murder.* London, 1653.

Donne, John. *Biathanatos.* London, [1644]. Edited by Michael Rudick and M. Pabst Battin. Garland English Texts 1. New York: Garland, 1982.

Dumas, Jean. *Traité du suicide, ou Du meurtre volontaire de soimême.* Amsterdam, 1773.

Durkheim, Émile. *Le suicide: Étude de sociologie.* Paris, 1897. In English translation as *Suicide: A Study in Sociology,* edited by George Simpson, translated by John A. Spaulding and George Simpson (Glencoe, Ill.: Free Press, 1951).

Duvergier de Hauranne, Jean. *Question royalle et sa decision.* Paris, 1609.

Encyclopédie méthodique, ou par ordre de matières: Par une société de gens de lettres, de savans et d'artistes. 200 vols. Paris and Liège, 1782–1832. *Jurisprudence,* vol. 7 (1787), s.v. "suicide."

Faber, M. D. *Suicide in Greek Tragedy.* New York: Sphinx Press, 1970.

Fedden, Henry Romilly. *Suicide: A Social and Historical Study.* London: P. Davies, 1938. Reprint, New York: B. Blom, 1972.

Fleming, Caleb. *A Dissertation upon the Unnatural Crime of Self-Murder.* London, 1773.

Frison-Roche, Marie-Anne. *Le suicide.* Paris: Presses Universitaires de France, 1994.

Garrisson, Gaston. *Le suicide dans l'Antiquité et dans les temps modernes.* Paris, 1885.

——. "Le suicide en droit romain et en droit français." Thèse d'État, Université de Toulouse, 1883.

Grisé, Yolande. *Le suicide dans la Rome antique.* Paris: Belles Lettres, 1982; Montreal: Bellarmin, 1983.

Haeberli, L. "Le suicide à Genève au XVIIIᵉ siècle." In *Pour une histoire quantitative* (Geneva, 1975).

Hair, P.E.H. "A Note on the Incidence of Tudor Suicide." *Local Population Studies* 5 (1970): 36–43.

Henley, John. *Cato Condemned, or, The Case and History of Self-Murder.* London, 1730.

Herries, John. *An Address to the Public, on the Frequent and Enormous Crime of Suicide.* London, 1774.

Higonnet, Patrice-Louis. "Du suicide sentimental au suicide politique." In *La Révolution et la mort: Actes du Colloque international, Toulouse, 9–10 mars 1989,* edited by Elisabeth Liris and Jean-Maurice Biziere (Toulouse: Presses Universitaires de Mirail-Toulouse).

Hume, David. *Essays on Suicide and on the Immortality of the Soul.* London, 1783. Facsimile reprint, edited by John Vladimir Price, Key Texts (Bristol: Thoemmes Press, 1992).

Jaccard, Roland, and Michel Thévoz. *Manifeste pour une mort douce.* Paris: Grasset, 1992.

Kany, J. "Le suicide politique à Rome et en particulier chez Tacite." Thèse de troisième cycle, Université de Reims, 1970.

Kushner, Howard I. *Self-Destruction in the Promised Land: A Psychocultural Biology of American Suicide.* New Brunswick, N.J.: Rutgers University Press, 1989.

Leech, Clifford. "Le dénouement par le suicide dans la tragédie élisabéthaine et jacobéenne." In *Le théâtre tragique,* edited by Jean Jacquot (Paris: Centre National de la Recherche Scientifique, 1962).

Lefay-Toury, Marie-Noëlle. *La tentation du suicide dans le roman français du XIIᵉ siècle.* Paris: Champion, 1979.

Legoyt, Alfred. *Le suicide ancien et moderne: Étude historique, philosophique, morale et statistique.* Paris, 1881.

MacDonald, Michael, and Terence R. Murphy. *Sleepless Souls: Suicide in Early Modern England.* New York: Oxford University Press, 1990.

Merian, Johann Bernhard. "Sur la crainte de la mort, sur le mépris de la mort, sur le suicide." In *Histoire de l'Académie Royale des Sciences et Belles-Lettres (1763).* Berlin, 1770.

Minois, Georges. "L'historien et la question du suicide." *L'histoire* 189 (1995).

Moore, Charles. *A Full Inquiry into the Subject of Suicide.* London, 1790.

O'Dea, James J. *Suicide: Studies on its Philosophy, Causes and Prevention.* New York, 1882.

Paulin, Bernard. *Du couteau à la plume: Le suicide dans la littérature anglaise de la Renaissance 1580–1625).* Lyons: Hermès; Saint-Étienne: Université de Saint-Étienne, 1977.

Philipot, Thomas. *Self-Homicide-Murther, or, Some Antidotes and Arguments Gleaned out of the Treasures of our Modern Casuists and Divines against that Horrid and Reigning Sin of Self-Murther.* London, 1674.

Prince, John. *Self-Murder Asserted to be a Very Heinous Crime.* London, 1709.

Rist, John M. "Suicide." In *Stoic Philosophy* (London: Cambridge University Press, 1969).

Romi. *Suicides passionnés, historiques, bizarres, littéraires.* Paris: Serg, 1964.

A Sad and Dreadful Account of the Self-Murther of Robert Long, alias Baker. London, 1685.

Schär, Markus. *Seelennöte der Untertanen: Selbstmord, Melancholie und Religion im alten Zürich, 1500–1800.* Zurich: Chronos-Verlag, 1985.

Schmitt, Jean-Claude. "Le suicide au Moyen Age." *Annales ESC* 31 (1976): 3–28.

Sena, John F. "The English Malady: The Idea of Melancholy from 1700 to 1760." Ph.D. dissertation, Princeton University, 1967.

Snyder, Susan. "The Left Hand of God: Despair in Medieval and Renaissance Tradition." *Studies in the Renaissance* 12 (1965): 18–59.

Sprott, Samuel Ernest. *The English Debate on Suicide: From Donne to Hume.* Lasalle, Ind.: Open Court, 1961.

Staël, Madame de. *Réflexions sur le suicide.* In *Œuvres complètes* (Paris, 1861).

Stevenson, S. J. "The Rise of Suicide Verdicts in South-East England, 1530–1590: The Legal Process." *Continuity and Change* 2, no. 1 (1987): 37–76.

Le suicide. Special issue. *L'histoire* 189 (June 1995).

Watts, Isaac. *A Defense Against the Temptation to Self-Murder, Wherein the Criminal Nature and Guilt of it are Display'd.* London, 1726.

Wenzel, Siegfried. *The Sin of Sloth: Acedia in Medieval Thought and Literature.* Chapel Hill: University of North Carolina Press, 1967.

Willie, R. "Views on Suicide and Freedom in Stoic Philosophy and Some Related Points of View." *Prudentia* 5 (1973).

Withers, W[illiam]. *Some Thoughts Concerning Suicide, or Self-Killing.* London, 1711.

Wymer, Rowland. *Suicide and Despair in Jacobean Drama.* New York: St. Martin's Press, 1986.

Zell, Michael. "Suicide in Pre-Industrial England." *Social History* 11 (1986): 303–17.

INDEX

The Library of Congress has cataloged the hardcover edition of this book
as follows:

Minois, Georges, 1946–
 [Histoire du suicide. English]
 History of suicide : voluntary death in Western culture / Georges
Minois ; translated by Lydia G. Cochrane.
   p.   cm.
 Includes bibliographical references (p.   ).
 ISBN 0-8018-5919-0 (alk. paper)
 1. Suicide—History.   2. Right to die.   I. Title.
 RC569.M55   1998
179.7—DC21   98-4069

ISBN 0-8018-6647-2 (pbk.)